MEDICAL MASTERCLASS

Gastroenterology and Hepatology

Disclaimer

Although every effort has been made to ensure that drug doses and other information are presented accurately in this publication, the ultimate responsibility rests with the prescribing physician. Neither the publishers nor the authors can be held responsible for any consequences arising from the use of information contained herein. Any product mentioned in this publication should be used in accordance with the prescribing information prepared by the manufacturers.

The information presented in this publication reflects the opinions of its contributors and should not be taken to represent the policy and views of the Royal College of Physicians of London, unless this is specifically stated.

Every effort has been made by the contributors to contact holders of copyright to obtain permission to reproduce copyright material. However, if any have been inadvertently overlooked, the publisher will be pleased to make the necessary arrangements at the first opportunity.

Medical Masterclass

EDITOR-IN-CHIEF

John D. Firth DM FRCP
Consultant Physician and Nephrologist
Addenbrooke's Hospital,
Cambridge

Gastroenterology and Hepatology

EDITOR

Jane D. Collier MBChB MD MRCP
Consultant
John Radcliffe Hospital
Oxford

**Blackwell
Science**

© 2001 Royal College of Physicians of London, 11 St Andrews Place, London NW1 4LE
Registered Charity No. 210508

Published by:
Blackwell Science Ltd
Editorial Offices:
Osney Mead, Oxford OX2 0EL
25 John Street, London WC1N 2BS
23 Ainslie Place, Edinburgh EH3 6AJ
350 Main Street, Malden
　MA 02148-5018, USA
54 University Street, Carlton
　Victoria 3053, Australia
10, rue Casimir Delavigne
　75006 Paris, France

Other Editorial Offices:
Blackwell Wissenschafts-Verlag GmbH
Kurfürstendamm 57
10707 Berlin, Germany

Blackwell Science KK
MG Kodenmacho Building
7–10 Kodenmacho Nihombashi
Chuo-ku, Tokyo 104, Japan

Iowa State University Press
A Blackwell Science Company
2121 S. State Avenue
Ames, Iowa 50014-8300, USA

First published 2001

Set by Graphicraft Limited, Hong Kong
Printed and bound in Italy by
Rotolito Lombarda SpA, Milan

Catalogue records for this title are available from the British Library and the Library of Congress

ISBN 0-632-05867-6 (this book)
　　　0-632-05567-7 (set)

Commissioning Editors: Mike Stein and
　Rachel Robson
Project Manager (RCP): Filipa Maia
Editorial Assistant (RCP): Katherine Bowker
Production: Charlie Hamlyn and Jonathan
　Rowley
Layout and Cover Design: Chris Stone

DISTRIBUTORS

Marston Book Services Ltd
PO Box 269
Abingdon, Oxon OX14 4YN
(*Orders*: Tel: 01235 465500
　　　　Fax: 01235 465555)

USA
Blackwell Science, Inc.
Commerce Place
350 Main Street
Malden, MA 02148-5018
(*Orders*: Tel: 800 759 6102
　　　　　781 388 8250
　　　　Fax: 781 388 8255)

Canada
Login Brothers Book Company
324 Saulteaux Crescent
Winnipeg, Manitoba R3J 3T2
(*Orders*: Tel: 204 837 2987)

Australia
Blackwell Science Pty Ltd
54 University Street
Carlton, Victoria 3053
(*Orders*: Tel: 3 9347 0300
　　　　Fax: 3 9347 5001)

For further information on
Blackwell Science, visit our website:
www.blackwell-science.com

Contents

List of contributors, vii
Foreword, viii
Preface, ix
Acknowledgements, x
Key features, xi

1 Clinical presentations, 3
  1.1 Chronic diarrhoea, 3
  1.2 Heartburn and dysphagia, 7
  1.3 Melaena and collapse, 9
  1.4 Haematemesis and jaundice, 13
  1.5 Abdominal mass, 17
  1.6 Jaundice and abdominal pain, 20
  1.7 Jaundice in a heavy drinker, 23
  1.8 Abdominal swelling, 27
  1.9 Abdominal pain and vomiting, 30
  1.10 Weight loss and tiredness, 31
  1.11 Diarrhoea and weight loss, 34
  1.12 Rectal bleeding, 36
  1.13 Severe abdominal pain and vomiting, 39
  1.14 Chronic abdominal pain, 41
  1.15 Change in bowel habit, 43
  1.16 Acute liver failure, 45
  1.17 Iron-deficiency anaemia, 48
  1.18 Abnormal liver function tests, 49
  1.19 Progressive decline, 53
  1.20 Factitious abdominal pain, 55
2 Diseases and treatments, 58
  2.1 Inflammatory bowel disease, 58
    2.1.1 Crohn's disease, 58
    2.1.2 Ulcerative colitis, 61
    2.1.3 Microscopic colitis, 63
  2.2 Oesophagus, 63
    2.2.1 Barrett's oesophagus, 63
    2.2.2 Oesophageal reflux and benign stricture, 65
    2.2.3 Oesophageal tumours, 67
    2.2.4 Achalasia, 69
    2.2.5 Diffuse oesophageal spasm, 70
  2.3 Gastric and duodenal disease, 70
    2.3.1 Peptic ulceration and *helicobacter pylori*, 70
    2.3.2 Gastric carcinoma, 73
    2.3.3 Rare gastric tumours, 74
    2.3.4 Rare causes of gastrointestinal haemorrhage, 74
  2.4 Pancreas, 75
    2.4.1 Acute pancreatitis, 75
    2.4.2 Chronic pancreatitis, 78

    2.4.3 Pancreatic cancer, 80
    2.4.4 Neuroendocrine tumours, 82
  2.5 Biliary tree, 82
    2.5.1 Choledocholithiasis, 82
    2.5.2 Cholangiocarcinoma, 84
    2.5.3 Primary sclerosing cholangitis, 86
    2.5.4 Primary biliary cirrhosis, 88
    2.5.5 Intrahepatic cholestasis, 90
  2.6 Small bowel, 90
    2.6.1 Coeliac disease, 90
    2.6.2 Bacterial overgrowth, 92
    2.6.3 Other causes of malabsorption, 93
  2.7 Large bowel, 94
    2.7.1 Adenomatous polyps of the colon, 94
    2.7.2 Colorectal carcinoma, 95
    2.7.3 Diverticular disease, 97
    2.7.4 Intestinal ischaemia, 99
    2.7.5 Anorectal disease, 100
  2.8 Irritable bowel, 101
  2.9 Acute liver disease, 103
    2.9.1 Hepatitis A, 103
    2.9.2 Hepatitis B, 104
    2.9.3 Other viral hepatitis, 106
    2.9.4 Alcohol and alcoholic hepatitis, 106
    2.9.5 Acute liver failure, 109
  2.10 Chronic liver disease, 110
  2.11 Focal liver lesions, 113
  2.12 Drugs and the liver, 116
    2.12.1 Hepatic drug toxicity, 116
    2.12.2 Drugs and chronic liver disease, 118
  2.13 Gastrointestinal infections, 118
    2.13.1 Campylobacter, 118
    2.13.2 Salmonella, 118
    2.13.3 Shigella, 119
    2.13.4 Clostridium difficile, 119
    2.13.5 Giardia lamblia, 119
    2.13.6 Yersinia enterocolitica, 120
    2.13.7 Escherichia coli, 120
    2.13.8 Entamoeba histolytica, 120
    2.13.9 Traveller's diarrhoea, 120
    2.13.10 Human immunodeficiency virus (HIV), 120
  2.14 Nutrition, 121
    2.14.1 Defining nutrition, 121
    2.14.2 Protein-calorie malnutrition, 123
    2.14.3 Obesity, 123
    2.14.4 Enteral and parenteral nutrition, 124
    2.14.5 Diets, 125

2.15 Liver transplantation, 125
2.16 Screening, case finding and surveillance, 127
    2.16.1 Surveillance, 127
    2.16.2 Case finding, 128
    2.16.3 Population screening, 128
3 Investigations and practical procedures, 129
    3.1 General investigations, 129
    3.2 Rigid sigmoidoscopy and rectal biopsy, 133

3.3 Paracentesis, 134
3.4 Liver biopsy, 135
4 Self-assessment, 138

Answers to self-assessment, 145
The Medical Masterclass series, 157
Index, 167

List of contributors

Jane D. Collier MBChB MD MRCP
Consultant
John Radcliffe Hospital
Oxford

John M. Hebden MBBS BSc MD MRCP
Consultant
Royal Hallamshire Hospital
Sheffield

Satish Keshav MBBCh DPhil MRCP
Senior Lecturer
Centre for Gastroenterology, Royal Free and University
College Medical School
London

Jeremy Shearman DPhil MRCP
Consultant
Warwick Hospital
Warwick

Foreword

Medical Masterclass is the most innovative and important educational development from the Royal College of Physicians in the last 100 years. Throughout our 480-year history we have pioneered and supported high-quality medicine, and while *Medical Masterclass* continues that tradition, it also represents a quantum leap for the College as it moves into the 21st century.

The effort that the College has put in to improve the Membership Examination, which started 150 years ago and is now run by all three UK Royal Colleges of Physicians, will now be matched by its attention to basic learning in general medicine—the grounding and preparation for the exam.

Teaching and learning for the exam have changed little over the past 50 years, relying on local courses, word-based teaching and commercial courses. *Medical Masterclass* is a completely new approach for those wishing to practise high-quality medicine. It is an imaginative multimedia programme with paper and CD modules covering the major areas of medicine, supported by a website which will provide summaries and links to the latest articles and guidelines, and self-assessment questionnaires with feedback. Its focus is on self-learning, self-assessment and dealing with realistic clinical problems—not just force-feeding facts. The series of interactive case studies on which the modules are based entail making diagnostic and treatment decisions, closely mimicking the situations found in the admission suite or outpatient clinic.

Medical Masterclass has been produced by the RCP's Education Department together with Blackwell Science. It represents a formidable amount of work by Dr John Firth and his team of authors and editors and is set to be the jewel in our crown. It also signals very clearly our intention to lead in the field of learning and to be supportive to our future members. I anticipate the package will also be invaluable for continued learning by our specialist registrars and consultants as part of continuing professional development.

I congratulate our colleagues for this superb product and commend it to you without reservation.

Professor Sir George Alberti
President of the Royal College of Physicians, London

Preface

Medical Masterclass comprises twelve paper-based modules, two CD-ROMs and a companion website. Its aim is to help doctors in their first few years of training to improve their medical skills and knowledge.

The twelve paper-based modules are divided as follows: two cover the scientific background to medicine, one is devoted to general clinical issues, one to emergency medicine and practical procedures, and eight cover the range of medical specialities. Medicine is often fairly straightforward when the diagnosis is clear, but patients rarely come to their doctor and say 'I've got Hodgkin's disease': they have lumps. The core material of each of the clinical specialities is defined by case presentations in the first part of each module: how do you approach the man who has lumps? Structured concise notes on specific diseases follow later. All practising doctors know that medicine is much more than knowing lots of facts about diseases: how do you tell someone they've got cancer? How do you decide when to stop treatment? Most medical texts say little about these issues: *Medical Masterclass* does not avoid them, nor does it talk in vague and abstract terms.

The two CD-ROMs each contain 30 interactive cases requiring diagnosis and treatment. The format is remarkably close to real life: you see the patient and are told the story; you have to decide how to investigate and treat; but you can't see all the results before you start to make decisions!

The companion website, which will be regularly updated, includes extended case material, literature and guideline updates and review, and self-assessment questions. How much do you know, and are you improving? You will see how your score compares with your previous attempts, and also how your performance compares with others who have logged on to the site.

The *Medical Masterclass* is produced by the Education Department of the Royal College of Physicians of London and published by Blackwell Science. It is not a crammer for the MRCP exam and not written by those who set the exam. However, I have no doubt that someone putting effort into learning through the *Medical Masterclass* would be in a strong position to impress the examiners, although I am afraid that success—like much else in medicine and in life—cannot be guaranteed.

John Firth
Editor-in-Chief

Acknowledgements

Medical Masterclass has been produced by a team. The names of those who have written and edited material are clearly indicated elsewhere, but without the efforts of many other people *Medical Masterclass* would not exist at all. These include Professor Lesley Rees and Mrs Winnie Wade from the Education Department of the Royal College of Physicians of London, who initiated the project; Dr Mike Stein and Dr Andy Robinson from Medschool.com and Blackwell Science, respectively, who have enthusiastically supported it from the beginning; and Ms Filipa Maia and Ms Katherine Bowker, who have run the office with splendid efficiency and induced authors and editors to perform to a schedule rarely achieved. I and the whole of the team of editors and authors are immensely grateful to all of these people for the energy that they have poured into *Medical Masterclass* in various ways.

John Firth
Editor-in-Chief

Key features

We have created a range of icon boxes to help you identify key information and to make learning easier and more enjoyable. Here is a brief explanation:

 Clinical pointer

This icon highlights important information to be noted.

 Further information

This icon indicates the source of further information and reference.

 Hints

This icon highlights useful hints, tips and mnemonics.

 Key points

This icon is used to highlight points of particular importance.

 Quote

This icon indicates useful or interesting citations from notable individuals, including well-known physicians.

 Think about

This icon indicates what the reader should reflect on after having read a passage from the text.

 Warning/Hazard

This icon is used to indicate common or important drug interactions, pitfalls of practical procedures, or when to take symptoms or signs particularly seriously.

Gastroenterology and Hepatology

AUTHORS:

J.D. Collier, J.M. Hebden, S. Keshav, J. Shearman

EDITOR:

J.D. Collier

EDITOR-IN-CHIEF:

J.D. Firth

1 Clinical presentations

1.1 Chronic diarrhoea

Case history

A 24-year-old married man presents with a 6-month history of watery diarrhoea with blood mixed in with the stool. He has lost some weight and also complains of arthralgia.

Clinical approach

This man is most likely to have idiopathic inflammatory bowel disease (IBD), but it is important to exclude chronic infection and to consider other causes of chronic diarrhoea (Table 1). In older patients it is particularly important to consider intestinal neoplasia and paradoxical 'overflow' diarrhoea caused by chronic constipation. Always check that the patient does actually have diarrhoea, i.e. increased daily stool volume. In any patient presenting with chronic diarrhoea ask specific questions to determine if there has been weight loss, a systemic response revealed by fevers and sweats, bloody diarrhoea or passage of pus or mucus, or steatorrhoea.

Coeliac disease is common and may present subtly with chronic diarrhoea (without steatorrhoea) and vague malaise.

History of the presenting problem

Stool character

The stool character is critical in formulating an appropriate differential diagnosis. Questions include:
- exact frequency of passing motions
- whether there is urgency
- pain on defecation
- tenesmus.

The nature of any rectal bleeding must be clarified:
- is the blood passed freely, sometimes without any stool?
- is it mixed with the stool?
- is it only present on the toilet paper when the anus is wiped? (suggests piles).

Ask about passage of mucus or pus.

Table 1 Differential diagnosis of chronic diarrhoea.

Intestinal inflammation
Idiopathic IBD: UC and CD
Microscopic/lymphocytic/collagenous colitis
NSAID enteropathy
Intestinal tuberculosis, which may be clinically indistinguishable from CD
Radiation enteritis, colitis and proctitis

Chronic infectious diarrhoea
In HIV infection, and other immunocompromised individuals. Organisms frequently encountered are microsporidia and cryptosporidium. Cytomegalovirus and atypical mycobacterial infections may occur. It is debatable whether a specific HIV enteropathy exists as a separate entity
Some enteric infections, such as giardiasis and amoebiasis, may produce prolonged symptoms even in immunocompetent individuals
Tropical sprue
Whipple's disease
Clostridium difficile-related diarrhoea is usually acute, but may be chronic and relapsing

Intestinal neoplasia
Intestinal lymphoma may complicate coeliac disease and chronic immunosuppressive therapy
Adenomas, particularly secretory villous adenomas of the colon can produce a secretory diarrhoea
Obstructing neoplastic lesions may produce chronic constipation and paradoxical 'overflow' diarrhoea

Malabsorption
Pancreatic insufficiency, e.g. in chronic pancreatitis
Coeliac disease (see Section 1.10, p. 31)
Bacterial overgrowth (see Section 1.11, p. 34)
Bile salt diarrhoea due to ileal disease and reduced absorption of bile salts

Systemic disorders and drug-related diarrhoea
Thyrotoxicosis
Secretory neuroendocrine tumours, such as carcinoid, phaeochromocytoma and VIPoma
Diarrhoea is a frequent side effect of some drugs, such as olsalazine, mycophenolate mofetil, misoprostol, colchicine and antibiotics

Factitious/fictitious
Laxative abuse
Patients assign their own meaning to technical terms: check what they mean by diarrhoea, constipation, 'runs', 'accident', etc.

IBD, inflammatory bowel disease; UC, ulcerative colitis; CD, Crohn's disease; NSAID, non-steroidal anti-inflammatory drug; PBC, primary biliary cirrhosis; PSC, primary sclerosing cholangitis; VIPoma, vasoactive intestinal peptide secreting tumour.

Exclude steatorrhoea by asking:
- is the stool bulky and light coloured?
- does it float on the water in the toilet?
- does it have an offensive odour?

In assessing the severity of the diarrhoea it is important to know:
- is the stool extremely watery, or passed in large volumes?
- does the patient feel faint or unwell when passing stool?
- is there undigested food in the stool?

Systemic symptoms

Non-specific malaise, with or without weight loss, is frequently present in uncomplicated ulcerative colitis and coeliac disease. Weight loss, fever, night sweats and malaise are usually prominent in patients with Crohn's disease and intestinal tuberculosis.

Pain

Cramping abdominal pain often accompanies diarrhoea of any cause. Deep-seated abdominal pain should alert one to the possibility of Crohn's disease, intestinal tuberculosis and neoplasia. Pain suggesting pancreatitis or cholelithiasis may provide a clue to the cause of steatorrhoea.

Relevant past history

Epidemiological considerations

Age is important in that neoplasia is unlikely in younger patients such as this man. Whipple's disease occurs almost exclusively in older men, and microscopic colitis occurs typically in older women. Inflammatory bowel disease (IBD) and coeliac disease, on the other hand, can present at any age. Tuberculosis is particularly common in Asia and Africa.

Risk factors

Apart from a positive family history, there are no known risk factors for IBD, although in some patients it appears to be triggered by an episode of infectious colitis. The main risks for chronic pancreatitis are excess alcohol use and cholelithiasis, although patients heterozygous for the cystic fibrosis mutation may be at increased risk of idiopathic chronic pancreatitis.

Systematic enquiry

Direct questions are usually needed to address possible endocrine disorders, carcinoid syndrome, HIV disease, travel (When did you last go abroad? How long were you there? What were you doing? And the time before that?), diet, and laxative and other drug use. If IBD is suspected, patients should be questioned about arthralgia, arthritis, skin rashes and visual symptoms.

Examination

 Consider hospitalization of anyone with a severe exacerbation of colitis, heralded by increased stool frequency (>10× per day), fever, tachycardia and abdominal pain. Fulminant colitis carries a high risk of morbidity and mortality, and requires combined medical and surgical management.

General

The most important immediate consideration is whether the patient is well, unwell or extremely unwell.
- Check vital signs—tachycardia, hypotension and fever may be present with severe colitis.
- Check carefully for signs of intravascular volume depletion—low JVP and postural hypotension (lying and sitting if standing is not prudent). If these are present, obtain venous access and begin resuscitation whilst completing the history and examination.
- It is also important to establish the nutritional status—how much does the patient weigh? What is their body mass index weight $(kg)/(height\ (m))^2$? Examine the hands, skin, eyes, mouth and joints for signs of systemic or multisystem disease. Aphthous ulceration may be present in Crohn's disease.

Gastroenterological

External examination of the abdomen may be unremarkable, or may reveal tender inflamed areas of underlying bowel. With ulcerative colitis, a thickened, fibrosed segment of sigmoid colon may be felt. Crohn's disease and ileocaecal tuberculosis may cause an ill-defined tender mass in the right iliac fossa. Generalized abdominal tenderness, scant bowel sounds or visible distension are generally signs of severe disease in acutely ill patients.

Rectal examination

This is mandatory. Examine the anal verge for signs of excoriation, which may result from excess secretions. Many patients with Crohn's disease will have anorectal involvement, with ulceration, fissuring and scarring. Insertion of the examining finger may be painful, so prepare the patient and obtain consent for the examination. Blood and pus may be detected on the glove on withdrawal.

Approach to investigations and management

Investigations

 Intercurrent infectious diarrhoea should always be considered, even in patients with known IBD, particularly before starting immunosuppression.

Examination of the stool

All patients should have stool examined for bacterial pathogens and for the ova, cysts and adult forms of various parasites. Amoebae may be difficult to detect if a fresh ('hot') stool sample is not examined. If the test is available, estimation of faecal leucocytes is invaluable in distinguishing inflammatory disease from other causes of diarrhoea.

In some cases it is necessary to measure the stool volume over a 24-h period or to estimate faecal fat excretion over a 72-h period.

Rigid sigmoidoscopy

This should be performed if at all feasible. Rectal involvement is almost universal in ulcerative colitis, while the rectum may be spared completely in Crohn's disease. Bleeding, ulceration and a mucopurulent exudate may be seen. In less severe inflammation there may simply be loss of vascular patterns and a granular, friable mucosa. A biopsy should be taken for histological examination.

Systemic inflammation

The ESR and serum C-reactive protein should be measured in all patients in whom IBD is suspected.

 Raised systemic inflammatory markers are unusual in ulcerative colitis unless the disease is severe, but Crohn's disease can produce a marked serum response with few clinical signs.

Nutritional assessment

Assessment and management of nutrition is a key feature of managing patients with chronic diarrhoea, particularly in IBD with small intestinal involvement. Check haemoglobin level, mean red cell volume, serum albumin, iron, ferritin, folic acid and vitamin B_{12} levels.
• Inflammation *per se* may affect the serum albumin and ferritin levels.
• Iron, folate and B_{12} are absorbed preferentially in different parts of the small intestine, and provide clues to localization of disease processes.
• In malabsorption due to pancreatic and biliary disease, fat and fat-soluble vitamin absorption are most affected: serum calcium, vitamin D and prothrombin time, which is prolonged by vitamin K deficiency, are informative in these cases.

Specialized diagnostic tests

PLAIN ABDOMINAL RADIOGRAPH

If severe colitis is suspected, the patient should be admitted

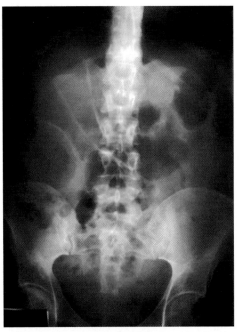

Fig. 1 Plain abdominal radiograph showing a very dilated colon (toxic megacolon).

and an abdominal radiograph obtained. What is the intestinal gas pattern? Visible dilatation of the large intestine may presage perforation and is an emergency (Fig. 1). Pancreatic calcification may help establish a diagnosis of chronic pancreatitis.

COLONOSCOPY

This allows direct visualization of the entire mucosa, and in many cases allows examination and biopsy of the terminal ileum. Colonoscopy should be performed in all patients with suspected colitis or Crohn's disease, and may be the most direct way of establishing a diagnosis in other patients (Fig. 2).

BLOOD AND URINE TESTS

The presence of IgA antibodies to endomysial antigens is virtually diagnostic of coeliac disease, although the test may be falsely negative in patients with IgA deficiency. Fasting gut hormone profiles may reveal abnormal concentrations of gastrin, glucagon and vasoactive intestinal peptide (VIP). The carcinoid syndrome may be diagnosed by increased urinary excretion of 5-HIAA.

Management

 Severe fulminant colitis is an emergency. It requires hospital treatment, intravenous steroids and consideration of emergency colectomy.

(a)

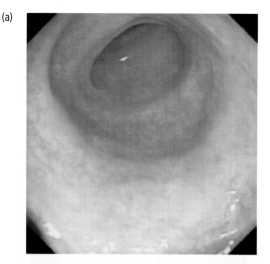

(b)

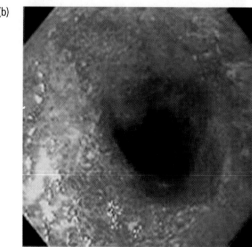

Fig. 2 Ulcerative colitis: (a) normal colonic mucosa; (b) inflamed colonic mucosa at endoscopy.

Table 2 The management of different causes of chronic diarrhoea.

Chronic intestinal infection and bacterial overgrowth
Amoebiasis and giardiasis respond to treatment with metronidazole
Whipple's disease and tropical sprue are treated by prolonged course of tetracycline
Chronic infections in patients with HIV disease can often only be adequately treated by measures which improve the patient's CD4 lymphocyte count
Chronic *C. difficile*-related diarrhoea may require prolonged or cyclical treatment with metronidazole, oral vancomycin and oral cholestyramine, which binds the enterotoxin of *C. difficile*. Reconstitution of the balance of normal enteric flora with orally administered lactobacilli is a promising alternative

Coeliac disease
(See Section 1.10, p. 32.)

Malabsorption
Pancreatic enzyme supplements should be tailored to the patient's symptoms

Secretory diarrhoea
Secretion of gut hormones may be inhibited by octreotide, which also improves diarrhoea in the carcinoid syndrome
Secretory diarrhoea caused by excess intestinal loss of bile salts, as in patients with ileal resection or terminal ileal disease, may be treated with a binding resin such as cholestyramine
Acid suppression with proton pump inhibitors may reduce intestinal secretion
Antidiarrhoeals such as loperamide and codeine phosphate may be used when infection or inflammation has been excluded

Resuscitation

If the patient is volume depleted then they require resuscitation, whatever the cause of their colitis. Give colloid or 0.9% saline rapidly i.v. until the JVP is at the upper end of the normal range and postural hypotension has been abolished.

Inflammatory bowel disease

CORTICOSTEROIDS AND 5-AMINOSALICYLIC ACID

Acute inflammatory exacerbations are controlled by intravenous or oral steroids. For colonic and terminal ileal disease, 5-aminosalicylic acid compounds have been shown to maintain remission. Local treatment of anorectal or distal colonic disease with steroid or 5-aminosalicylic acid enemas is feasible.

CYCLOSPORIN AND OTHER IMMUNOSUPPRESSANTS

Cyclosporin given orally or intravenously may induce remission in severe colitis but is not useful in maintenance treatment. Long-term immunosuppression with azathioprine and other agents is often used to maintain remission in both Crohn's colitis and ulcerative colitis.

SURGERY

Emergency colectomy is indicated for toxic megacolon and severe disease that does not improve with medical therapy. In cases of severe colitis joint surgical/medical liaison is essential. (See *Emergency medicine*, Section 1.12.)

NUTRITION

Attention to nutrition is essential. In severe colitis patients may require total parenteral nutrition (see Section 2.14.4, p. 124).

Other causes of chronic diarrhoea

The specific management of other causes of chronic diarrhoea is shown in Table 2.

 The management of patients with inflammatory bowel disease requires a long-term, multidisciplinary approach, including dieticians, specialist nurses, physicians and surgeons.

See *Emergency medicine*, Section 1.12.

See *Infectious diseases*, Section 1.23.

Afzalpurkar RG, Schiller LR, Little KH, Santangelo WC, Fordtran JS. The self-limited nature of chronic idiopathic diarrhoea. *N Engl J Med* 1992; 327: 1849–1852. [Outcome of diarrhoea in which a cause is not found.]

Alam MJ. Chronic refractory diarrhoea: A manifestation of endocrine disorders. *Dig Dis* 1994; 12: 46–61. [Endocrine causes of diarrhoea.]

Donowitz M, Kokke FT, Saidi R. Evaluation of patients with chronic diarrhoea. *N Engl J Med* 1995; 332: 725–729. [Review of chronic diarrhoea.]

Langholz E, Munkholm P, Davidsen M, Binder V. Course of ulcerative colitis: analysis of changes in disease activity over years. *Gastroenterol* 1994; 107: 3–11. [Natural history of ulcerative colitis.]

Website for National Association for Crohn's and Ulcerative Colitis. http://www.nacc.org.uk

Stack WA, Long RG, Hawkey CJ. Short and long-term outcome of patients treated with cyclosporin for severe acute ulcerative colitis. *Aliment Pharmacol Ther* 1998; 12: 973–978. [The role of cyclosporin in the treatment of ulcerative colitis.]

1.2 Heartburn and dysphagia

Case history

A 60-year-old woman presents to outpatients with progressive dysphagia for solids over the last 6 months. She has had retrosternal burning pain for many years and regularly uses over-the-counter antacids.

Clinical approach

Dysphagia is an 'alarm' symptom and should be investigated rapidly. Causes are listed in Table 3, but the obvious concern is that it is due to a carcinoma of the oesophagus or gastric cardia, and this should be the working diagnosis until proven otherwise.

History of the presenting problem

Pain

The obvious assumption in this case is that the pain is due to reflux oesophagitis. However, it is always important to take a careful history when assessing chest pain.
• Reflux oesophagitis typically produces retrosternal burning pain radiating upwards into the throat.
• Angina typically produces central, tight, heavy chest pain that radiates into the left arm.
It can often be very difficult to differentiate between the two conditions, and in the patient presenting with acute chest pain the default position must be to assume that the pain is cardiac.

Table 3 Differential diagnosis of dysphagia.

Common	Less common	Rare
Benign oesophageal stricture	Pharyngeal pouch	Scleroderma
Oesophageal carcinoma		Motor neurone disease
Oesophageal dysmotility		Achalasia

See *Emergency medicine*, Section 1.3 and *Cardiology*, Section 1.5 for further discussion. In this case the pain has been present for many years and the dominant symptom is dysphagia.

Dysphagia

Type of dysphagia

Dysphagia means difficulty swallowing. It may be due to causes in the mouth, pharynx or oesophagus (Table 3). The history usually identifies oral problems.
• Strictures (benign or malignant) usually cause dysphagia first for food (particularly bread and meat), and later for liquids.
• Dysphagia for solids and liquids from the outset is more typical of achalasia.
• Dysphagia for liquids (more so than solids) often indicates a pharyngeal problem, e.g. stroke, motor neurone disease (see *Neurology*, Section 1.10).
• Odynophagia, pain on swallowing, occurs in reflux oesophagitis, achalasia, oesophageal candidiasis and herpetic oesophagitis, and with benign and malignant strictures.

 Although the patient will often indicate the apparent level of obstruction on the sternum, there is very poor correlation with the actual site of blockage.

Length of history of dysphagia

Rapidly progressive dysphagia is suggestive of a malignant stricture. A gradual onset of symptoms stretching back over 6 months or more, as in this case, is typical of a benign stricture.

Weight loss

Any mechanical blockage to the passage of food into the stomach will restrict calorie intake and therefore result in weight loss. Severe and rapid weight loss tends to point to a malignant process.

Relevant past history

Drugs

NSAIDs, potassium salts, bisphosphonates and tetracyclines have all been implicated as causes of oesophagitis and oesophageal stricture formation.

Gastro-oesophageal reflux disease

Gradual onset of dysphagia in a patient with longstanding gastro-oesophageal reflux disease suggests the development of a benign oesophageal stricture. A past history of a peptic oesophageal stricture is clearly relevant because these frequently recur following dilatation, even after many years.

Radiation-induced oesophagitis

May occur weeks or months after irradiation treatment for malignancies (e.g. bronchial carcinoma).

Oesophageal candidiasis

Oesophageal candidiasis may be asymptomatic or cause symptoms of heartburn and dysphagia. Predisposing factors include diabetes mellitus, inhaled corticosteroids and immunosuppression due to chemotherapy, therapeutic immunosuppression or HIV infection.

Examination

Examination of the patient with heartburn and dysphagia

- General impression: is the patient well or cachectic?
- Careful and thorough abdominal examination.

General

What does the patient look like? Although benign and malignant strictures can both limit food intake, it is unusual to see marked cachexia in the context of benign peptic strictures. How much does the woman weigh? What is her BMI? Is the skin on the fingers and around the mouth rather tight and shiny? Could this be a case of scleroderma? (See *Rheumatology and clinical immunology*, Section 1.13.)

Abdominal examination

Take particular note of the following:
- Is the patient anaemic or jaundiced?
- Are any supraclavicular nodes palpable (Virchow's node in gastric adenocarcinoma)?
- Is there an epigastric mass?
- Is there hepatomegaly?

Differential diagnosis

In the patient with dysphagia, consider the following:
- *Pharyngeal pouch.* Usually presents in elderly people. Patients may sense a lump in the throat on or after swallowing.

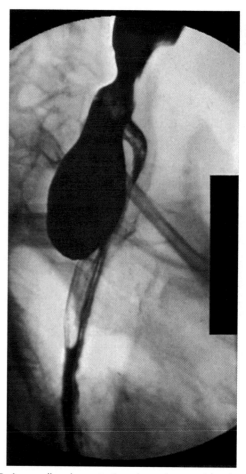

Fig. 3 Barium swallow demonstrating a large pharyngeal pouch.

Differential diagnosis (continued)

Occasionally causes a palpable swelling in the neck, which can be emptied by pressure. Barium swallow is essential, because endoscopy can easily result in perforation as scope passes into blind sac (Fig. 3).
- *Motor neurone disease.* Ask about choking and coughing on swallowing, with fluids occasionally coming back through the nose. Look for tongue fasciculation.
- *Globus syndrome.* Patients get a sensation of a lump in the throat, but this seldom interferes with swallowing. Associated with psychiatric disorders.

Approach to investigations and management

Investigations

Investigation of dysphagia
- Barium swallow—urgent
- Endoscopy—biopsy and brushings if any stricture identified
- Manometry.

No matter how likely the diagnosis of a benign stricture, the patient still requires investigation with a barium swallow and endoscopy to rule out malignancy.

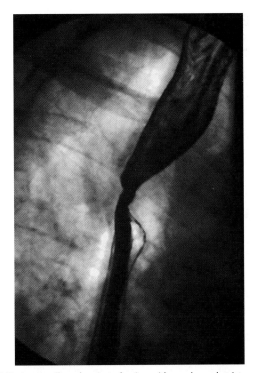

Fig. 4 Barium swallow showing a benign midoesophageal stricture.

Blood tests and plain radiology

Check blood tests for evidence of iron-deficiency anaemia and malnutrition (see Section 1.1, p. 3). Look very carefully at the chest radiograph (PA and lateral) for hiatus hernia or evidence of carcinoma (primaries or secondaries).

Examination of the oesophagus

BARIUM SWALLOW

This is usually the initial investigation. It allows the site of pathology to be identified and forewarns of any pitfalls, such as a pharyngeal pouch (Fig. 3). If dysphagia is minor, or a stricture has been previously diagnosed (Fig. 4), then endoscopy may be the initial investigation.

ENDOSCOPY

Any stricture must be brushed and biopsied to exclude malignancy. If the stricture is impassable and dysphagia severe, then dilatation is performed.

MANOMETRY

If barium swallow and/or endoscopy are normal, oesophageal manometry may be useful in diagnosing a motility disorder, e.g. oesophageal spasm. It may also provide additional confirmatory evidence of achalasia (hypertensive lower oesophageal sphincter which fails to relax on swallowing) following a suggestive barium study.

Other tests

Other investigations may be required in some cases, e.g. serological tests in suspected scleroderma; electromyography (EMG) in suspected motor neurone disease.

Management

Benign oesophageal stricture

Ensure the patient is on a proton pump inhibitor. Oesophageal dilatation may be required (see Section 2.2, p. 63).

Oesophageal carcinoma or motility disorder

See Section 2.2, p. 63.

See Section 2.2, p. 63.
Barbezat OC, Schlup M, Lubcke R. Omeprazole therapy decreases the need for dilatation of peptic oesophageal strictures. *Aliment Pharmacol Ther* 1999; 13: 1041–1043. [Role of proton pump inhibitors in reflux oesophagitis.]

1.3 Melaena and collapse

Case history

A 55-year-old man presents with a 3-day history of melaena. He had collapsed while walking to the bathroom.

Clinical approach

The history of melaena indicates the patient has had a gastrointestinal haemorrhage from a lesion anywhere from the oesophagus to the terminal ileum; more distal haemorrhage results in fresh rectal bleeding (Table 4). The most

Table 4 Differential diagnosis of melaena.

Common	Less common	Rare
Duodenal ulceration	Oesophageal/gastric	Aorto-enteric
Gastric ulceration/erosions	varices	fistulae
Gastric carcinoma	Dieulafoy lesion	Small bowel
NSAID-induced enteropathy	Angiodysplasia	tumour
Oesophagitis		

NSAID, non-steroidal anti-inflammatory drug.

likely cause of melaena in this case is peptic ulceration. It is important to try and determine the likely cause of bleeding, the severity of the haemorrhage and whether there is continual bleeding. It is also important to assess for the presence of comorbidity such as a chronic liver disease and ischaemic heart disease, which increase the mortality associated with gastrointestinal bleeding.

History of the presenting problem

Blood loss

When did the melaena start?

Sudden onset with haemodynamic compromise indicates a large bleed.

Haematemesis

Has he vomited? And if so, what? Be particular:
• Did he vomit fresh blood? This suggests either a proximal source of bleeding, e.g. the oesophagus (see Section 1.4, p. 13), a large gastrointestinal haemorrhage, or persistent bleeding. But remember that persistent life-threatening bleeding can occur with melaena in the absence of a haematemesis.
• Was the vomit 'coffee grounds'? (suggestive of altered and therefore old blood).

Dizziness or syncope

Syncope suggests a significant gastrointestinal haemorrhage or a large bleed against the background of chronic anaemia. A history of shortness of breath on exertion or worsening of angina in the weeks preceding presentation suggests that chronic iron-deficiency anaemia is likely.

Underlying source of bleeding

Vomiting

The presence of recurrent or forceful vomiting followed by a haematemesis typically occurs with a Mallory–Weiss tear. If vomiting after eating precedes melaena, this may suggest a peptic ulcer in the pyloric canal causing gastric outflow obstruction.

Abdominal pain

• There may have been recent retrosternal discomfort and acid reflux into the mouth due to oesophagitis.
• Gastric and duodenal ulcers may be associated with recent epigastric discomfort or 'indigestion'.

• Pain radiating through to the back typically occurs with a deep posterior duodenal ulcer.
• The possibility of perforation must be considered if pain is severe.

Weight loss

Weight loss can occur as a result of anorexia with an underlying carcinoma, or through reduced oral intake due to pain from a peptic ulcer.

Relevant past history

Drugs

Non-steroidal anti-inflammatory drugs (NSAIDs) and aspirin can cause either ulceration or erosions in the stomach, duodenum or small bowel. Establish if there has been a recent change in the type of NSAID used or change in dose of aspirin. Anticoagulation with warfarin clearly has the potential to make any bleeding worse. Beta blockers may mask a tachycardia associated with hypovolaemia.

Liver disease

Most important is to establish if the patient has a history of chronic liver disease that would increase the risk of oesophageal or gastric varices. Ask the patient:
• Have you ever been told you have cirrhosis, liver disease or a scarred liver?
• Have you ever been jaundiced?
• Have you ever had a distended abdomen due to fluid (ascites)?
• How much alcohol do you normally drink? When did you last have a drink, and what was it? Have you ever been a heavy drinker in the past? You've never been a '10 pint' or a 'bottle of whisky a day man' (or woman in another case)?
• Have you ever previously had bleeding from the gut?

Previous peptic ulcer surgery

Historically, a partial gastrectomy with or without a gastroenterostomy (Bilroth I or II) used to be performed for bleeding gastric or duodenal ulcers (Figs 5 and 6): now they are usually just oversewn. There is an increased incidence of stomal ulceration and carcinoma of the stoma following partial gastrectomy.

Comorbidity

Ask specifically about ischaemic heart disease, chronic pulmonary disease, and organ failure (renal, cardiac or liver). The presence of these factors increases the morbidity associated with gastrointestinal bleeding.

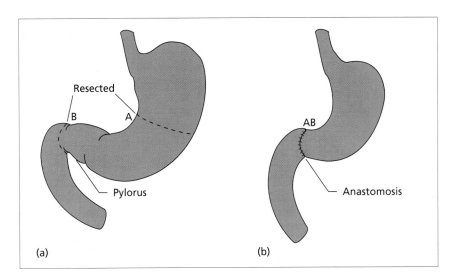

Fig. 5 Schematic diagram of the anatomy following a partial gastrectomy (Bilroth I).

(a)   (b)

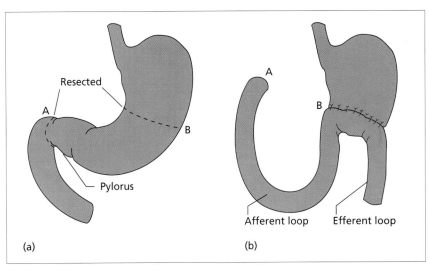

Fig. 6 Schematic diagram of the anatomy following a partial gastrectomy with a gastroenterostomy (Bilroth II).

(a)   (b)

Differential diagnosis

When taking a history from a patient presenting with melaena, consider:
- *Gastric carcinoma*, particularly in an elderly person with a history of anorexia and weight loss.
- *Oesophagitis*. Must be considered in any age group, particularly if there is a history of reflux symptoms or dysphagia. Aspirin and NSAIDs can lodge in the oesophagus if there is a pre-existing benign peptic stricture.
- *Oesophageal or gastric varices*. Can occur at any age. Does the patient have any history of liver disease, or anything that would put them at risk of liver disease (alcohol, drugs, etc.)?

Examination

Examination of the patient with melaena

- General impression—is the patient well, ill, very ill or nearly dead: if nearly dead call for ICU help immediately. If ill or very ill, then start resuscitation immediately, before completing the history and examination.
- Assessment of hypovolaemia—pulse, BP (lying and sitting), are the peripheries cold and clammy?
- Careful abdominal examination.

General

Does the patient look well or unwell, and if unwell—how bad? Check vital signs, in particular pulse and BP: the severity of the bleeding and risk of death can be assessed clinically on the basis of the patient's age, pulse, systolic BP and comorbidity (Table 5).

Look specifically for evidence of chronic liver disease (see Sections 1.4, p. 13 and 1.8, p. 27).

Abdominal and rectal examination

Take note of the following:
- jaundice
- epigastric mass
- hepatomegaly and/or splenomegaly
- tenderness
- rebound or guarding
- abdominal distention (ascites, aortic aneurysm)
- presence of melaena.

Table 5 Clinical assessment of the severity of the gastrointestinal haemorrhage based on initial clinical findings prior to endoscopy (Rockall score).

Clinical parameter	Score			
	0	1	2	3
Age (yrs)	<60	60–79	80+	
Shock				
Systolic BP (mmHg)	>100	>100	<100	
Pulse (/min)	<100	>100		
Comorbidity	Nil	Other	Cardiac failure IHD	Renal failure Liver failure
Total score	0	2	4	6
Mortality (%)	0.2	5	24	49

BP, blood pressure; IHD, ischaemic heart disease.

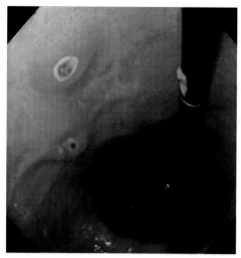

Fig. 7 Small gastric ulcer and adjacent erosion viewed at gastroscopy.

Differential diagnosis

When examining a patient presenting with melaena, consider:
- *Oesophageal/gastric varices.* Can cause major haemorrhage and must always be considered.
- Look for cutaneous stigmata of chronic liver disease, hepatomegaly, splenomegaly and ascites.
- *Gastric carcinoma.* There may be an abdominal mass, left subclavian lymph node and cachexia.
- *Aortoenteric fistulae.* Suspect if back pain and a tense distended abdomen with hypotension. Always consider if a history of abdominal aneurysm: urgent surgery rather than endoscopy is indicated.

Approach to investigations and management

Investigation of melaena

- Full blood count
- Electrolytes and renal function
- Liver biochemistry and clotting screen
- Endoscopy—within 24–48 h.

Immediate Investigation

Blood tests

- Check full blood count: what is the haemoglobin? What is the MCV? (reduced in chronic iron-deficiency anaemia). Repeat after 12 h.
- Check electrolytes and renal function: in upper GI bleeding urea is elevated out of proportion to creatinine due to blood in bowel.
- Prothrombin time and liver function tests.
- Cross match at least 4 units of blood for anyone who

appears to have had a substantial GI bleed, as in this case.

 The haemoglobin may initially be normal following an acute GI bleed.

Erect chest radiograph

Required if a perforation is suspected to look for free air under the diaphragm, or the patient has vomited and there is the possibility of aspiration pneumonia.

Endoscopy

This should ideally be performed within 24 h of admission in anyone with a substantial GI bleed. Urgent endoscopy is indicated if oesophageal varices are suspected, or the patient is actively bleeding or remains hypotensive. It may be necessary for this to be performed in theatre with the surgical team on 'standby', when endoscopy will exclude variceal haemorrhage and an inoperable gastric cancer as well as defining the lesion (Fig. 7). Note whether the following stigmata of recent haemorrhage are seen:
- blood in the stomach
- clot over an ulcer
- an actively bleeding vessel.

These endoscopic findings help in stratifying patients' risk of rebleeding and mortality (see Section 2.3, p. 70).

 It is dangerous to perform endoscopy on a patient who is hypovolaemic.

Abdominal CT with contrast

Required if an aortoenteric fistula is suspected.

Initial management

Management of the patient with gastrointestinal haemorrhage
- Resuscitate first: ask questions afterwards
- Do not attempt to insert an internal jugular or subclavian central line into someone who is obviously hypovolaemic, i.e. until they are resuscitated.
- Early liaison with the surgical team is essential.

Resuscitation

If the patient is shocked, i.e. has cool peripheries, tachycardia, hypotension or severe postural hypotension (lying and sitting) and a low JVP, then give high-flow oxygen and:
- Insert large-bore cannulae into both antecubital fossae: if not possible, insert large-bore central venous catheter into femoral vein using Seldinger technique.
- Give blood (if available), colloid or 0.9% saline: 1 litre i.v. as fast as possible.
- Check peripheral perfusion, pulse rate, BP and JVP.
- If there is still evidence of shock give another litre of fluid as fast as possible.
- Keep doing so until peripheries are warming, pulse is settling, BP is restored (without postural drop) and JVP can be seen.

Do not attempt to insert a central venous line (internal jugular or subclavian) into someone who is clearly hypovolaemic because:
- A central line never made anyone better, but has killed quite a few—insertion is difficult when veins are constricted, making the chance of complications much higher.
- Knowing exactly how low the CVP is will not alter management.
- Time spent trying to insert a line can be better spent doing other things.

When intravascular volume has been restored then a central line should be inserted in most cases to allow early detection of rebleeding.

See *Emergency medicine*, Section 1.11.

Other aspects

- Inform surgical colleagues sooner rather than later.
- Acid suppression for ulcer healing—there is now evidence that use of a high dose intravenous proton pump inhibitor reduces rebleeding after endoscopic treatment of bleeding peptic ulcers.
- Endoscopic therapy—see Section 2.3, p. 70.
- Eradication of *H. pylori*—this is indicated if infection is present with a gastric or duodenal ulcer (see Section 2.3, p. 70).

See *Emergency medicine*, Section 1.11.

Cook DJ, Guyatt GH, Salena BJ, Laine LA. Endoscopic therapy for acute non-variceal upper gastrointestinal haemorrhage: a meta-analysis. *Gastroenterol* 1992; 102: 139–148. [Reduction in mortality with endoscopic therapy of bleeding peptic ulcers.]

Rockall TA, Logan RFA, Delvin HB, Northfield TC. Risk assessment after acute upper gastrointestinal haemorrhage. *Gut* 1996; 38: 316–321. [Assessment of mortality and risk of rebleeding following a gastrointestinal haemorrhage based on both clinical and endoscopic parameters.]

Lau JY, Sung JJ, Lee KK, Yung MY *et al.* Effect of intravenous omeprazole on recurrent bleeding after endoscopic treatment of bleeding peptic ulcers. *N Engl J Med* 2000; 343: 310–316.

1.4 Haematemesis and jaundice

Case history

A 51-year-old man presents with a brisk, painless, large-volume haematemesis. He is tachycardic, hypotensive and jaundiced.

Clinical approach

A large-volume painless haematemesis is very suspicious of oesophageal variceal bleeding, particularly if there is any indication of chronic liver disease. This should be the working diagnosis in this case, and the management should be undertaken with the help of an appropriately skilled specialist. Portal hypertension and variceal haemorrhage may also occur in non-cirrhotic patients, e.g. as a result of portal vein thrombosis. Furthermore, other causes of bleeding, particularly peptic ulcer disease, can and do occur in the context of portal hypertension (Table 6).

History of the presenting problem

Typical history

Unlike the history of blood-stained vomitus following prolonged retching, or fresh blood and 'coffee grounds' associated with oozing from peptic ulceration, variceal haemorrhage usually occurs with minimal warning, although it may be preceded by nausea, and is characterized by fairly

Table 6 The most common causes of haematemesis in patients with liver cirrhosis.

Bleeding oesophageal varices	60%
Bleeding peptic ulcer	20%
Portal hypertensive gastropathy	5%
Bleeding gastric varices	5%
Other causes and undiagnosed	10%

large volumes of fresh blood with or without clots. The patient may feel faint or light-headed as a result of massive blood loss, or may be in circulatory shock. If there has been time for blood to pass through the gut, melaena or even apparently fresh rectal bleeding may occur following brisk upper gastrointestinal bleeding.

 Significant gastrointestinal haemorrhage from oesophageal varices can present with melaena in the absence of haematemesis.

Relevant past history

Alcohol

Alcohol is the most common cause of chronic liver disease, and patients with cirrhosis of any aetiology who continue to drink are particularly at risk from variceal haemorrhage as alcohol exacerbates portal hypertension. How much alcohol does the patient drink? When did they last have a drink? Have they ever been a heavy drinker in the past (see *General clinical issues*, Section 3)?

Chronic liver disease

Has the patient had, or are they at risk of, chronic viral hepatitis, primary biliary cirrhosis, primary sclerosing cholangitis, genetic haemochromatosis or autoimmune hepatitis? In about 20% of cases of chronic liver disease, no cause is found (idiopathic cirrhosis). See Section 2.10, p. 110.

 Variceal haemorrhage may be a presenting feature of previously undiagnosed liver disease.

Other evidence of hepatic decompensation

There is an association of variceal haemorrhage with the development of ascites in previously compensated chronic liver disease: has the patient's belly swollen up recently? A preceding history of variceal haemorrhage, ascites or hepatic encephalopathy increase the likelihood of variceal bleeding. See Section 1.8, p. 27.

Examination

General

As described in Section 1.3, p. 9, the first priority is to assess how unwell the patient is and to call immediately for help if this is required, then to assess intravascular volume and to initiate resuscitation.

Remember that obtunded patients are at high risk of aspiration of vomitus, also that those with liver disease are at risk of sepsis, and there may be evidence of this on presentation.

Gastroenterological

Portal hypertension and hepatic decompensation

Look specifically for splenomegaly, prominent anterior abdominal wall veins with flow away from the umbilicus, ascites and hepatic encephalopathy.

Chronic liver disease

This man is jaundiced. Check in addition for wasting, palmar erythema, leukonychia, finger clubbing, spider naevi, loss of body hair, gynaecomastia and testicular atrophy. Subacute liver disease with portal hypertension may also present with variceal haemorrhage, particularly in Budd–Chiari syndrome, when ascites, jaundice and hepatomegaly are usually prominent.

 Examine for signs of liver failure or decompensation: hepatic fetor, flapping tremor, altered consciousness, bruising, petechiae, jaundice, ascites and peripheral oedema.

Approach to investigations and management

Initial investigation

As described in Section 1.3, p. 9. Blood tests for infective causes of chronic liver disease (hepatitis B and C) should be requested urgently (when appropriate), with samples also sent for non-urgent screen for other causes of chronic liver disease (e.g. serological tests for autoantibodies).

Initial management

Although up to half of cases of variceal haemorrhage may stop bleeding spontaneously, and the use of pharmacological measures may increase this percentage, variceal haemorrhage remains a life-threatening emergency requiring urgent fluid resuscitation. Patients remain at risk of further bleeding, particularly immediately following the initial haemorrhage, and the overall mortality in the short and long term is high.

Fluid resuscitation

See Section 1.3, p. 9 and *Emergency medicine*, Section 1.11. Use blood or packed cells as soon as they are available: overenthusiastic use of other colloids or crystalloids may significantly impair tissue oxygenation.

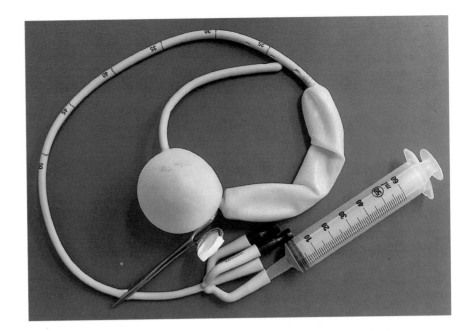

Fig. 8 Sengstaken–Blakemore tube. This particular tube has a gastric (inflated) and an oesophageal (deflated) balloon, but in most cases tamponade can be achieved by just inflating the gastric balloon. There is also a gastric aspiration channel and an oesophageal aspiration channel. The gastro-oesophageal junction is 40 cm from the mouth.

Pharmacological measures to reduce variceal haemorrhage

The use of octreotide and vasopressin analogues, which reduce splanchnic blood flow, have been shown to be at least as effective as emergency endoscopic therapy, and these should be used when variceal haemorrhage is suspected.

Correction of coagulopathy

Patients with decompensated cirrhosis typically have low platelet counts and a prolonged prothrombin time. There is little evidence to suggest that correcting these abnormalities is beneficial, although this may change with the availability of powerful new agents, such as recombinant activated factor VII, which can correct the prothrombin time without requiring large volumes of fresh frozen plasma (FFP). It is the usual practice to attempt to correct any concomitant vitamin K deficiency, to maintain platelet counts above 25, and to transfuse 2 units of FFP for every 4 units of blood or packed cells.

Prophylactic use of antibiotics

There is an association of bleeding oesophageal varices with sepsis, and patients are at risk of aspiration pneumonia, so it is standard practice to administer broad-spectrum antibiotics.

 Ascites frequently develops over a period of 3–5 days in patients who have had a variceal haemorrhage. Prophylactic antibiotics on admission reduce the risk of spontaneous bacterial peritonitis.

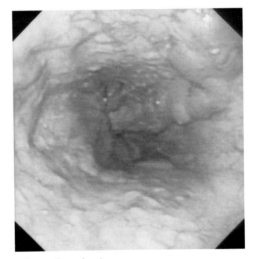

Fig. 9 Small oesophageal varices.

Balloon tamponade

When haemorrhage is torrential, or other factors prevent effective and safe emergency endoscopy, balloon tamponade of the gastric fundus and oesophagus may achieve haemostasis. A Sengstaken–Blakemore or Minnesota tube is employed as a temporary measure, which should not be used continuously for longer than 24 h. The clinician should be aware of the risk of oesophageal perforation and inadvertent intubation of the trachea (Fig. 8).

Emergency upper GI endoscopy

This may be diagnostic and therapeutic and should be performed as soon as it is safe to do so (Fig. 9). Bleeding oesophageal varices may be injected with sclerosant or ligated with rubber bands to stem bleeding. Banding varices

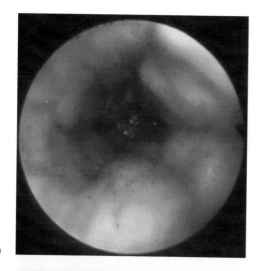

(a)

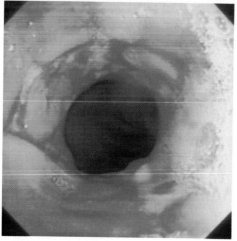

(b)

Fig. 10 Oesophageal varices: (a) large varices; (b) banded varices with superficial banding ulcers.

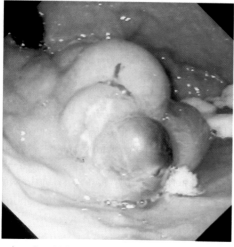

Fig. 11 Gastric varices. Varices at the gastro-oesophageal junction with surface ulceration and clot.

is associated with less secondary oesophageal ulceration than injection sclerotherapy (Fig. 10). As a significant number of patients with chronic liver disease may bleed from other causes, including gastric varices, diagnostic endoscopy is usually indicated (Table 6 and Fig. 11).

Emergency transjugular intrahepatic portosystemic shunt (TIPSS)

Portal hypertension can be reduced by deploying a stent to maintain a shunt between the portal vein and a major hepatic vein. The procedure is performed with radiological guidance and is particularly valuable for cases where bleeding is from gastric varices or portal hypertensive gastropathy, which can be difficult or impossible to control by other means.

Emergency surgery

Surgical transection of the oesophagus can be used to halt oesophageal variceal haemorrhage.

Further investigations

Abdominal ultrasound scan

This should address the questions of whether the liver is abnormal and whether there is any focal lesion, whether the spleen is enlarged, and whether there is subclinical ascites. Doppler venography should be used to assess portal vein patency and flow.

Elective endoscopy

More complete examination of the upper GI tract is possible when active bleeding has ceased.

Evaluation of the underlying liver disease

Investigations, including a liver biopsy, may be helpful in establishing a prognosis and deciding on long-term treatment options, such as liver transplantation. In alcoholic cirrhosis significant reduction in portal pressure may be achieved by abstinence from alcohol. Portal venous pressure may be determined by wedged hepatic venous pressure measurement, which can be performed at the same time as transjugular liver biopsy (see Section 3.4, p. 135).

Further management

Assessment of rebleeding

Close monitoring and transfusion to maintain circulatory volume are required.

Prevention of hepatic encephalopathy

Early use of laxatives (lactulose) and enemas are essential to reduce the risk of hepatic encephalopathy, which is aggravated by the enteric protein load of blood.

Nutrition

Patients with chronic liver disease are often malnourished, and should be allowed to eat as soon as possible. Thiamine replacement should be used where there is a history of excess alcohol use.

 Protein restriction is rarely indicated in patients with chronic liver disease. Sodium intake should be less than 100 mmol/day, which can be achieved most simply by not adding salt to food at the table.

Other

If there is a risk of withdrawal from alcohol, a reducing regimen of chlormethiazole or a benzodiazepine should be prescribed (see Section 1.7, p. 23).

Variceal bleeding

Patients remain at increased risk of rebleeding for about 7 days, when their risk returns to that of any patient with chronic liver disease and portal hypertension. It is therefore usual to monitor patients in hospital, and to maintain infusions of octreotide or a vasopressin analogue for 48 h after acute haemorrhage has been controlled.

 Variceal haemorrhage may precipitate more widespread hepatic decompensation with ascites, jaundice, coagulopathy and encephalopathy. The clinician should be alert to these potential risks.

Prevention of rebleeding

Abstinence from alcohol, anti-inflammatory or immuno-suppressive therapy in autoimmune hepatitis, and treatment of chronic viral hepatitis may help to arrest progression of chronic liver disease and reduce portal hypertension. Where haemorrhage is due to oesophageal varices, patients should be enrolled in a programme of endoscopic variceal obliteration, using sclerotherapy or band ligation. Where these measures fail, surgical or radiological (TIPSS) shunting should be considered, also liver transplantation in selected cases.

 See *Emergency medicine*, Sections 1.11 and 1.26.
Gimson AE, Ramage JK, Panos MZ *et al*. Randomised trial of variceal banding ligation versus injection sclerotherapy for bleeding oesophageal varices. *Lancet* 1993; 342: 391–394.
Jalan R, Liu HF, Readhead DN, Hayes PC. TIPPS 10 years on. *Gut* 2000; 46: 578–581.
Jalan R, Hayes PC. UK guidelines on the management of variceal haemorrhage in cirrhotic patients. *Gut* 2000; 46 (Suppl. 3).
Stanley AJ, Hayes PC. Portal hypertension and variceal haemorrhage. *Lancet* 1997; 350: 1235–1239.

1.5 Abdominal mass

Case history

A 28-year-old man is referred as an emergency. He has been unwell for a month with anorexia, nausea and weight loss and is awaiting a gastroenterology clinic appointment. His GP is now concerned because the patient has developed abdominal pain, vomiting and a tender palpable mass in his right lower abdomen.

Clinical approach

 The two major questions to ask in the setting of an abdominal mass are:
- Is the mass related to the gut (including liver and pancreas) or another intra-abdominal organ (e.g. ovary, kidney, etc.)?
- Is the mass part of a more generalized disease process?

The story presented above describes some important gastrointestinal symptoms (i.e. vomiting) but also suggests there is probably a systemic component to the illness (i.e. anorexia, weight loss). This is a frequent clinical presentation of an inflammatory mass from ileocaecal Crohn's disease (Table 7). In many instances the combination of weight loss and a palpable abdominal mass will suggest the presence of a cancer: the patient may well be concerned about this, even if in their particular circumstances this is a remote possibility.

History of the presenting problem

A careful clinical history should obtain answers to the following questions if the details do not emerge spontaneously:
- Are there symptoms to suggest intestinal obstruction? Central (periumbilical) colicky abdominal pain with nausea and vomiting suggest partial intestinal obstruction.
- Has there been a significant change in bowel habit? Nocturnal diarrhoea and the presence of rectal bleeding should be noted.
- Has the patient experienced anorexia and/or weight loss?

Table 7 Differential diagnosis of a right iliac fossa mass.

Common	Uncommon	Rare
Ileal Crohn's—younger patients, clinical features of inflammatory disease	Appendix mass (abscess, mucocoele)	TB—although TB may cause an ileitis and regional lymphadenopathy
Caecal carcinoma—older patients, anaemia, subacute bowel obstruction	Ovarian carcinoma	this rarely causes a palpable mass. Lymphoma

TB, tuberculosis.

These features may be non-specific but may considerably predate the pain and development of the mass.

• Has the patient experienced any systemic symptoms? Fever may be vague and at best non-specific, but reports of mouth ulcers, arthralgia and gritty eyes are common in patients with Crohn's disease.

• Have there been any symptoms of perianal/pelvic disease? Ask explicitly about rectal bleeding, discharge and pneumaturia, which means that there must be a fistula between bladder and bowel.

Relevant past history

The information gleaned from past medical history is often limited in young people, but ask about the following:

• Has there been previous abdominal surgery or admissions to hospital.

• A family history of inflammatory bowel disease (particularly Crohn's disease) may be relevant. Also note that many patients are now very much aware of the inherited component to colorectal carcinoma and this can influence their own thoughts regarding the nature of any illness that they suffer.

Examination

General

The first part of the general examination is to determine whether the patient looks unwell or not. This may be subjective, but its importance must not be underestimated: a pale clammy patient with a drawn face and sunken eyes is unwell! Someone who has been vomiting may be volume depleted.

• Check pulse, BP (lying and standing) and JVP to assess intravascular volume.

• Check skin turgor and mucous membranes to assess dehydration (reduction in total body water): these signs are often unreliable in elderly people, but in young patients—such as this man—low skin turgor would be a significant finding. Note the following:

• *Fever*. Even a low-grade pyrexia might be significant.

• *Nutritional state*. What is the patient's weight and BMI? What did they weigh 6 months ago? Look for specific physical signs of malnutrition (e.g. clubbing, angular stomatitis, glossitis, etc.), but these are often absent in young patients with a relatively short history.

• *Lymphadenopathy.*

• *Arthropathy.* May be evident in patients with acute Crohn's disease, usually those with colonic disease.

> **Lymph node enlargement**
>
> Generalized lymph node enlargement should be sought as lymphoma may present with abdominal pain. Although gastrointestinal malignancy is rare in this age group, Virchow's node behind the medial head of the left clavicle should be palpated.

Abdominal

Examine for:

• *Scars* from previous surgery.

• *Signs of peritonism*. Tenderness with guarding and rebound may be localized to the site of an inflammatory mass, but generalized peritonism (i.e. elicited away from the mass) suggests peritonitis and a perforated viscus.

• *Position and character of the mass*. An inflammatory mass may be rather diffuse (i.e. without distinct limits) and is usually tender.

• Are there *other physical signs* of inflammatory bowel disease (i.e. Crohn's)? Look carefully for mouth ulcers, perianal disease and skin lesions (erythema nodosum, pyoderma gangrenosum)—you will not notice these unless you do.

Approach to investigations and management

Investigations and management have to be considered in two stages. Firstly, those aspects required immediately; secondly, those to establish and treat the definitive diagnosis.

Investigations

Blood tests

Check full blood count, electrolytes, renal and liver function, clotting and blood cultures (if febrile)—anaemia may be normocytic (anaemia of chronic disease) or microcytic (secondary to iron deficiency from chronic gastrointestinal blood loss). A raised platelet count suggests chronic inflammation (see *Haematology*, Section 1.18). Hypokalaemia may result from chronic diarrhoea and volume depletion may lead to renal failure. A low serum albumin may be due to a combination of protein loss from the gut and chronic inflammation.

Radiological imaging

Check plain abdominal radiograph, looking for pneumoperitoneum and for inflamed loops of bowel that may appear as soft-tissue shadowing containing gas. Abdominal ultrasound is increasingly used in the acute evaluation of lower abdominal masses: thickened bowel loops may be seen; is there an associated abscess?

Definitive diagnostic tests

After the immediate management there are various ways in which the diagnosis may be confirmed:

• *Small bowel enema/enteroclysis*. This is probably the best way to evaluate distal small bowel Crohn's. It gives information relating to the extent of mucosal disease in addition to assessment to the degree of small bowel obstruction.

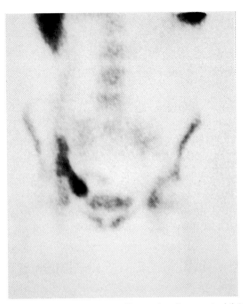

Fig. 12 Indium-111-labelled white cell scan showing terminal ileitis in a patient with active Crohn's disease. Note at the top of the scan the normal intense uptake in the liver and spleen and fainter uptake in the vertebrae and iliac crests.

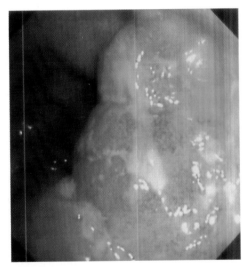

Fig. 13 Endoscopic appearance of Crohn's disease.

- *Radiolabelled leucocyte scan.* This may show uptake of isotope in the right iliac fossa, although this is relatively non-specific (Fig. 12).
- *Colonoscopy/barium enema.* An alternative approach is to consider colonoscopy with intubation of the terminal ileum, or barium enema with reflux of barium into the terminal ileum. This approach is useful in patients with colonic Crohn's disease but may not fully delineate the extent of small bowel disease (Fig. 13).
- *Abdominal CT.* CT may be useful if there is fistulating disease and an associated abscess is suspected.
- *MRI.* MRI is useful for pelvic disease such as fistulae (Fig. 14).
- *Laparotomy/laparoscopy.* These 'surgical' approaches are often forgotten as a form of investigation but are useful

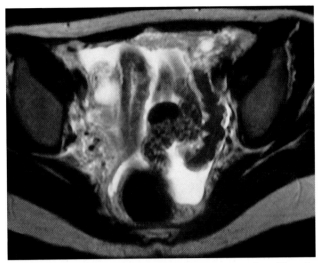

Fig. 14 Crohn's disease. MRI scan showing thickened loop of small bowel with adjacent inflammatory mass (on the left) containing fluid.

when diagnostic uncertainty persists or when patients fail to improve with initial medical management.

Management

If the patient is severely ill with evidence of volume depletion, they require immediate resuscitation (see Section 1.3, p. 9). If there are signs of generalized peritonism, seek experienced surgical advice immediately—but, whilst maintaining cordial relations, do not allow inexperienced surgeons to 'dive into' the abdomen of someone that you think probably has inflammatory bowel disease.

General symptom relief

The most effective way to relieve subacute obstructive symptoms is to rest the gut. Opiates will probably be required initially, and the patient should certainly be given adequate doses to relieve their pain, but where possible avoid giving these for days on end—they undoubtedly inhibit the return of normal intestinal function. Intravenous fluids are commonly used in the first instance, but oral rehydration and nutrition should be instituted early where possible (see below).

Nutrition

Although gut rest is often the first line of symptomatic therapy, patients presenting with inflammatory bowel disease often have very high metabolic demands and early consideration of nutrition is vital. Although total parenteral nutrition is still relied upon in some circumstances it is now possible to maintain nutritional status in acute Crohn's disease with the early use of elemental (i.e. amino acid-based) or polymeric (i.e. peptide-based) liquid diets. This approach addresses the nutritional needs of the patient whilst providing no residue to the gut. There is evidence that this approach alone is as efficacious as steroids in acute Crohn's. The two treatments are complementary (see Section 2.14.5, p. 125).

Specific therapies

The specific drug therapy for acute Crohn's disease is steroids. These may initially be given intravenously, converting to oral therapy once the symptoms have settled, and gradually reduced and withdrawn over a period of 6–8 weeks. Azathioprine may be introduced subsequently if there is an early breakthrough of symptoms or early relapse. This may take 4–6 weeks to have an effect.

Surgery

The surgical management of Crohn's disease tends to be as conservative as possible. Broadly, the indications for surgical intervention are failure of medical therapy and the presence of secondary complications (i.e. fistulae, abscesses).

Further management

See Section 2.6, p. 90.
See *Emergency medicine*, Section 1.13.
Kapoor VK. Abdominal tuberculosis. *Postgrad Med J* 1998; 74: 459–467. [The variable clinical presentation of abdominal TB.]
National Association for Crohn's and Ulcerative Colitis.
Present DH, Rutgeerts P, Targan S *et al.* Infliximab for the treatment of fistulas in patients with Crohn's disease. *N Engl J Med* 1999; 340: 1398–1405. [Role of anti-TNF antibody in Crohn's fistula.]

1.6 Jaundice and abdominal pain

Case history

A 75-year-old woman presents with mild right upper quadrant pain, fever and jaundice. She has a previous medical history of fatty food intolerance but otherwise has been fit and well.

Clinical approach

In any jaundiced patient the initial step is to decide whether this is due to hepatic (parenchymal) disease, or whether it is due to posthepatic (biliary) obstruction (Table 8). More rarely the problem is prehepatic (e.g. haemolysis, Gilbert's syndrome). History, examination and liver function tests usually give a good indication of which category the patient fits into, but liver ultrasound is virtually mandatory. Dilated common and intrahepatic bile ducts indicate obstruction

Table 8 Differential diagnosis of obstructive jaundice.

Common	Less common	Rare
Choledocholithiasis	Cholangiocarcinoma	Primary
Carcinoma of pancreas	External compression from	sclerosing
Chronic pancreatitis	malignant hilar lymph nodes	cholangitis

and endoscopic retrograde pancreaticocholangiography (ERCP) is required. If the ducts are a normal size (in the absence of pain), parenchymal liver disease is more likely, and a screen of liver blood tests (Hepatitis B surface antigen (HBsAg), autoimmune profile, etc.) is indicated, often with progression to a liver biopsy.

History of the presenting problem

Painful or painless jaundice

Pain usually indicates obstruction of the common bile duct (CBD) with a stone; pancreatic carcinoma classically gives rise to painless jaundice. Note, however, that parenchymal liver disease can result in right upper quadrant discomfort due to stretching of the liver capsule.

- Pain is unusual in obstructive jaundice not due to common bile duct stones.
- Biliary pain must be differentiated from abdominal discomfort that can occur in a hepatitis.

Weight loss

Weight loss is an ominous symptom, and is usually due to pancreatic carcinoma or cholangiocarcinoma.

Change in urine/stool colour

In obstructive jaundice, the stool becomes paler (because bile is unable to flow into the intestine and colour the stool) and the urine darker (excess conjugated bilirubin). Similar (though less extreme) changes can also occur in parenchymal disease, since inflammation of the liver parenchyma can cause local obstruction of the bile canaliculi and interlobular bile ducts.

Fevers or rigors

Fever, pain and jaundice (Charcot's triad) are characteristics of ascending cholangitis due to bacterial infection in the biliary system. This is usually a complication of common bile duct stones and rarely occurs with pancreatic carcinoma.

Cholangitis may present as confusion or 'off legs' in the absence of fever in an elderly person (see *Medicine for the elderly*, Section 1.2).

Recent travel/contact with jaundiced people

Has the patient been abroad to a country where hepatitis A is endemic? Have they been in contact with anyone else with viral hepatitis?

Alcohol consumption

Alcohol not only causes parenchymal liver disease, but may also produce jaundice by triggering pancreatitis. Focal pancreatitis or pseudocysts can externally compress the common bile duct.

Relevant past history

Gallstones

Is the patient known to have gallstones?

Choledocholithiasis may present some time after previous cholecystectomy for gallstones. This may be due to stones that have been missed (silent) in the common bile duct at the time of operation, or possibly formation of stones *in situ*.

Examination

Examination of the patient with jaundice

- General impression—well, septicaemic, cachectic?
- Are there peripheral stigmata of chronic liver disease, indicating parenchymal liver disease?
- Are there excoriations—indicating pruritus of obstructive jaundice?
- Full abdominal examination—hepatomegaly/splenomegaly indicate chronic liver disease; a palpable gall bladder is unusual with gallstones (Courvoisier's law) and classically found in pancreatic carcinoma.

General

Most patients with gallstones causing obstructive jaundice are not very unwell, presenting as in this case with a relatively short history of increasing jaundice, with or without abdominal pain.

Are there features of chronic liver disease? This woman is jaundiced, so check in addition:
- hands for clubbing, leukonychia, Dupytren's contracture, palmar erythema
- skin for bruising, spider naevi
- parotid swelling (pseudocushingoid)
- peripheral oedema
- possibility of hepatic encephalopathy, suggesting acute hepatic decompensation (see Section 2.10, p. 110)

- anaemia which would not be expected in jaundice due to gallstones
- signs of feminization in a man (loss of body hair, gynaecomastia and testicular atrophy).

Abdominal

Assess for the presence of tenderness, palpable masses and peritonism, taking particular note of the following:
- hepatosplenomegaly
- palpable gall bladder
- ascites
- caput medusae.

Differential diagnosis

In the patient presenting with obstructive jaundice, consider the following:
- *Pancreatic carcinoma/cholangiocarcinoma.* Usually painless, but CBD stones may also be painless. Pain from pancreatic carcinoma is a deep, boring pain in the epigastrium radiating through to the back.
- *Pancreatitis.* Pancreatitis (from alcohol for example) may result in oedema and swelling in the head of the pancreas and cause extrinsic compression of the bile duct and jaundice. It can often be very difficult to distinguish between such focal pancreatitis and pancreatic cancer. Brushings at ERCP or needle biopsy may be required.
- *Budd–Chiari.* Obstruction of the hepatic vein results in rapid engorgement of the liver, producing pain, jaundice (often mild or absent) and ascites. Associated with haematological disorders (primary polycythaemia, protein C and S deficiency, antithrombin III deficiency and anticardiolipin antibody), malignancy and the oral contraceptive pill. Ultrasound with Doppler studies to look at portal and hepatic vein flow. Liver biopsy shows characteristic changes.

Approach to investigations and management

Investigation of jaundice

- Test urine for bilirubin and urobilinogen
- Blood tests ('liver screen')
- Ultrasound scan of liver, gall bladder, bile ducts and pancreas (if this can be seen)
- ERCP or liver biopsy.

Investigation

Urine tests

Check urine with dipstick for bilirubin and urobilinogen:
- Presence of bilirubin indicates obstructive jaundice, either intra- or posthepatic.
- Excess of urobilinogen indicates prehepatic jaundice or (sometimes) liver damage.
- Urobilinogen is absent when there is complete obstruction to bile flow.

Blood tests

Check full blood count, electroytes, renal and liver function tests, amylase and clotting screen. Predominantly raised alkaline phosphatase (ALP)/gammaglutamyl transferase (GGT) point to an obstructive cause of jaundice, whilst predominantly elevated aspartate transaminase (AST)/alanine transferase (ALT) favour hepatocellular inflammation. Often the picture is 'mixed'. A common bile duct stone, for example, may cause an obstructive picture, but a superadded ascending cholangitis may cause marked elevation of the hepatocellular enzymes.

It is prudent to check hepatitis A serology in all patients presenting with jaundice. Further blood tests will be required if ultrasound does not confirm the clinical suspicion of biliary obstruction, e.g. liver autoantibodies (i.e. antimitochondrial antibody), immunoglobulins, hepatitis B and C serology and ferritin; also α_1-antitrypsin, copper and caeruloplasmin in those under 45 years old.

Abdominal ultrasound

Dilated common bile and intrahepatic ducts confirm obstructive aetiology. The ultrasound may show a cause for obstruction, but common bile duct stones are often missed, and the pancreas may be difficult to visualize due to overlying bowel. Dilated ducts are an indication for ERCP; if the biliary system is not dilated, then consider liver biopsy.

Endoscopic retrograde pancreaticocholangiography (ERCP)

Injection of contrast into the biliary system will readily show whether obstruction is due to stones or a biliary stricture (Fig. 15). Malignant strictures due to pancreatic carcinoma or cholangiocarcinoma are usually obvious, but positive cytology from brushings is desirable. Differentiating focal pancreatic inflammation from pancreatic carcinoma can be very difficult. If cannulation of the CBD is not possible at ERCP, the bile system can be accessed by percutaneous transhepatic cholangiography (PTC).

Magnetic resonance cholangiopancreatogram (MRCP)

This is a non-invasive method of diagnosing common bile duct stones (Fig. 16).

Management

Management depends upon the setting. If the patient has a high fever or rigors or is obviously septicaemic, then treat for septicaemia with the working diagnosis of ascending

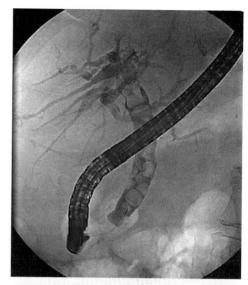

(a)

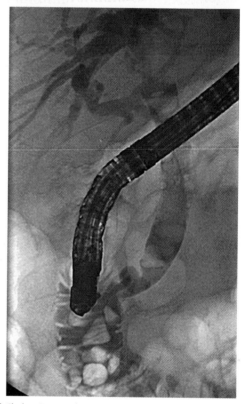

(b)

Fig. 15 (a) Cholangiogram showing common bile duct packed with stones. (b) The stones are seen within the duodenum following a sphincterotomy and trawling of the common bile duct with a balloon.

cholangitis (see *Emergency medicine*, Section 1.28; *Infectious diseases*, Section 1.2).

In acute ascending cholangitis with obstruction, urgent drainage of the biliary system is required. In the ill patient with deranged clotting, insertion of a stent allows drainage around stones, with temporary clinical improvement. Alternatively, sphincterotomy and stone extraction may be achieved at initial endoscopy. Cholecystectomy is usual at a later date to remove the focus, unless comorbidity/frailty dictates otherwise. Few problems seem to arise in those in whom the gall bladder is left *in situ*.

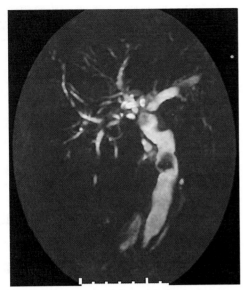

Fig. 16 Magnetic resonance cholangiogram. A stone can be seen in the common bile duct.

Further management

For management of the non-urgent case, see Section 2.5, p. 83.

See *Biochemistry and metabolism*, Section 2.6.
Chopra KB, Peters RA, O'Toole PA *et al.* Randomised study of endoscopic biliary endoprosthesis versus duct clearance of bile duct stones in high-risk patients. *Lancet* 1996; 348: 791–793. [The effectiveness of stenting the CBD in the presence of common bile duct stones.]
Freeman ML, Nelson DB, Sherman S *et al.* Complications of endoscopic biliary sphincterotomy. *N Engl J Med* 1996; 335: 909–918. [Complications of sphincterotomy for common bile duct stones.]

1.7 Jaundice in a heavy drinker

Case history

A 45-year-old publican presents with a 2-month history of anorexia, some weight loss and a 1-week history of painless jaundice. The referral note says that 'he admits to liking a few drinks'.

Clinical approach

The most likely diagnosis is alcoholic hepatitis, but it is clearly important to establish a history of excess alcohol use. In the absence of this other hepatic causes of jaundice including acute hepatitis, chronic liver disease and malignant infiltration of the liver need to be excluded (Table 9), as would painless causes of obstructive jaundice (Table 8).

Table 9 Differential diagnosis of jaundice due to liver disease.

Common	Less common	Rare
Acute alcoholic hepatitis	Acute hepatitis B	Hepatic venous outflow obstruction (Budd–Chiari, right heart failure)
Acute hepatitis A	Autoimmune chronic active hepatitis	
Drug-induced hepatotoxicity		Weil's disease
Intrahepatic cholestasis due to sepsis		Wilson's disease
Chronic liver disease		Pregnancy-associated liver disease

It is important to assess the recent daily alcohol intake to evaluate the risk of alcohol withdrawal.

Remember that alcoholic hepatitis may occur against the background of chronic alcoholic liver disease (which includes cirrhosis) and that it is not unusual for alcoholic hepatitis to be the initial presentation. Alcohol excess also causes chronic pancreatitis, which can lead to a lower common bile duct stricture and obstructive jaundice.

History of the presenting problem

Alcohol history

A detailed alcohol history is required to assess likelihood of alcohol damage and risk of withdrawal. This must be approached without causing offence (see *General clinical issues*, Section 3), but you do need answers to the following questions if the information does not emerge without prompting:
- When did you last drink any alcohol?
- Do you drink daily or binge drink (have months alcohol free)?
- What type of alcohol do you drink (spirits, beer)?
- How much do you drink each week now, and how much in the past? Figure 17 allows you to calculate the number of units.
- Have you ever been told you have an alcohol problem and told to stop drinking?
- Have you ever undergone alcohol detoxification in or out of hospital?

The CAGE questionnaire is useful in confirming a suspicion of alcohol excess if the patient denies having an alcohol problem. One point is given for every 'yes' response: two or more points suggests an alcohol problem. Have you ever:
C—felt a need to *C*ut down?
A—been *A*nnoyed at the suggestion of a drinking problem?
G—felt *G*uilty about your drinking?
E—had to have a drink (*E*ye opener) in the morning?

Is the jaundice due to acute alcoholic hepatitis?

Onset of jaundice

Jaundice often occurs between a few days and 4 weeks after stopping alcohol. Patients often stop drinking because

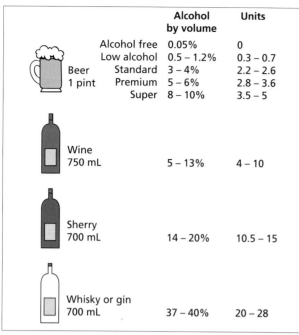

		Alcohol by volume	Units
Beer 1 pint	Alcohol free	0.05%	0
	Low alcohol	0.5 – 1.2%	0.3 – 0.7
	Standard	3 – 4%	2.2 – 2.6
	Premium	5 – 6%	2.8 – 3.6
	Super	8 – 10%	3.5 – 5
Wine 750 mL		5 – 13%	4 – 10
Sherry 700 mL		14 – 20%	10.5 – 15
Whisky or gin 700 mL		37 – 40%	20 – 28

Fig. 17 Number of units of alcohol present in various alcoholic beverages (10 g of alcohol = 1 unit).

they feel unwell. The jaundice may or may not be accompanied by pale stools and dark urine.

Pain

Mild upper abdominal discomfort is common but severe abdominal pain does not occur. Abdominal discomfort also occurs if there is ascites.

Weight loss

The amount and rate of weight loss need to be gauged. Alcoholics lose weight due to:
• malabsorption (chronic pancreatitis)
• poor oral intake. Take a dietary history: What did you eat yesterday? What did you have for breakfast, lunch, tea, supper? Was that a normal day for you?
• the hypermetabolic state of chronic liver disease.
Rapid weight loss in the absence of steatorrhoea suggests malignancy.

Other issues

Ask specifically:
• Has there been any abdominal distention (ascites), suggesting chronic liver disease?
• Has there been any change in his ability to concentrate, e.g. ability to read the newspaper or do the crossword, perhaps suggesting hepatic encephalopathy?
• Has he had any black loose stool (melaena), indicating GI bleeding, which could be from a variety of sources (see Section 1.4, p. 13)?

• Has he ever had a liver biopsy?
• Has he been told he has cirrhosis or a scarred liver or liver disease?

 If a patient with chronic liver disease is jaundiced, ask yourself the following questions:
• Is this acute liver injury on top of chronic liver disease (e.g. alcoholic hepatitis)?
• Is this a biliary disease (e.g. primary biliary cirrhosis, primary sclerosing cholangitis)?
• Is this end-stage progressive chronic liver disease?
• Is there a complication (e.g. hepatocellular carcinoma, bacterial peritonitis)?

Relevant past history

Find out if there is a history to suggest alcohol excess:
• Previous head injuries?
• Previous rib or other peripheral fractures?
• Fits associated with alcohol withdrawal?
• Previous history of recurrent acute pancreatitis?

Drug history

A comprehensive drug history is required, including drugs that have been recently stopped. This should include details of herbal remedies, medications bought over the counter, non-prescribed drugs, as well as any given by the general practitioner.

Social history

You must exclude coinfection with hepatitis B and C. Check for:
• History of recent or previous intravenous drug use?
• Exposure to sexual partner with hepatitis B or multiple partners without using barrier methods of contraception?

 Differential diagnosis

In the alcohol abuser presenting with jaundice, in addition to alcoholic hepatitis consider the following:
• *Alcoholic chronic pancreatitis.* If there is a history of back pain, weight loss, steatorrhoea or previous episodes of acute pancreatitis.
• *Acute viral hepatitis.* Particularly in a young person. Often a prodromal illness of lethargy and arthralgia and nausea. There may be a history of intravenous drug use.
• *Acute hepatitis from drug toxicity.* This may be clinically indistinguishable from alcoholic hepatitis unless a detailed drug history including use of non-proprietary medication is taken.
• *Hepatic metastases.* In older patients with a rapid history of weight loss.
• *Chronic liver disease.* Particularly if a history of previous jaundice, confusion, melaena and abdominal distention.
• *Autoimmune chronic active hepatitis.* Particularly in women with a personal or family history of other autoimmune conditions.

Examination

Examination of a patient with jaundice

- General impression
- Full abdominal examination
- Are there cutaneous stigmata to suggest chronic liver disease?
- Is there marked cachexia and/or lymphadenopathy to suggest malignancy?

General

Is the patient confused, which may be due to alcohol withdrawal, Wernicke's encephalopathy, hepatic encephalopathy or infection? Alcohol withdrawal is suggested by agitation, hallucinations and tremor. Look for nystagmus and ophthalmoplegia (Wernicke's encephalopathy).

Look for features of chronic liver disease (see Section 1.6, p. 20).

Fever is common in the presence of alcoholic hepatitis, but infection must always be excluded (urine, blood, ascites). TB is uncommon, but alcoholism is a risk factor.

Abdominal

Look in particular for:
- *Liver edge.* Usually enlarged up to 10 cm in acute alcoholic hepatitis and firm and tender. May be irregular if associated cirrhosis.
- *Hepatic bruit.* Present in severe alcoholic hepatitis as well as with hepatocellular carcinoma.
- *Splenomegaly.*
- *Ascites.*
- *Melaena* on rectal examination.

Differential diagnosis

If the liver is enlarged in a patient with jaundice, consider the following:
- *Acute viral hepatitis.* Tender mildly enlarged 2–3-cm smooth-edged hepatomegaly.
- *Liver metastases.* In all patients with firm irregular hepatomegaly with or without ascites.
- *Chronic liver disease.* Cutaneous stigmata of chronic liver disease, firm or irregular hepatomegaly of any size.
- *Evidence of portal hypertension* i.e. splenomegaly and ascites.

Approach to investigations and management

Investigation

Blood tests

As in Section 1.6, p. 20; also including blood cultures and random ethanol level. The prothrombin time and albumin are important prognostic markers. Macrocytosis is unusual in liver disease not due to alcohol (see *Haematology*, Section 1.4).

Severity of alcoholic hepatitis can be assessed by the Maddrey's criteria [1]. (4.6 × increase in PT in s over normal) + bilirubin (mg/dL) (1 mg/dL = 17 μmol/L). A value >32 indicates a poor prognosis.

Ultrasound of abdomen

Exclude biliary obstruction with common bile duct dilatation. Confirm evidence of portal hypertension. Exclude focal liver lesions (metastases and hepatocellular carcinoma).

Further blood tests

Remember that not everyone who drinks will have alcoholic liver disease.

Exclude other causes of an acute hepatitis; hepatitis A IgM, hepatitis Bs Ag and eAg, liver autoantibodies (antinuclear antibody, smooth muscle and antimitochondrial antibody) and immunoglobulins. In a patient of less than 40 with no alcohol excess exclude Wilson's disease with a copper, caeuroplasmin and unconjugated bilirubin level (haemolysis contributes to the elevated bilirubin level).

Check α-fetoprotein (AFP) to exclude hepatocellular carcinoma if the patient is likely to have cirrhosis.

Management

Nutrition

Give 5% intravenous dextrose if not hyponatraemic. Give thiamine and pyridoxine, intravenously for the first 48 h and then orally.

Alcohol withdrawal

Treatment for alcohol withdrawal should be initiated before the patient develops signs of withdrawal (Table 10). See *Emergency Medicine*, Section 1.14 and *Psychiatry*, Section 1.7.

In the presence of alcoholic hepatitis and/or cirrhosis accumulation of sedatives occurs and there is a risk of precipitating encephalopathy. Review dosing on a daily basis and stop if patient becomes drowsy.

Table 10 Suggested initial dose regime for treatment of mild to moderate alcohol withdrawal with chlordiazepoxide.

Time	Dose
Day 1 (first 24 h)	30 mg q.d.s.
Day 2	20 mg t.d.s. 30 mg nocte
Day 3	10 mg t.d.s. 20 mg nocte
Day 4	5 mg t.d.s. 10 mg nocte
Day 5	5 mg mane 10 mg nocte
Day 6 THEN STOP	5 mg nocte

Infection

Have a low threshold for giving broad-spectrum antibiotics once cultures have been taken: it can be difficult to distinguish clinically between infection and alcoholic hepatitis.

Corticosteroids

Consider giving corticosteroids: these are controversial in this context, but may be beneficial in severe alcoholic hepatitis.

Alcoholic with jaundice

If the patient deteriorates in hospital, prognosis is poor. Early active treatment is essential. Do not wait until they have developed hepatorenal failure before you refer to a liver unit.

Alcoholic with liver disease who is deteriorating

Progressive liver failure may develop with rising PT, increasing jaundice, encephalopathy, gastrointestinal haemorrhage (varices or gastropathy) and hepatorenal failure despite abstinence and good supportive medical care. Treatment is supportive for patients with alcoholic hepatitis who are not candidates for liver transplantation as their survival after this procedure is poor.

Acute liver failure

See Section 1.16, p. 45 and *Emergency medicine*, Section 1.14.

Complications of chronic liver disease

These include ascites, variceal haemorrhage, encephalopathy and hepatocellular carcinoma: see Sections 1.4, p. 13 and 1.8, p. 27.

Ethics of alcoholic liver disease

The treatment of alcoholics raises difficult ethical issues. In part these are based around the cost and resources needed to treat a self-induced disease, especially if the individual is still drinking despite advice to abstain. In part they stem from concern that the doctor should not offer treatments that are not likely to be effective, i.e. do lasting good, in the particular patient under consideration. Ethical issues that are commonly encountered include:

• Should a man who presents with his first episode of alcoholic hepatitis be treated actively? The answer to this must be 'yes'. If this is the patient's first admission with alcohol-related liver disease and there has been no medical input into their alcohol problem in the past, they may be able to stop drinking, particularly if good social support is obtainable; and if someone recovers from alcoholic hepatitis and remains abstinent, a good 10-year life expectancy can be expected, even in the presence of cirrhosis.

• Should a woman who has had repeated admissions with decompensated alcoholic liver disease be transfused and endoscoped when she presents again with a variceal haemorrhage? There is no right answer to this question: there comes a point when to continue seems futile and may be cruel, but judging this point is not easy. All involved in the patient's care should discuss matters, and the patient's views (if known) and those of the relatives should be taken into account, but the decision should be made by the doctor in charge (see *General clinical issues*, Section 3).

• Should a patient with worsening liver failure from alcoholic cirrhosis who has stopped drinking for over 6 months be offered liver transplantation? Different liver transplant units take different views on this. How aggressive should the transplant unit be in determining whether the patient has actually stopped? If you thought you were dying in this context, and someone asked you if you'd stopped drinking, would you say 'yes' or 'no'?

• Should patients with repeated withdrawal fits be admitted for inpatient detoxification? Different drug and alcohol detoxification units take different views on this: how should they use their scarce resources?

See *Emergency medicine*, Sections 1.13 and 1.14.
See *Psychiatry*, Section 1.7.
Christensen E, Gludd C. Glucocorticoids are ineffective in alcoholic hepatitis: a meta-analysis adjusting for confounding variables. *Gut* 1995; 37: 113–118. [Role of glucocorticoids in alcoholic hepatitis.]
Lieber CS. Alcoholic liver disease: new insights in pathogenesis lead to new treatments. *J Hepatol* 2000; 32 (Suppl. 1): 113–128.
Sherlock S. Alcoholic liver disease. *Lancet* 1995; 345: 227–229.
Website of Medical Council on alcoholism: http://www.medicouncilalcol.demon.co.uk
1 Carithers RL. Methylprednisolone therapy in patients with severe alcoholic hepatitis. A randomised multicentred trial. *Ann Intern Med* 1989; 110: 685. [Prognostic factors in alcoholic hepatitis.]

1.8 Abdominal swelling

Case history

A 60-year-old woman presents with a 2-week history of abdominal swelling on a 3-year background of increasing lethargy.

Clinical approach

Abdominal swelling is an unusual presenting problem, and ascites is the most important diagnostic consideration, the causes of which are shown in Table 11. Chronic constipation in elderly people and Hirschsprung's disease in younger patients may lead to progressive abdominal swelling, while with intestinal obstruction and paralytic ileus anorexia and vomiting are prominent. Occasionally the diagnosis is simply one of obesity or pregnancy! Swelling must be distinguished from the sensation of bloating, which is part of the irritable bowel syndrome symptom complex.

History of the presenting problem

Ask about the following if the details do not emerge spontaneously:
- How long have you had the swelling? Intestinal obstruction and paralytic ileus typically develop rapidly, while most cases of ascites develop over days and weeks. Fat, faeces, foetal tissue and tumours accumulate over months.
- Have you had any pain? Abdominal discomfort due to distention with ascites is common: pain may indicate inflammation or malignancy. Colicky abdominal pain suggests intestinal disease, particularly obstruction. Pain radiating to the back is typical of pancreatitis, a rare but important cause of ascites.
- Any vomiting? If persistent, large volume, faeculent or projectile, then intestinal obstruction is likely.
- Any jaundice? Suggests a hepatic causes of ascites.

 Absence of jaundice does not exclude chronic liver disease.

Relevant past history

Alcohol

Alcohol remains the commonest cause of chronic liver disease in the western world. Progression to cirrhosis requires decades of excess intake, but may occur earlier if there are concurrent risks, e.g. (α_1-antitrypsin deficiency, hepatitis C infection). See Section 1.7, p. 23 for details about how to take a history of alcohol consumption.

Chronic viral hepatitis

Ask about the following risk factors:
- *Blood product transfusion.* Fifteen years previously this woman was involved in a road traffic accident and required a blood transfusion.
- *Needle sharing.* Intravenous drug use and tattoos.
- *High-risk sexual behaviour.*
See *General clinical issues*, Section 3.

Disease associations

Has the patient had inflammatory bowel disease, associated with primary sclerosing cholangitis (PSC); or coeliac disease or any autoimmune disease, associated with primary biliary cirrhosis (PBC)?

Examination

General

The most important consideration is whether the patient is well, unwell or extremely unwell. Intestinal obstruction, paralytic ileus and intestinal pseudo-obstruction typically occur in patients who are unwell, and soon become extremely unwell. Acute hepatitis and acute Budd–Chiari syndrome may present with abdominal pain, swelling and jaundice, and can progress rapidly to liver failure, coma and death.

Examine for signs of liver failure such as:
- hepatic fetor
- flapping tremor
- altered consciousness

Table 11 Differential diagnosis of ascites.

Chronic liver disease with decompensation
Has ascites developed simply as a result of progressive decline in liver function?
Has there been an acute precipitant, e.g. infection, hepatocellular carcinoma, portal vein thrombosis, alcoholic hepatitis?

Other causes of portal hypertension
Veno-occlusive disease of the liver and Budd–Chiari syndrome

Peritoneal disease
Peritoneal carcinomatosis
Peritoneal tuberculosis and other infections

Other causes (less common)
Right-sided heart disease, especially constrictive pericarditis
Ovarian carcinoma: Meig's syndrome, pseudomyxoma peritoni
Acute pancreatitis with pancreatic ascites
Peritoneal dialysis fluid
Nephrotic syndrome
Myxoedema

- bruising or petechiae
- jaundice.

Examine for signs of chronic liver disease (see Sections 1.4, p. 13, 1.6, p. 20 and 1.7, p. 23).

Abdominal

Is the swelling due to fluid, gas, doughy faeces or solid tissue? Check for shifting dullness. Is the liver enlarged, and what is the consistency? Is it tender, pulsatile, hard and craggy? Does it have a bruit? Is the spleen enlarged? Are there other abdominal masses? Are bowel sounds present and normal? Does the rectum contain solidly impacted faeces?

Other features

Examine carefully for evidence of:
- *Right heart failure*. Where is the JVP? Could it be grossly elevated?
- *Hypothyroidism*. What does the patient look like? Are the tendon jerks slow relaxing?
- *Nephrotic syndrome*. What does stick testing of the urine reveal?

Approach to investigations and management

This will be guided by the findings on history and examination. If the patient is unwell with a tender abdomen they may require resuscitation (see Section 1.3, p. 10) and urgent investigation/surgical opinion. This woman was not in that category: the clinical diagnosis of her abdominal distension was ascites.

Investigations

Blood tests

ASSESS LIVER FUNCTION

These include prothrombin time, serum albumin and bilirubin.

ASSESS TYPE OF LIVER DAMAGE

These should include transaminases, alkaline phosphatase and γ-glutamyl transferase (see Sections 1.6, p. 20 and 1.18, p. 49).

DETERMINE THE CAUSE OF THE UNDERLYING LIVER DISEASE

Useful tests include:
- *Viral serology*. Hepatitis B and C. This woman had evidence of hepatitis C infection, presumably transmitted by her

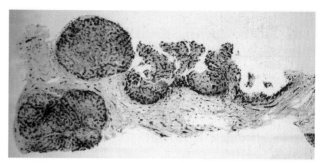

Fig. 18 Macronodular cirrhosis secondary to haemochromatosis. Iron in hepatocytes within the nodules is stained blue.

blood transfusion 15 years previously (before screening for hepatitis C was available).
- *Antimitochondrial antibody*. PBC.
- *Autoimmune serology*. Autoimmune chronic active hepatitis.
- *Serum ferritin and haematinics*. Haemochromatosis (see Section 2.10, p. 110 and see *Endocrinology*, Sections 1.5 and 2.5.3; *Rheumatology and clinical immunology*, Section 1.18).
- Serum α_1-antitrypsin deficiency and tests for Wilson's disease.
- *Percutaneous or transjugular liver biopsy* (Fig. 18).

ALPHA-FETOPROTEIN

Elevated in about 60% of cases of hepatocellular carcinoma. Often normal with small tumours.

Imaging studies

PLAIN ABDOMINAL RADIOGRAPH

If gastrointestinal obstruction is suspected.

ABDOMINAL ULTRASOUND SCAN

To establish the extent of fluid and its distribution, e.g. loculated or free. To examine the texture and size of the liver and identify hepatocellular carcinoma, which was unfortunately revealed in this woman (Fig. 19). Also to look for evidence of portal hypertension, such as splenomegaly, and to perform Doppler studies of the portal vein and hepatic veins.

Diagnostic aspiration of ascitic fluid

Test for total leucocytes, microorganisms, neoplastic cells, albumin and amylase.

If the serum albumin to ascites albumin gradient is greater than 11 g/L, portal hypertension is the cause of the ascites; if the gradient is less than 11 g/L, the ascites is exudative (e.g. caused by neoplasia, infection or pancreatitis).

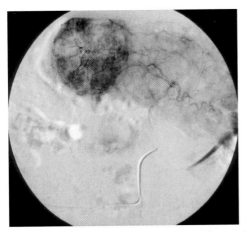

Fig. 19 Hepatic angiogram demonstrating a large, typically vascular, hepatocellular carcinoma with a feeding vessel.

A third of patients admitted with chronic liver disease and ascites develop spontaneous bacterial peritonitis, which carries a poor prognosis and is diagnosed by a neutrophil count in ascitic fluid of greater than 250 cells/mL.

 Spontaneous bacterial peritonitis is fatal if left untreated. A diagnostic ascitic tap is essential in all patients admitted with ascites.

Management

The underlying condition may be treatable, e.g. auto-immune hepatitis with steroids, acute hepatitis B infection with antiviral agents. For details see the relevant sections of this module.

 Decompensation in cirrhosis is partially reversible if the hepatic insult is removed, e.g. abstinence from alcohol.

Diuretics

Ninety per cent of cases of ascites can be controlled with spironolactone and (sometimes) frusemide.

 Diuretics can precipitate hepatorenal failure. It is essential to monitor renal function and stop diuretics if the serum creatinine starts to rise. (See *Nephrology*, Section 2.7.10.)

Diuretic-resistant ascites

Diuretic-resistant ascites may require therapeutic paracentesis (see Section 3.3, p. 134). Portosystemic shunting procedures, e.g. TIPSS (transjugular intrahepatic portosystemic shunt) may also have a role in managing diuretic-resistant ascites. Selected patients may benefit from a Levine shunt, where ascites is shunted from the peritoneal cavity into a jugular vein.

Antibiotics

Spontaneous bacterial peritonitis is life threatening and early diagnosis, treatment and prevention are critical. Cephalosporins and the quinolone antibiotics are effective.

Liver transplantation

Diuretic-resistant ascites and an episode of spontaneous bacterial peritonitis are both indications for consideration of elective liver transplantation (see Section 2.15, p. 125).

Communication

This case raises many issues. First, find out if the woman wants a full explanation. At the end of a first meeting you might say, 'It looks as though there might be something serious to explain all this … are you the sort of person who likes to know exactly what's going on?' It is likely that she will say 'yes', which will pave the way for discussion, when the diagnosis has been confirmed, of:
- the prognosis and treatment of hepatocellular carcinoma (see Section 2.11, p. 113)
- the role of blood transfusion in causing the problem (see Section 2.10, p. 110).

She will inevitably be very upset at learning of the diagnosis, and it is more than likely that she—or her relatives—will be angry at the reason: 'The doctors did this to me/her'. This anger may manifest itself as a formal complaint against the hospital that treated her following her road traffic accident 15 years ago, also as aggression directed towards yourself and others trying to look after her now. Although it is unpleasant to be on the receiving end, this reaction is understandable: speak quietly and calmly; don't be evasive; write clear notes; don't take it personally (see *General clinical issues*, Section 3).

 See *Pain relief and palliative care*, Section 1.2.
See *Oncology*, Section 2.10.
Okuda K. Hepatocellular carcinoma. *J Hepatol* 2000; 32 (Suppl.1): S25–S37.
Rimola A, Garcia-Tsao G, Navasa M *et al.* Diagnosis, treatment and prophylaxis of spontaneous bacterial peritonitis: a consensus document. *J Hepatol* 2000; 32: 142–153. [Guidelines on management of ascites and spontaneous bacterial peritonitis.]
Rossle M, Ochs A, Gulberg V *et al.* A comparison of paracentesis and transjugular intrahepatic portosystemic shunting in patients with ascites. *N Engl J Med* 2000; 342: 1701–1707. [Role of TIPPS in management of diuretic-resistant ascites.]
Runyon, BA. Care of patients with ascites. *N Engl J Med* 1994; 330: 337–342.
Website for the British Liver Trust.
http://www.britishlivertrust.org.uk

1.9 Abdominal pain and vomiting

Case history

You are asked to see a 79-year-old man on the ward. He had been admitted to hospital with heart failure and was noted to be anaemic. He has been receiving sodium pico-sulphate in preparation for a barium enema examination when he develops severe abdominal pain and vomiting.

Clinical approach

The history given is very suggestive of colonic obstruction precipitated by the bowel preparation (Table 12).

 Patients do not always know which ward they are on! Although large bowel obstruction has traditionally been considered a surgical matter, problems such as this may present themselves whilst patients are in hospital for other reasons.

History of the presenting problem

Find out:
• What is the nature of the pain?
• When did the patient last pass stool or wind?

 The nature of the pain is not very discriminatory, although constant as opposed to colicky pain should alert the clinician to the possibility of bowel infarction and/or perforation.

Relevant past history

Find out if:
• the patient has had any previous abdominal surgery?
• there has been a change in bowel habit or rectal bleeding prior to admission? There may be features to suggest the presence of a colorectal tumour.

It is also important to determine the presence of significant comorbidity and medications. This man was admitted with 'heart failure', which might be entirely attributable to his anaemia, but since acute intestinal obstruction will commonly require surgical intervention it is very important

Table 12 Differential diagnosis of colonic obstruction.

Common	Uncommon	Rare
Colorectal carcinoma	Sigmoid volvulus	Intussuception—
Adhesional obstruction— history of, or scars from, previous surgery	Benign colonic stricture (e.g. related to diverticular disease) Pseudo-obstruction or paralytic ileus	rare and usually due to an underlying tumour

to identify comorbid risks such as ischaemic heart disease and treatments such as anticoagulants at an early stage.

Examination

Is the patient well, ill, very ill or nearly dead? If the man is nearly dead, call for immediate help from the ICU. If he is peripherally shut down and hypotensive, start resuscitation immediately (see Section 1.3, p. 9), whilst completing the history and examination.

In addition to seeking signs consistent with the clinical diagnosis of intestinal obstruction it is important to look for evidence of an incurable underlying disease or significant comorbidity that might influence/preclude subsequent investigations or treatments.

General

Assess the circulatory state: check peripheral perfusion, pulse, BP (lying and sitting), JVP. Elderly patients with vomiting may easily become hypovolaemic. Check respiratory rate and listen to the lungs: could he have aspirated?

Abdominal

Look for:
• *Abdominal scars* from previous surgery.
• *Distension*. The abdomen may be distended and tender. There may be signs of peritonitis with guarding and (possibly) rebound.
• *Bowel sounds*. Active (high-pitched) bowel sounds are consistent with intestinal obstruction, whereas a silent abdomen would be more in keeping with either a pseudo-obstruction or a complicating perforation.
• *Faecal impaction or melaena* on rectal examination.

Approach to investigations and management

The pace of investigation will be determined by the clinical state: if the patient is very ill then resuscitation, ordering of blood tests and radiological investigations (abdominal radiograph and perhaps CT scan of the abdomen) and request for a surgical opinion should happen concurrently.

Investigations

Blood tests

Check full blood count, electrolytes, renal and hepatic function, amylase, clotting and Group and Save. If his anaemia is due to iron deficiency, this raises the probability of an underlying colonic carcinoma. Abnormal liver blood tests (particularly elevated alkaline phosphatase and GGT) may suggest metastatic disease.

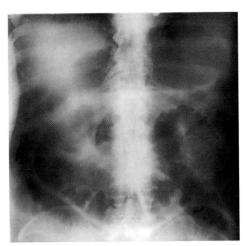

Fig. 20 Plain abdominal radiograph showing stomach and small bowel in patient with colonic obstruction.

Radiological

ABDOMINAL RADIOGRAPH

This may demonstrate features of colonic obstruction and may even demonstrate a pneumoperitoneum secondary to a complicating perforation (Fig. 20).

CONTRAST RADIOLOGY

An unprepared (or instant) enema is probably the safest way to demonstrate a colonic obstruction and to clearly distinguish this from a pseudo-obstruction.

CT SCANNING

CT scanning of the abdomen is increasingly used in the investigation of patients with an acute abdomen and can be very informative. Those who are very ill with obvious peritonitis require urgent resuscitation and laparotomy. Those who are less ill, or in whom the diagnosis of an intra-abdominal surgical catastrophe is not obvious, need an urgent CT scan of the abdomen.

Rectal examination/sigmoidoscopy

A significant number of colonic neoplasms arise within the rectosigmoid. Flexible sigmoidoscopy and colonoscopy (Fig. 21) do not have a role in acute colonic obstruction, but should be considered if the acute problem resolves with conservative management.

Management

General measures

Nasogastric aspiration with a large-bore tube (e.g. Ryles) relieves vomiting and to a lesser extent, pain. Give adequate

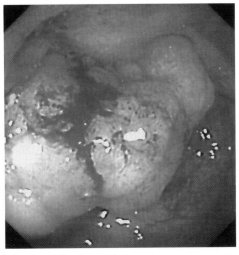

Fig. 21 Colonoscopy showing a colonic carcinoma.

analgesia. Resuscitate as needed (see Section 1.3, p. 9). Doctors are often reluctant to give fluids to someone labelled as having 'heart failure', as in this case, but the rules remain simple:
• Give IV fluid (blood, colloid, 0.9% saline) rapidly until postural hypotension is abolished and the JVP can be seen easily.
• Stop giving fluid rapidly when JVP has risen to 2–4 cm above the angle of Louis, or CVP has risen to 8–10 cm above the midaxillary line, or if tachypnoea, crackles in the lungs or falling oxygen saturation (pulse oximetry) develop before then.

Surgical opinion

A senior surgical opinion should be sought at the earliest opportunity.

Further management

Further management will depend on the specific diagnosis: see Section 2.7, p. 94.

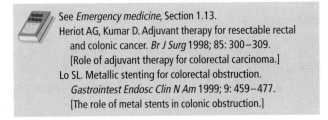

See *Emergency medicine*, Section 1.13.
Heriot AG, Kumar D. Adjuvant therapy for resectable rectal and colonic cancer. *Br J Surg* 1998; 85: 300–309.
[Role of adjuvant therapy for colorectal carcinoma.]
Lo SL. Metallic stenting for colorectal obstruction. *Gastrointest Endosc Clin N Am* 1999; 9: 459–477.
[The role of metal stents in colonic obstruction.]

1.10 Weight loss and tiredness

Case history

A 24-year-old woman presents with a history of weight loss and tiredness.

Clinical approach

Tiredness is a common and non-specific symptom. Weight loss must be taken seriously. Although malignancy is usually high on the differential diagnosis, in a young patient malabsorption, thyrotoxicosis, diabetes mellitus and intentional weight loss should probably be above this on the list of possibilities. Weight is usually fairly constant, loss of 5% or more of the usual body weight being significant. A detailed history is important in gaining clues.

History of the presenting problem

Weight loss

It is vitally important to actually document weight loss (on the same scales if at all possible): patient perceptions are sometimes misleading, and to embark on a protracted series of investigations for a problem that does not exist is clearly not sensible! If the patient has not weighed themselves, ask if clothes/trousers have become looser. Rapid weight loss, particularly in middle-aged or elderly patients, is often associated with malignancy.

 Rapid weight loss over the course of days is usually due to loss of fluid, hence daily weights are useful in assessing the response of the patient with heart failure or ascites to diuretic therapy.

Appetite

Decreased appetite invariably leads to weight loss and is a feature of many diseases. Weight loss in the context of a good or increased appetite is suggestive of thyrotoxicosis or diabetes mellitus.

 Diabetes and thyrotoxicosis are very common. Diabetes affects 1–2% of the population, and thyrotoxicosis affects 1–2% of women at some time in their lives.

Diarrhoea

Diarrhoea may be a feature of thyrotoxicosis. Is there steatorrhoea—a sign of malabsorption characterized by loose, oily, bulky, offensive stools that are difficult to flush away? This might be due to:
• mucosal disease, e.g. coeliac, Crohn's disease (see Sections 1.1, p. 3 and 1.5, p. 17)
• pancreatic insufficiency, e.g. chronic pancreatitis, cystic fibrosis (see Section 2.4, p. 75).

Abdominal pain

Abdominal pain does not occur in coeliac disease. Pain, particularly in the right iliac fossa, together with weight loss should alert the clinician to the possibility of Crohn's disease. Repeated attacks of central/epigastric pain, especially in the context of high alcohol intake, should raise the possibility of chronic pancreatitis.

Intentional weight loss

Is the patient trying to lose weight? How does their weight now compare with that 5 and 10 years ago? Have they been on a diet recently, or at any other time? Have they had problems with anorexia nervosa or bulimia in the past? See *Psychiatry*, Section 1.5.

Relevant past history

Malignancy

Is there a past history of malignancy? If so, onset of weight loss is highly suspicious of recurrence or metastatic disease.

Other

Are there features to suggest diabetes mellitus (polyuria, polydipsia) or thyrotoxicisis (tremor, agitation)? (See *Endocrinology*, Sections 1.3 and 1.13).

Family history

There is a 10% risk of coeliac disease in the offspring of an affected patient. Diabetes and thyroid disease also have a genetic component.

Examination

 Examination of the patient with weight loss and tiredness

• General impression—is the patient well or ill?
• Is there evidence of marked weight loss/cachexia?
• Are they anaemic?
• Are lymph nodes palpable?
• Is there any evidence of thyrotoxicosis?
• Are there any abdominal masses, suggesting colonic carcinoma, or a Crohn's inflammatory mass?

General

Profound weight loss or cachexia is usually obvious. Anaemia can be difficult to detect, especially if mild. Look carefully for any of the following:
• *Hands.* Clubbing (Crohn's disease, coeliac disease, bronchial carcinoma—the latter most unusual in a woman of this age); koilonychia (iron-deficiency anaemia);

pigmentation in palmar creases (Addison's disease); calluses on knuckles (self-induced vomiting).
- *Blood pressure.* Hypotension suggesting anorexia nervosa or Addison's disease.
- *Face and neck.* Goitre, exophthalmos, lid lag indicating thyrotoxicosis.
- *Mouth.* Aphthous ulceration (Crohn's disease, coeliac disease); eroded teeth (self-induced vomiting).
- *Lymphadenopathy.* (Lymphoproliferative disease or regional lymphatic spread from carcinoma—the latter unlikely in a woman of this age.)
- *Abdomen.* Hepatomegaly/splenomegaly (suggesting a lymphoproliferative disorder) or abdominal masses (Crohn's).

Differential diagnosis

In a young woman presenting with weight loss, consider the following:
- *Crohn's disease.* Peak incidence in young (teens and twenties), with second peak in 60s and 70s. Classically presents with abdominal pain, diarrhoea and weight loss.
- *Thyrotoxicosis.* Fairly common, especially in women. Is there a family history of Graves' disease? Look for resting fine tremor of outstretched hands, warm sweaty hands, tachycardia, fidgety behaviour, palmar erythema, exophthalmos, lid lag and goitre. Usually ravenous but still losing weight.
- *Addison's disease.* Rare, and easily missed. Suspect if past or family history of autoimmune disease. Insidious onset, weakness, lethargy, weight loss, light-headedness on standing, nausea or vomiting. May complain of abdominal pain. Look for pigmentation in palmar creases and buccal mucosa, hypotension, hyponatraemia, hyperkalaemia and raised urea.
- *Pancreatic insufficiency.* Usually secondary to chronic pancreatitis (chiefly alcohol induced). Steatorrhoea may be massive.
- *Diabetes mellitus.* Diagnosis usually obvious with polydipsia, polyuria, good appetite and weight loss.
- *Eating disorders.* Deliberate dieting and anorexia nervosa need to be kept in mind.
- *Chronic infection and malignancy.* Be alert to the possibility of tuberculosis (cough, night sweats) especially in debilitated, alcoholic or Asian patients. A pyrexia of unknown origin may be due to malignancy, autoimmune disease or chronic infection. Site of malignancy often suggested by history. Don't forget haematological malignancies, especially in the younger patient.

Approach to investigations and management

Investigation

The following tests may be indicated in the investigation of tiredness and weight loss, but often the history and examination mean that only a few of them are necessary.

A diagnosis is usually evident after the history, examination and relevant blood tests.

Blood and urine tests

Check urine with dipstix for glucose, blood and protein. Check full blood count, electrolytes, renal and liver function tests, inflammatory markers (ESR and CRP), glucose, thyroid function tests, 'malabsorption' markers (ferritin, folate, B_{12}, calcium). Consider short Synacthen test. Check antiendomysial antibodies: coeliac disease often presents as iron-deficiency anaemia without any other symptoms.

 A raised platelet count may be found with chronic GI blood loss, but also regard it as an 'inflammatory marker'. It is often raised in active inflammatory bowel disease, especially Crohn's disease.

Imaging

A chest radiograph is useful, looking for tuberculosis, bronchial neoplasm or mediastinal lymphadenopathy. Abdominal ultrasound or abdominal CT scanning are non-invasive and may detect inflammatory masses or thickened oedematous loops of small bowel in Crohn's disease, intra-abdominal collections, lymphadenopathy or renal carcinoma.

Further investigation

If no clear diagnostic leads have emerged from the blood tests described, chest radiography and abdominal imaging, then further investigation is almost certainly not warranted and it is likely that attention can most fruitfully be directed towards psychological causes of tiredness and weight loss, e.g. eating disorder or depression (see *Psychiatry*, Sections 1.5 and 2.11).

If iron-deficiency anaemia is present both the upper and lower GI tract should be investigated since there may be dual pathology. Barium follow-through or small bowel enema may reveal Crohn's disease. Coeliac disease is confirmed by total or subtotal villous atrophy on duodenal biopsies (Fig. 22). Further specific tests may be clinically indicated, e.g. lymph node biopsy.

 Don't forget that the radiological appearances of intestinal tuberculosis may look identical to Crohn's disease, so keep a high index of suspicion, particularly in Asian patients.

Management

The management is clearly dictated by the specific diagnosis made. This woman had coeliac disease, with positive

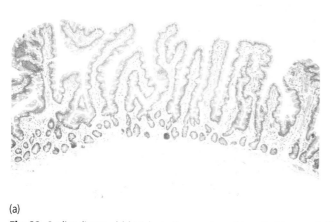

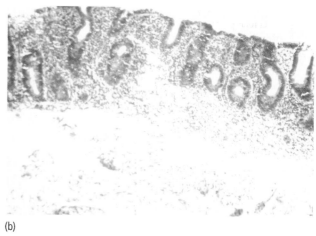

(a)
(b)

Fig. 22 Coeliac disease: (a) histologically normal small bowel with normal villi contrasts with (b) total villous atrophy of coeliac disease.

antiendomysial antibodies and appropriate findings on duodenal biopsy. The management of coeliac disease is described in Section 2.6.1; consultation with a dietician is required, the condition responding to a lifelong gluten-free diet. It is usual to rebiopsy after 12 months on gluten-free diet to demonstrate improvement.

 Persistence of anti-endomysial antibodies 6 weeks after starting a diet suggests poor dietary compliance or dietary-resistant coeliac (the latter is rare).

For management of:
- thyrotoxicosis see *Endocrinology*, Section 2.3.2
- diabetes mellitus see *Endocrinology*, Section 2.6
- eating disorders see *Psychiatry*, Section 1.5.

Coeliac Society and British Digestion Foundation.
http://www.digestivedisorders.org.uk
http://www.coeliac.co.uk
Collin P, Kaukinen K, Maki M. Clinical features of celiac disease today. *Dig Dis* 1999; 17: 100–106.
Feighery C. Coeliac disease. *BMJ* 1999; 319: 236–239.
Scott EM, Gaywood I, Scott BB for the British Society of Gastroenterology. Guidelines for osteoporosis in coeliac disease and inflammatory bowel disease. *Gut* 2000 (Suppl. 1): 46. [Guidelines on prevention and treatment of osteoporosis associated with coeliac disease.]

1.11 Diarrhoea and weight loss

Case history

A 72-year-old woman presents with a 6-month history of increasing diarrhoea and tiredness associated with weight loss. She has had no constipation. She has also noticed increasingly frequent angina on exertion.

Clinical approach

In any elderly patient the first priority is to exclude a colonic neoplasm as a cause of change in bowel habit associated with weight loss. The next most common cause of diarrhoea is malabsorption, particularly if there is a history of steator-rhoea and symptoms to suggest anaemia. In an older patient the most likely cause for this is bacterial overgrowth, which can occur as a result of jejunal diverticula or surgical blind loops (see Section 2.6).

History of presenting problem

As always, it is important to establish the facts right at the beginning: when the woman says that she has diarrhoea, what does she mean? How many times has she opened her bowels today? What is the consistency of her stools? (See Section 1.1.) What is her weight now, and what was it 6 months ago? (See Section 1.10.)

Colonic malignancy

Has there been any blood in the motions? Bright red blood on the paper suggests piles; blood mixed in with the stool suggests sinister pathology in this context.

Malabsorption

Ask specifically:
- Is the stool pale?
- Is the stool difficult to flush away?
- Any abdominal bloating?
- Any mouth ulcers?

Abdominal pain

This is unusual in malabsorption from bacterial overgrowth alone and suggests intermittent small bowel obstruction as may occur with Crohn's strictures.

Chronic pancreatic insufficiency can occur in elderly people with the development of an atrophic pancreas. Unlike alcoholic chronic pancreatitis this is usually painless.

Relevant past history

Is she at risk of bacterial overgrowth? Predisposing factors include:
• systemic sclerosis or diabetes mellitus that impair gastrointestinal motility
• previous gastric surgery, where bacterial colonization can occur in blind loops, such as an afferent loop following a gastroenterostomy (see Fig. 6)
• use of proton pump inhibitors, which lead to hypochlorhydria.
There were no such factors in this woman.

 Proton pump inhibitors can cause diarrhoea without steatorrhoea.

Examination

There was no blood in the motions in this case, and the history suggested that this woman had malabsorption, when few abnormal signs are expected.

General

Look for:
• *weight loss*
• *pallor* suggesting anaemia
• *angular stomatitis and koilonychia* suggesting iron deficiency
• *leuconychia* which is uncommon unless malabsorption is severe
• a *smooth tongue*
• *ankle swelling* which occurs in the presence of severe hypoalbuminaemia.

Abdominal

Examine for:
• *Abdominal scars*
• *Masses*
• *Ascites*. Only likely to be due to malabsorption if this is severe
• *Perform rectal examination* to confirm steatorrhoea.

Approach to investigation and management

Investigations

These are clearly dictated by the clinical findings, but where bacterial overgrowth is the most likely diagnosis, as in this case, then proceed as follows:

Malabsorption

BLOOD TESTS

Check full blood count (looking particularly for macrocytic anaemia), electrolytes, renal and liver function (albumin will be low in severe malabsorption), serum B_{12} (deficiency is common), folate (deficiency is common, particularly in the presence of a blind intestinal loop), serum iron/TIBC (usually normal). Note that the pattern of a high alkaline phosphatase, normal GGT and low corrected serum calcium would suggest vitamin D deficiency, which is uncommon.

STOOL ANALYSIS

Confirm steatorrhoea by microscopy of a single sample for fat globules. Many gastroenterologists recommend a 3-day faecal fat collection, but they do not perform the test themselves and many laboratories refuse to do so (check before you send one: they may send it back!).

Bacterial overgrowth

BREATH TESTS

Bacterial fermentation of an oral dose of carbohydrate releases hydrogen, and of an oral dose of conjugated bile acid, radiolabelled in the amino portion with ^{13}C, yields radiolabelled carbon dioxide. If there is an increase in bacteria in the upper small bowel an early peak in hydrogen or carbon dioxide can be detected in expired air (see Section 3.1, pp. 132–138).

ENDOSCOPY AND DUODENAL ASPIRATE

The diagnosis of bacterial overgrowth is confirmed if there are $>10^5$/mL of mixed bacteria. The test can also be helpful if subsequent antibiotic resistance occurs.

SMALL BOWEL ENEMA

To look for small bowel diverticula or small bowel strictures as a cause for overgrowth (Fig. 23). Diverticula were present in this woman.

Management

In cases of bacterial overgrowth:
• Replace deficient B_{12} intramuscularly and folate orally.
• Give antibiotics: tetracycline or augmentin for 10 days. Prolonged courses (1–2 months) may be needed. Recurrence occurs, and cyclical antibiotics for 1 week in every 4 may be required.

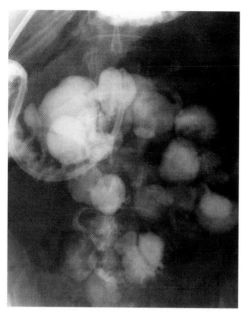

Fig. 23 A small bowel enema showing multiple diverticula.

- If there is a clear localized anatomical reason for bacterial overgrowth, then surgical correction may be appropriate if there is poor response to medical therapy.

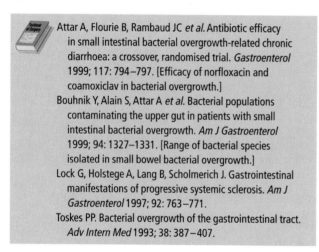

Attar A, Flourie B, Rambaud JC *et al.* Antibiotic efficacy in small intestinal bacterial overgrowth-related chronic diarrhoea: a crossover, randomised trial. *Gastroenterol* 1999; 117: 794–797. [Efficacy of norfloxacin and coamoxiclav in bacterial overgrowth.]

Bouhnik Y, Alain S, Attar A *et al.* Bacterial populations contaminating the upper gut in patients with small intestinal bacterial overgrowth. *Am J Gastroenterol* 1999; 94: 1327–1331. [Range of bacterial species isolated in small bowel bacterial overgrowth.]

Lock G, Holstege A, Lang B, Scholmerich J. Gastrointestinal manifestations of progressive systemic sclerosis. *Am J Gastroenterol* 1997; 92: 763–771.

Toskes PP. Bacterial overgrowth of the gastrointestinal tract. *Adv Intern Med* 1993; 38: 387–407.

1.12 Rectal bleeding

Case history

A 65-year-old man gives a history of persistent lower abdominal pain and an episode of bright red rectal bleeding.

Clinical approach

Passing more than small amounts of blood per rectum usually signifies substantial lower gastrointestinal pathology and the symptom must be investigated. There is a wide differential diagnosis (Table 13), but the main possibilities are:

Table 13 Differential diagnosis of rectal bleeding.

Haemorrhoids
The most common cause. The bleeding is usually minor, at the end of defaecation, and manifested by blood on the toilet paper or coating the stool. Occasionally bleeding is more brisk
Haemorrhoids are common, and commonly coexist with other pathology

Colorectal carcinoma
May bleed briskly or occultly. Benign polyps rarely bleed

Diverticular disease
Diverticula increase with age, and may be entirely asymptomatic, or may cause chronic or episodic pain, possibly associated with infective episodes (diverticulitis). Occasionally, erosion into the feeding artery of a diverticulum may cause brisk lower gastrointestinal haemorrhage that may be life-threatening. Diverticula rarely bleed chronically

Angiodysplasia and other vascular lesions
Ectatic, dysplastic blood vessels in the colonic mucosa occur in older patients, when they may bleed episodically and briskly. They may also bleed slowly, causing iron deficiency
Telangiectasias of hereditary haemorrhagic telangiectasia (Osler–Weber–Rendu syndrome) increase with age, and rectal bleeding may be the first manifestation in some patients

Mucosal inflammation
Florid mucosal ulceration in ulcerative colitis and Crohn's disease may present with predominant rectal bleeding, with the blood mixed in with stool, or flowing freely
Similarly, bleeding may be prominent in bacterial or amoebic colitis, and NSAID-associated colitis
Radiation enteritis, colitis or proctitis may present with brisk rectal bleeding

Mesenteric ischaemia
See Section 1.14, pp. 41–43

Miscellaneous causes
Occasionally patients will mistake food pigments or dyes for blood (e.g. after eating beetroot)
Intussusception, volvulus, intestinal trauma and bleeding disorders (including warfarin) may cause rectal bleeding
Patients with portal hypertension may develop rectal varices that can bleed catastrophically

NSAID, non-steroidal anti-inflammatory drug.

- colorectal carcinoma
- diverticular disease
- bleeding angiodysplastic lesions.

All of these are particularly common in older patients.

 Although haemorrhoids may occasionally bleed briskly, symptoms should not be attributed to haemorrhoids without investigation.

History of the presenting problem

Nature of the bleeding

Brisk episodic haemorrhage is typical of bleeding diverticula. Blood mixed with stool over many days is very suspicious of a neoplastic lesion, whilst blood predominantly seen on wiping the anus is typical of bleeding haemorrhoids. None of these features are diagnostic.

Pain

The abdominal pain of diverticular disease is typically felt in the left iliac fossa. Cramping pain may occur in colitis. Pain from neoplasia is a late sign. Severe abdominal pain accompanying bleeding in an ill patient is highly suggestive of mesenteric ischaemia. Perianal pain is typical of haemorrhoids. Internal haemorrhoids may cause anal discomfort, pain and pruritus.

Change in bowel habit

Recent change in bowel habit should alert the clinician to the possibility of neoplasia.

Weight loss

This is a sinister symptom, suggesting chronic intestinal inflammation or neoplasia.

Relevant past history

Enquire regarding chronic liver disease with portal hypertension resulting in rectal haemorrhoids, bleeding diathesis, local radiotherapy (e.g. for bladder or (in a woman) cervical neoplasia), inflammatory bowel disease. Also take note of previous cardiovascular, cerebrovascular or peripheral vascular disease, both because they are relevant to treatment options that might be considered (e.g. assessment of surgical risk) and because the presence of vascular disease would increase the likelihood of symptoms being due to mesenteric ischaemia. Angiodysplastic bleeding from the colon is said to be more common in patients with aortic valve stenosis.

Drug history

Ask particularly about the use of non-steroidal anti-inflammatory agents, warfarin and vasoactive drugs such as ergotamine.

Family history

A family history of colorectal carcinoma or colonic polyps should be sought, and strengthens the case for thorough investigation, particularly in a younger patient. Hereditary haemorrhagic telangiectasia is an autosomal dominant disorder.

Examination

General

Following brisk bleeding, the patient may be in circulatory shock: check for cool peripheries, tachycardia, hypotension (lying and sitting) and low JVP. If present, commence resuscitation as described in Section 1.3, p. 13. If there is also fever, prostration and abdominal pain and tenderness, the probability of intestinal ischaemia is increased.

Most patients (as this man) with this history are not haemodynamically compromised, but do they appear well, or ill, suggesting chronic illness? Look for signs to indicate likely pathology:
- Do they look as though they have lost weight? Clearly suspicious of carcinoma in this context.
- Are they pale? Suggesting anaemia and long-term bleeding.
- Are they jaundiced? Suggesting malignancy, but also chronic liver disease.
- Do they have lymphadenopathy? Strongly suggesting malignancy.
- Do they have signs of chronic liver disease and/or portal hypertension? (See Sections 1.6, p. 20 and 1.7, p. 23.)
- Do they have generalized vascular disease (absent pulses, vascular bruits, abdominal aortic aneurysm)? Increases the chances of mesenteric ischaemia.
- Check the skin and mucosae for telangiectasia. This is 'small print': but if you don't do it you'll never make the diagnosis!

Abdominal

Abdominal examination may reveal a tender, palpable sigmoid colon, suggesting sigmoid diverticular disease. Other colonic masses are usually impalpable or only vaguely felt. Rectal examination must be performed, preferably with proctoscopy and rigid sigmoidoscopy. Digital rectal examination can detect masses up to 10 cm from the anal verge. Any blood or pus on the gloved finger should be noted. Are there thrombosed external piles, bleeding or ulcerated prolapsed haemorrhoids, or skin tags relating to anal Crohn's disease? Occasionally an anal carcinoma may be the cause of symptoms.

Approach to investigations and management

Investigations

Blood tests and chest radiography

These are performed to determine whether the patient is anaemic, and whether there are any clues to the cause of rectal bleeding. Check full blood count (is there microcytic anaemia?; a raised platelet count may occur in inflammation or brisk bleeding), electrolytes, renal and liver function

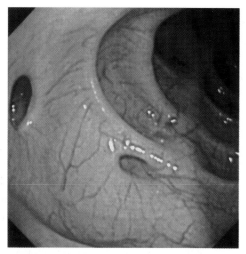

Fig. 24 Two sigmoid diverticula seen at colonoscopy.

(abnormal liver function tests may be an early indicator of metastatic neoplasia), clotting, inflammatory markers (ESR and CRP may be substantially raised in diverticulitis and intestinal inflammation) and iron status. Group and save or cross match blood as appropriate.

Source of the bleeding

Frank rectal bleeding can originate anywhere in the gastrointestinal tract, including the upper tract (oesophagus and stomach) if the bleeding is brisk enough. Therefore, depending on the circumstances, it may be necessary to examine both upper and lower ends of the bowel (see Sections 1.3, p. 9 and 1.4, p. 13). Usually, however, only the lower tract needs to be examined, and there is a choice of modalities. Tests should be selected in the light of the clinical picture, potential benefit, local availability and acceptability to the patient.

COLONOSCOPY

This offers direct visualization of the entire colon, and usually of the terminal ileum. Some bleeding mucosal lesions such as angiodysplasia can only be detected by colonoscopy. In addition, colonoscopy offers the possibility of diagnostic biopsy and therapeutic haemostasis (by electrocautery) or removal of small tumours (by snaring and cautery). On the other hand, there is a small risk of intestinal perforation, particularly in cases of florid inflammation, obstructing tumours and severe diverticulosis, which can make colonoscopy difficult and dangerous. Nonetheless, colonoscopy is the preferred investigation in most cases (Fig. 24).

BARIUM ENEMA

This is as effective as colonoscopy in detecting colonic neoplasia and diverticular disease (the diagnosis in this man),

carries a smaller risk of complications, and may be preferred by some patients.

AIR-CONTRAST CT SCAN AND VIRTUAL COLONOSCOPY

High-speed spiral CT scanners and computer equipment enable these rapidly evolving tests. They allow visualization of the intestinal wall with an accuracy approaching that of colonoscopy, and cause minimal discomfort to patients.

MESENTERIC ANGIOGRAPHY AND RED CELL SCANNING

Brisk bleeding from a source that cannot be identified by the other tests can sometimes be identified if the patient can be investigated during the bleeding episode.

Management

As in all cases of bleeding, resuscitation and replacement of circulating volume take precedence in the acute situation (see Section 1.3, p. 13). Torrential lower gastrointestinal haemorrhage should always be treated in cooperation with a surgical team. Endoscopy in this situation is difficult, dangerous and unrewarding: emergency angiography and embolization of a bleeding vessel should be considered as an option. A single episode of diverticular haemorrhage may not recur, but persistent pain, infection or bleeding may necessitate surgery.

See Table 14 and Section 2.7, pp. 95–100 for management options in other causes of rectal bleeding.

Table 14 Diagnosis-specific treatment of rectal bleeding.

Vascular lesions
Local treatment with electrocautery or laser coagulation may control symptoms
Oral oestrogen treatment is said to reduce bleeding episodes
In some patients, a pragmatic approach with chronic oral iron
  supplementation and occasional 'top-up' blood transfusion may be
  indicated

Radiation colitis and proctitis
Symptoms may be intractable although some patients improve spontaneously
Local anti-inflammatory treatment with 5-aminosalicylic acid compounds
  may produce some benefit
Surgery is usually unsatisfactory in the relatively avascular postradiation tissue

 See *Emergency medicine*, Section 1.11.
1 Reinus JF, Brandt LJ. Vascular ectasias and diverticulosis: common causes of lower intestinal bleeding. *Gastrointest Endosc Clin N Am* 1994; 23: 1–20.
2 Miller LS, Barbarevech C, Friedman, LS. Less frequent causes of lower gastrointestinal bleeding. *Gastrointest Endosc Clin N Am* 1994; 23: 21–30.

1.13 Severe abdominal pain and vomiting

Case history

A 34-year-old man is referred to you from the local military base with severe upper abdominal pain and vomiting. The problem had initially been put down to 'overindulgence' but the referring medical officer has become concerned that after 24 h of observation in the medical unit he has got worse and has started vomiting 'coffee grounds'.

Clinical approach

 Young patients with severe acute illness can be a substantial challenge, especially when alcohol plays a part in the presentation. In situations like this the true contribution of alcohol may only become apparent at a later date and from third parties.

In the acute situation information is often scanty and it is important to focus on the basics: Does the patient look ill, very ill or nearly dead? What are the vital signs? Are there signs of peritonitis? Is the patient beginning to show signs of alcohol withdrawal?

The progressive nature of the problem in the context of the history suggests acute pancreatitis, although other diagnoses should be considered (Table 15).

History of the presenting problem

It is likely that you will only be able to obtain a limited history from the patient, who will probably not be able or willing to cooperate with extensive interrogation. Concentrate on the key features.

Nature of the pain

Acute pancreatic pain is usually constant, epigastric and radiates through to the back. That from a peptic ulcer can be indistinguishable, but is usually less severe, and except for a posterior penetrating ulcer does not usually radiate to the back. Biliary colic typically causes pain in the right upper quadrant and epigastrium, the key distinguishing feature from pancreatic or ulcer pain being that it is colicky, i.e. comes in waves with periods of respite in between.

Table 15 Differential diagnosis of severe acute upper abdominal pain with vomiting.

Common	Uncommon	Rare
Acute pancreatitis	Myocardial infarction	Acute porphyria
Peptic ulcer	Gastric volvulus	
Biliary colic	Intestinal infarction	

It is most unlikely that this man's pain is cardiac, but take 10 s to ask about radiation in a cardiac distribution: it is a very bad mistake to miss an acute coronary syndrome—especially if you proceed to laparotomy, which is not the normal treatment for cases of myocardial infarction!

Nature of the vomitus

The presence of obvious haematemesis is clearly significant, being a feature of peptic ulceration but not pancreatitis or biliary colic (see Section 1.3, p. 9). 'Coffee grounds' are produced by the vomiting of blood that has been present in the stomach for some time, but—unless you see a reasonable quantity of this yourself—do not attach too much weight to the patient's description or second- or third-hand reports: it is almost impossible for vomiting to occur without someone reporting that there 'might have been coffee grounds in it'.

Relevant past history

Try to find out if the patient has had:
• a history of heavy alcohol consumption (see Section 1.4, p. 14)
• previous admissions to hospital with similar problems or for other problems that might be related to excess alcohol consumption
• features to suggest pre-existing gallstones such as recurrent biliary colic
• a history of indigestion: Do they take antacids or any over-the-counter medications for indigestion? Have they ever had a barium meal or an endoscopy test?
• previous abdominal surgery
• angina or heart attacks in the past.

Examination

General

Is the patient ill, very ill or nearly dead? If nearly dead, call for help from the ICU immediately.
• Assess the circulation: peripheral perfusion, pulse, BP (lying and sitting), JVP. If compromised, begin resuscitation immediately (see Section 1.3, p. 13).
• What is the temperature? Are the sclerae icteric? Jaundice at presentation is an important clinical sign as it implies biliary obstruction and cholangitis: jaundice developing after admission is less discriminating.

Abdominal

Focus in particular on:
• *Epigastric tenderness*. This is non-specific. There may be features of localized peritonitis with guarding and rebound.

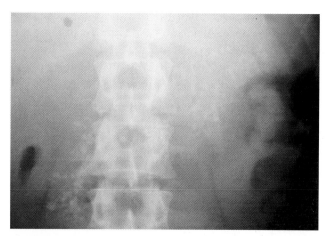

Fig. 25 Plain abdominal radiograph showing pancreatic calcification in a patient with chronic pancreatitis.

- *Bowel sounds*. Absent bowel sounds indicate paralytic ileus.
- *Abdominal wall bruising*. This may be periumbilical (Cullen's sign) or present in the flanks (Grey–Turner's sign). It occurs with severe acute pancreatitis.
- *Rectal examination* for melaena.

Approach to investigations and management

Investigations

 In acute pancreatitis it is important to:
- make the diagnosis
- assess severity
- determine aetiology
- identify complications.

Blood tests and plain radiology

Check:
- *Full blood count, electrolytes (including calcium), renal and hepatic function, amylase, clotting and Group and Save*. The serum amylase is diagnostic of pancreatitis if more than three times the upper limit of normal for the laboratory. Alternatives include serum lipase and possibly urinary trypsinogen.
- *Arterial blood gases*. Important in any severely ill patient, and used in grading the severity of pancreatitis (see Section 2.4.1, p. 75).
- *Chest and abdominal radiograph*. The chest radiograph may show effusions. The abdominal film may demonstrate a localized ileus ('sentinel loop'). Rarely calcified gallstones may be visible. Pancreatic calcification indicates chronic (usually alcoholic) pancreatitis (Fig. 25).

Other imaging

ABDOMINAL ULTRASOUND

An abdominal ultrasound should be performed within 24 h of admission. This will determine whether there are gallstones present and may demonstrate biliary dilatation, suggesting common bile duct obstruction.

ABDOMINAL CT

A CT with contrast should be performed in cases of severe pancreatitis between 3 and 10 days after admission (Fig. 26). This can identify secondary complications such as pseudocyst formation and the extent of pancreatic necrosis carries prognostic value (Balthazar score).

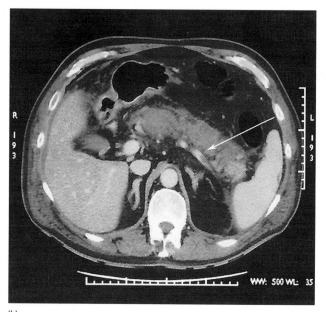

(a)

(b)

Fig. 26 CT scans of (a) normal pancreas (arrow) and (b) acute pancreatitis: the pancreas swollen and oedematous (arrow), and a thrombus is seen in the splenic vein behind the pancreas.

Management

Resuscitation

The first priority is to resuscitate the patient with the aim of reducing the chances of secondary organ failure (renal impairment, acute respiratory disease syndrome (ARDS)) (see Section 1.3, p. 13).

> Patients with severe acute pancreatitis (including organ failure) should be managed on an HDU/ICU.

Analgesia

Pain should be relieved. The preferred opiate is pethidine: morphine can cause spasm of the sphincter of Oddi and thereby exacerbate matters.

Alcohol withdrawal

If there is a clear history of alcohol dependence or you suspect that alcohol withdrawal is developing (due to increasing agitation and tremor) then start treatment with chlordiazepoxide (see Section 1.7, pp. 25–26 and Table 10, p. 26; also see *Psychiatry*, Section 1.7).

ERCP

An early ERCP (i.e. within the first 24 h) should be considered if gallstones are present on the ultrasound, or if the patient has clinical features of cholangitis (fever, jaundice), on the principle that relief of biliary obstruction will allow drainage of the biliary system and reduce complications. If this is not performed within 24–48 h then oedema of the papilla makes ERCP technically difficult.

Antibiotics

The role of antibiotics in acute pancreatitis is controversial. Antibiotics should be used in cases of proven infection or organ failure, and many would give broad-spectrum cover to any who are severely ill.

Nutrition

Consider early enteral feeding via a nasogastric or nasojejunal feeding tube. If this is not possible, then intravenous feeding should be considered sooner rather than later.

Treatment of complications

Persistent pain, fever and raised markers of inflammation (CRP) all raise the possibility of the development of infected necrosis of the pancreas and/or the development of a pancreatic abscess. These might require radiological or surgical drainage.

Further management

Treatment of underlying cause

Abstinence from alcohol or cholecystectomy. See Section 2.4, pp. 75–77 for further details.

> See *Emergency medicine*, Sections 1.13 and 1.14.
> See *Psychiatry*, Section 1.7.
> British Society of Gastroenterology. United Kingdom guidelines for the management of acute pancreatitis. *Gut* 1998; 42 (Suppl. 2): S1–13. [Guidelines on the management of acute pancreatitis.]

1.14 Chronic abdominal pain

Case history

A 77-year-old man presents with a 3-month history of crampy abdominal pain, occurring about 20 min after meals, together with 1 stone weight loss. His past history includes hypertension, angina and intermittent claudication.

Clinical approach

Common things being common, it would be important to consider biliary colic or peptic ulceration with this presentation. Colicky abdominal pain can also be due to mechanical obstruction of the intestine, and therefore adhesions, incarcerated hernias and strictures in the bowel due to carcinoma, Crohn's disease or lymphoma should all be thought about. Weight loss always raises concerns about a diagnosis of carcinoma, and gastric, pancreatic and colonic neoplasia need to be borne in mind, particularly if the pain is not particularly colicky in nature. A diagnosis of mesenteric ischaemia is almost one of exclusion, since it is rare, but it should be considered in those with atheromatous disease, such as this man.

History of the presenting problem

Origin of pain

Typically pain from the stomach is located in the epigastrium, pain from the small bowel is centred around the umbilicus, and pain from the large bowel is felt in the suprapubic region. Colicky (waxing and waning) pain indicates obstruction of a lumen, be it intestine, bile duct or ureter.

Other features

Are there any features to support a particular diagnosis? Vomiting would suggest small bowel obstruction or biliary colic. Change in urine or stool colour may be seen if gallstones have caused biliary obstruction; change in bowel habit or rectal bleeding would strongly support the diagnosis of colonic carcinoma; fevers would indicate that a systemic or inflammatory condition such as lymphoma or Crohn's disease was likely.

Weight loss does not necessarily imply malignant disease: it occurs in most illnesses where eating is associated with pain.

Relevant past history

Abdominal surgery

If the patient has had surgery, what was it for? They may not know, in which case it is extremely important to track down the relevant notes. In those who have had previous abdominal operations, always consider adhesions in cases of obstruction/subacute obstruction.

Atherosclerotic disease

Mesenteric ischaemia/infarction should be considered, particularly in the elderly patient—such as this man—with atherosclerotic disease (myocardial infarction, angina, intermittent claudication, TIA, CVA) or at high risk of this (diabetes mellitus). In those presenting with a single episode of severe abdominal pain the chance of mesenteric ischaemia is increased if there is a potential source of emboli, e.g. atrial fibrillation or structural cardiac abnormality.

Examination

General

This man is not presenting with an acute abdominal emergency, but does he look well or ill? Note in particular the presence of:
- *Fever*, suggesting an inflammatory (e.g. Crohn's) or systemic (e.g. lymphoma) process.
- *Lymphadenopathy*, suggesting carcinoma or lymphoma.
- *Signs of atherosclerotic vascular disease*, e.g. absent pulses, vascular bruits, abdominal aortic aneurysm, suggesting that mesenteric ischaemia is possible.

Abdominal examination

Take careful note of the following:

- abdominal scars and herniae—has the man got a femoral hernia (these are easy to miss)?
- visible peristalsis
- bowel sounds
- localized tenderness.

Rectal examination—are there fissures or other features to suggest Crohn's?

Signs of an acute abdomen are unlikely to be present.

Mesenteric infarction manifests as an acute abdomen in its later stages, but earlier on there may be severe abdominal pain with little in the way of abdominal signs.

Differential diagnosis

In the patient with crampy abdominal pain, consider the following:

- *Gastroenteritis.* Viral or bacterial infections of the gastrointestinal tract may present with colicky abdominal pain, usually with vomiting ± diarrhoea. The symptoms are short-lived, and this diagnosis can therefore be excluded in this case.
- *Biliary colic.* Tends to be located in the right upper quadrant, but may occur in the epigastrium. Usually builds up over 15–45 min following a meal (typically fatty). There may be associated nausea or vomiting. Referred pain to the shoulder tip makes biliary pain very likely.
- *Adhesions.* Take note of any previous abdominal operations/scars. Colicky pain typically follows some time after meals, with sudden relief after a variable time. Occasionally there may be visible peristalsis of the small bowel in thin subjects.
- *Incarcerated or strangulated herniae.* All hernial orifices must be examined carefully. Check for heat, tenderness, reducibility and cough impulse in any hernia present, as well as for bowel sounds.
- *Diverticular disease.* Diverticular disease may cause intermittent left iliac fossa pain, together with altered bowel habit. Acute diverticulitis, 'left-sided appendicitis', is manifest by fever, constitutional upset and marked local pain and tenderness.
- *Crohn's disease.* Central colicky abdominal pain or right iliac fossa pain together with diarrhoea and weight loss are characteristic features of Crohn's disease. Think of this in the young patient, especially if inflammatory markers or platelet count are raised, but remember that it can present for the first time in the 7th and 8th decades and cannot be completely discounted, even in a man who is 77 years old.
- *Peptic ulcer disease.* Gastric and duodenal ulcers may cause epigastric pain that is related to food. Typically, food relieves pain from duodenal ulcers. Gastric outlet obstruction with associated fullness and vomiting may occur secondary to scarring of the pyloric canal by peptic ulceration or by encroachment by gastric carcinoma.
- *Mesenteric ischaemia.* Causes pain after meals. There are usually no abnormal abdominal signs. Look for evidence of atheromatous vascular disease on history and examination.
- *Addison's disease.* This is a very rare cause of abdominal pain, but you will never make the diagnosis unless you think of it! Consider in any patient with undiagnosed abdominal pain, particularly if other endocrine disease is present. What is the blood pressure (hypotension is invariable)? Are the palmar creases hyperpigmented?
- Pancreatitis (see Section 1.13).

Approach to investigations and management

This will be obviously dictated by clues gleaned from the history and examination. In the absence of any clear leads, proceed as follows.

Investigations

Blood tests

Check full blood count, electrolytes, renal and liver function tests, amylase. Iron-deficiency anaemia would obviously suggest gastroinestinal blood loss in this context, perhaps from peptic ulcer disease or colonic malignancy. Vomiting (not present in this case) often causes hypokalaemia. If there is hyperkalaemia, hyponatraemia and mildly raised urea, then suspect Addison's disease. Amylase and liver function tests may be abnormal with choledocholithiasis.

> In the patient presenting with an acute abdomen, but relatively little in the way of abdominal signs, remember that a high white cell count ($20-30 \times 10^9$/L) and haematocrit (>50%, due to fluid loss into the gut) should raise suspicion of mesenteric ischaemia. Hyperkalaemia and acidosis are often associated with infarcted bowel in this context.

Abdominal radiograph and ultrasound

In obstruction the plain abdominal radiograph will reveal dilated loops of small bowel (and fluid levels if erect). In ischaemic colitis, 'thumb printing' may be seen, particularly at the splenic flexure and in the descending colon. Ultrasound may detect gallstones, also liver metastases or a pancreatic mass.

Barium studies

Barium follow-through or small bowel enema may show strictures in ischaemic colitis, typically affecting the splenic region, and with a segmental nature that mimics Crohn's.

Angiography

The definitive test for making the diagnosis of chronic mesenteric ischaemia is mesenteric angiography, although even this will not always provide a clear-cut answer. In the patient with generalized atheromatous vascular disease the mesenteric vessels are almost bound to be affected: how tight does a narrowing have to be to be significant?

Management

Further management will depend on the specific diagnosis: see relevant sections of this module.

Acute intestinal infarction is an indication for emergency surgery and small bowel resection. It seems reasonable to give those with chronic mesenteric ischaemia maximal medical treatment for atheromatous vascular disease: they should be told to stop smoking and be given aspirin and lipid-lowering therapy. Surgical bypass of angiographically proven mesenteric stenoses may be helpful, but patients with this condition are invariably high-risk candidates due to their widespread vascular disease and success from surgery cannot be guaranteed. Advice to take frequent small meals may be helpful.

> See *Emergency medicine*, Section 1.13.
> See *Endocrinology*, Section 2.2.2.
> Mansour MA. Management of acute mesenteric ischaemia.
> *Arch Surg* 1999; 134: 328–330.

1.15 Change in bowel habit

Case history

While you are telling a 40-year-old woman that her exercise tolerance test was reassuringly negative she tells you that she has been worried by a change in bowel habit over the preceding 6 months. Her aunt has recently been diagnosed as having bowel cancer and she has read in the *Daily Mail* that this is now recognized as being hereditary.

Clinical approach

The obvious likelihood is that this woman's complaint does not indicate significant gastrointestinal pathology, but is due to anxiety. However, it can be a bad mistake to assume this immediately, without the benefit of a thorough history and examination, but take care to explain the situation and not to compound it ('the doctor must have been worried—they asked all those questions').

History of the presenting problem

Let the patient talk about their symptoms, then ask specifically about the following if the information has not emerged spontaneously:
• How long has the problem been present, and have you had it before? Patients with functional bowel disease will often have a history of previous episodes, often occurring at times of stress.
• Has there been abdominal pain? Diffuse discomfort or bloating are common complaints in functional bowel disorder. But are there features to suggest another diagnosis? (See Section 1.14, p. 41.)

- Has there been 'diarrhoea'? This must be qualified (i.e. frequency of defecation or change in stool consistency—see Section 1.1, p. 3).
- Have there been identifiable dietary precipitants of the symptoms (fatty foods, dairy products, alcohol)? If there are, then avoidance may be helpful for symptom control.
- Has there been weight loss or loss of appetite? Anxiety/functional bowel disorder may be associated with some weight loss, but if this is a prominent feature then other diagnoses should be considered.

Ask also:

- Has sleep been disturbed (by either pain or diarrhoea)?
- Has there been rectal bleeding?

These would not be features of functional bowel disease.

Relevant past history

It is clearly important to find out if there is a history of previous abdominal problems. Often, however, there is nothing of note, but it is worth exploring the patient's concerns to understand their fears and concerns. This woman is obviously worried because an aunt has bowel cancer, but if any patient seems to have anxieties disproportionate to their symptoms, then always explore these. In a case such as this, ask:

- Is there any special reason that you are worried about your bowels?
- Have you had any serious trouble with them in the past?
- Have any of your family or friends got any severe bowel problems?
- Is there anything that you are particularly worried about?

This woman, at the age of 40 years, when her risk of ischaemic heart disease must be low, has had an exercise tolerance test. Ask any patient presenting with bowel symptoms that might be due to a functional disorder about other symptoms that might have the same origin.

- Have you ever had chest pains or been investigated for these?
- Have you ever had dizzy spells or funny turns or been investigated for these?

Examination

A thorough physical examination is very important, even if the symptoms do not in themselves raise alarm. It is impossible to reassure a patient with confidence without the benefit of a complete and normal physical examination.

General

A subjective sense of whether the patient looks unwell or not is important. Note in particular:

- Are there any signs in the hands? Look for clubbing, leuconychia, koilonychia.

- Could the woman be thyrotoxic? Look for fine tremor, associated eye signs, goitre, vitiligo.
- Is she pale?
- Is there palpable lymphadenopathy?

Abdominal

Are there any scars from previous abdominal surgery? Is there organomegaly? None is expected; a palpable loop of sigmoid colon in the left iliac fossa is not necessarily pathological but may elicit some tenderness. Examination of the hernial orifices is often forgotten by physicians but may be revealing in patients with longstanding and apparently obscure symptoms.

A rectal examination and rigid sigmoidoscopy should be performed. In patients with symptoms of colonic spasm, these may be reproduced by the insufflation of air. If there is loss of the vascular pattern on sigmoidoscopy or a history of persistent diarrhoea, then consideration should be given to performing a rectal biopsy.

Approach to investigation and management

As with the history and physical examination, a pragmatic but thorough approach to investigations should be adopted.

If you think it likely that investigations might prove to be normal, as in this case, it is always worth discussing this with the patient at the outset. You might say something along the following lines:

- I am pleased to say that I do not think there is anything terrible going on here …
- I have examined you thoroughly and cannot find anything wrong …
- This is good news …
- I think it would be worthwhile to check a few simple tests, including (list these) …
- I think it is likely that all of these will be normal, but would like to check them out …
- If they are normal, then I would not plan to do any more tests, but we will need to talk about how we might help the symptoms that you are getting from your bowels.
- Is that OK … do you have any questions about things?

If your suspicions that tests will be normal are fulfilled, then subsequent consultations are likely to be much easier if you have taken time to explain your clinical approach at the initial contact.

Investigations

Blood tests

Check full blood count, electrolytes, renal and liver function, inflammatory markers (CRP or ESR) and thyroid function. In patients that report weight loss, it is worth measuring iron indices, serum B_{12} and folate and antiendomysial antibody (see Section 1.10, p. 33).

Barium enema or colonoscopy

A patient over the age of 50 years presenting with change in bowel habit undoubtedly requires investigation of the colon to exclude malignancy. The likelihood of malignancy below this age is less, but in a woman of 40 years, as in this case, it would be the practice of most physicians to investigate a new symptom, but not a recurrence of long-standing symptoms.

- Colonoscopy has the advantage that if polyps are found they can be removed immediately, also that if the patient has true diarrhoea a series of colonic biopsies can be taken to exclude a microscopic or collagenous colitis.
- The disadvantage of colonoscopy is that in a small number of patients it is technically difficult to reach the caecum.

Barium enema is often as useful for the exclusion of colon cancer, which is the issue that most often lies behind the presentation of the patient's symptoms.

Management

If all the investigations are normal and the presenting symptom complex is characteristic, as in this case, the patient can be said to have a functional gastrointestinal disorder. The management of so-called irritable bowel depends very much on the patient's perceptions and understanding of the nature of their symptoms.

Reassurance

For many patients the 'qualified reassurance' of normal investigations is sufficient. For others specific approaches need to be considered.

Symptomatic treatment

If postprandial spasm/pain is the dominant symptom associated with a chaotic bowel habit, then antispasmodics such as mebeverine or alverine may be useful. If bloating is the major symptom many patients find peppermint preparations such as colpermin beneficial.

Dietary approaches

For those who can clearly identify specific dietary precipitants, then sensible changes to the diet may improve things considerably. The commonest dietary change to improve symptoms is probably an increase in non-fermenting fibre (e.g. bran). Commercial supplements of fibre such as Fybogel may help, although in those with bloating and wind these may actually make things worse. In patients with difficult symptoms an empirical low-lactose diet may be beneficial, and some who are resistant to all other measures might need to undertake an exclusion diet.

See *Psychiatry*, Section 1.6.
Francis CY, Whorwell PJ. The irritable bowel syndrome. *Postgrad Med J* 1997; 73: 1–7.
Nanda R, James R, Smith H, Dudley CR, Jewell DP. Food intolerance and the irritable bowel syndrome. *Gut* 1989; 30: 1099–1104. [Role of exclusion diet in management.]
Whithead WE. Patient subgroups in irritable bowel that can be defined by symptom evaluation and physical examination. *Am J Med* 1999; 107: 335–405. [Defining patient groups for specific treatment.]

1.16 Acute liver failure

Case history

A 36-year-old man presents with a 1-day history of increasing confusion, drowsiness and jaundice. He has been suffering from depression for the last 6 months but has otherwise been previously well.

Clinical approach

The presence of confusion and change in conscious level in the presence of jaundice is most likely due to hepatic encephalopathy, but alcohol withdrawal and bacterial infection also need to be considered. It is important to differentiate hepatic encephalopathy due to acute liver disease from chronic liver disease as the causes, management and outcome are different. Other symptoms of acute liver failure are often non-specific and in practice the diagnosis is often made following the finding of abnormal liver biochemistry and a prolonged prothrombin time, after which it is then necessary to retake the history and reassess examination findings. The causes of acute liver failure are shown in Table 16: in a man with a history of depression who presents with acute liver failure the first priority is to exclude the possibility of a late presentation of a paracetamol overdose.

It is crucial to recognize acute liver failure early so that the patient can be transferred to a liver unit that has the facility for liver transplantation when appropriate.

Table 16 Differential diagnosis of acute liver failure.

Common	Less common	Rare
Paracetamol (acetaminophen) overdose	Hepatitis A Hepatitis B Wilson's disease	Venous outflow obstruction Hepatic veins (Budd–Chiari) Hepatic venules
Non-A non-B non-C viral hepatitis (cryptogenic)	Autoimmune chronic active hepatitis	(veno-occlusive disease) Weil's disease (leptospirosis)
Drug induced		Halothane Acute fatty liver of pregnancy

History of the presenting problem

Hepatic encephalopathy

It is likely that only a limited history will be available from the patient, but try to obtain (from him or from relatives or friends) answers to the following specific questions:
• Has he had any visual hallucinations associated with the confusion? This suggests alcohol withdrawal.
• Has he had a fit? This is unusual in hepatic encephalopathy and would suggest alcohol withdrawal or focal cerebral pathology.
• When did the confusion start in relation to the jaundice? Hepatic encephalopathy usually follows jaundice, and the time from the onset of jaundice to encephalopathy is of prognostic significance. In paracetamol hepatotoxicity encephalopathy typically occurs within 24–48 h of jaundice and within 48–96 h of the overdose.
• Is there a history of chronic confusion and/or poor concentration? This does not occur in acute liver failure and suggests chronic liver disease in this context.

Acute or chronic liver damage

Has the patient got chronic liver disease, or is he at risk of this? Ask specifically for the following information:
• Has he previously been told he has liver disease?
• Has he been jaundiced in the past?
• Has he ever had a liver biopsy?
• Has he ever had hepatitis?
• How much alcohol does he drink a day now, and how much was he drinking a year ago?
• Has he had any abdominal swelling?

If he has acute liver failure, what is the likely cause? The possibility of paracetamol overdose or toxicity must be considered so ask:
• Is there any possibility he may have taken paracetamol in the last 48–72 h?
• Has he recently been suicidal?
• Has he taken previous overdoses?

Also consider the other diagnoses listed in Table 16: is the patient at risk of any of these? A full drug history is required. What medications (prescribed and over-the-counter) have been taken in the last few weeks? Is the patient at risk of viral hepatitis? (See *General clinical issues*, Section 3.)

 Occasionally paracetamol overdose can occur unintentionally with the drug taken over several days for medicinal purposes. Liver failure due to paracetamol is potentiated by the presence of alcoholic liver disease, also by some regular medications, e.g. phenytoin.

Pain or fever

Acute liver failure rarely causes pain, but there may be mild right-sided abdominal discomfort. If pain is prominent, consider hepatic vein occlusion (Budd–Chiari). Fever is unusual unless there is a complicating infection.

 Differential diagnosis

In the patient with acute liver failure, consider the following:
• *Drug hepatotoxicity* if there has been exposure to any new drug, particularly an NSAID, in the 2 weeks preceding onset of jaundice. Remember that it is important to exclude non-proprietary drugs such as herbal remedies.
• *Viral hepatitis* if there are risk factors for exposure to hepatitis B, e.g. in prostitutes, homosexuals, intravenous drug abusers and with use of potentially infected blood products from abroad.
• *Wilson's disease* if less than 40 years old. There may be a family history and/or chronic neurological symptoms, e.g. tremor, change in handwriting.
• *Autoimmune chronic active hepatitis*. Must always be excluded, particularly in middle-aged women. Look for a previous medical history or family history of other autoimmune conditions, e.g. thyroid disease, rheumatoid arthritis.
• *Leptospirosis (Weil's disease)* if occupational or recreational exposure to stagnant water. Look for myalgia/tender muscles and red eyes.

Examination

 Examination of a patient with acute liver failure

• General impression—how unwell is the patient? Check vital signs and Glasgow coma score/hepatic encephalopathy score.
• Are there features to suggest chronic liver disease?
• Is there hepatomegaly, indicating hepatic venous outflow obstruction, malignant infiltration or chronic liver disease?

Vital signs

In the early stages of acute hepatic failure vital signs are normal: late features include tachycardia and hypotension. Blood pressure rising and pulse falling are very late signs of cerebral oedema and associated with a poor prognosis.

General

Look carefully for:
• Jaundice—invariably present by the time that hepatic encephalopathy occurs: it is virtually impossible not to notice deep jaundice, but you will miss mild jaundice unless you look deliberately for it.
• Cutaneous stigmata of chronic liver disease (see Sections 1.4, p. 14 and 1.6, p. 20).

Table 17 Grade of hepatic encephalopathy.

Grade 1	Mild confusion, irritability, decreased attention
Grade 2	Drowsiness, lethargy, inappropriate behaviour
Grade 3	Somnolent but rousable. Disorientated
Grade 4	Coma

Abdominal

Take a careful note of:
- *Hepatomegaly.* The liver is usually normal size or small: enlargement should lead you to think of infiltration, hepatic vein occlusion (Budd–Chiari) or chronic liver disease.
- *Ascites.* This is unusual in paracetamol poisoning but may occur with more gradual onset of acute hepatic insufficiency, i.e. as it occurs over weeks rather than days.

Neurological

Grade the encephalopathy (Table 17). Decorticate and decerebrate posture and fixed pupils are late signs of irreversible cerebral oedema. Note that focal neurological signs are not expected and their presence should alert to the possibility of a focal cerebral lesion, with intracerebral haemorrhage likely in this context.

In acute liver failure rapid progression from grade 1 to grade 4 encephalopathy can occur within an hour or two.

Look for subconjunctival haemorrhages. These characteristically occur following a paracetamol overdose.

Less common causes of acute liver failure
- *Hepatic venous outflow obstruction (Budd–Chiari).* Consider if sudden onset of painful hepatomegaly and ascites.
- *Malignant infiltration of the liver.* Consider if more gradual onset of ascites and hepatomegaly, particularly if associated weight loss.

Approach to investigations and management

Investigations

Blood tests

SEVERITY

Check full blood count, prothrombin time, glucose, electrolytes, renal and liver function, amylase, blood cultures and arterial blood gases. Note that the transaminase level is of no prognostic significance and just indicates liver cell damage.

Patients with acute liver failure
- Where the prothrombin time (in seconds) is greater than the time after a paracetamol overdose (in hours), e.g. a PT of 40 s 30 h after the overdose, as opposed to a PT of 50 s 60 h after the overdose, there is a particular risk of developing liver failure.
- Paracetamol also causes pancreatitis and acute tubular necrosis.
- If renal failure occurs early, consider leptospirosis.

AETIOLOGY

If there is no history of paracetamol overdose, check hepatitis B core IgM, Hepatitis A IgM, liver autoantibodies (antinuclear antibody (ANA) smooth muscle antibody), and immunoglobulins. If patient is less than 40 years old, organize ophthalmic slit lamp examination for Kayser–Fleischer rings of Wilson's disease.

The presence of haemolysis (unconjugated bilirubin, anaemia and a low alkaline phosphatase) in a young person is suggestive of Wilson's disease.

Abdominal ultrasound

To look for hepatomegaly, ascites and splenomegaly. Perform Doppler of hepatic veins if Budd–Chiari syndrome is suspected. Tap ascites (if present) and send for microscopy, culture and sensitivity.

Management

Do not correct coagulopathy. Bleeding is rare in acute liver failure and the prothrombin time is an important prognostic indicator.

N-acetylcysteine

In cases of paracetamol overdose, this improves prognosis even in patients who present over 16 h afterwards. Following loading (see *Emergency medicine*, Section 2.1) continue maintenance dose of 100 mg/kg/24 h intravenously, which can be given as a concentrated solution if there is a problem with fluid overload.

Discussion with liver unit

Guidelines for referral to a liver unit are shown in Table 18. Early transfer is essential. Once hepatic encephalopathy develops, progression from grade 1 to 4 and development of cerebral oedema may occur in less than an hour.

Table 18 Guidelines for referral to specialist centres in cases of paracetamol toxicity according to findings on days 2–4 following the overdose.

Day 2 (24–48 h)	Day 3 (48–72 h)	Day 4 (72–96 h)
Arterial pH <7.3 INR >3 Encephalopathy Creatinine > 200 µmol/L Hypoglycaemia	Arterial pH <7.3 INR >4.5 Encephalopathy Creatinine >200 µmol/L	Any rise in INR Encephalopathy Creatinine >250 µmol/L

INR, international normalized ratio.

Ventilation

This is indicated in grade 3/4 hepatic encephalopathy. Elective intubation may be required to allow safe transfer to a liver unit.

Other complications

Treat as follows:
- *Hypoglycaemia*. 50% dextrose 5–10 mL/h given centrally.
- *Infection*. Prophylactic intravenous cephalosporins and fluconazole are commonly used, refined in the event of positive cultures from blood, ascites or elsewhere.
- *Hypovolaemia*. 4.5% albumin to restore CVP to +10 cm.

> Do not give narcotics, sedatives or non-steroidal anti-inflammatory drugs.

See *Emergency medicine*, Sections 1.14, 1.26 and 2.1.
Harrison PM, Keays R, Bray GP, Alexander GJM, Williams R. Improved outcome in paracetamol-induced fulminant hepatic failure following late administration of *N*-acetylcysteine. *Lancet* 1990; 335: 1572–1573. [Efficiency of administration of *N*-acetylcysteine 16 h after the overdose.]
Makin AJ, Wendon J, Williams R. A 7-year experience of severe acetaminophen-induced hepatotoxicity (1987–1993). *Gastroenterol* 1998; 94: 1186–1192. [Outcome following paracetamol overdose in the United Kingdom.]
O'Grady J. Paracetamol-induced liver failure: prevention and management. *J Hepatol* 1997; 26: 41–46.

1.17 Iron-deficiency anaemia

Case history

A 72-year-old woman with rheumatoid arthritis is referred to you for investigation of an iron-deficiency anaemia. She has no overt intestinal symptoms.

Clinical approach

The first issue is to determine that the woman does indeed have iron-deficiency anaemia, then to find out why, and in particular to exclude bowel malignancy.

History of the presenting problem

In this common clinical scenario there is often very little relevant history, but it is important to document the following:
- Has the patient ever been noted to be anaemic previously? Occasionally patients will admit to having been turned down by the Blood Transfusion Service on the basis of mild anaemia. They may also recall periods of iron replacement therapy, especially women during pregnancy.
- Are there any gastrointestinal symptoms at all? If present, these might expedite the subsequent investigations. Many patients regard their indigestion as part of normal life and forget to mention it, even when asked 'Do you get indigestion?', so follow this up with 'Do you take antacids or other medicines for your stomach? … Have you ever done this in the past?'
- What drugs is the patient taking and what have they had previously? Document in particular the use of non-steroidal anti-inflammatories (NSAIDs) and other drugs that might suppress bone marrow (e.g. methotrexate, azathioprine, etc.).
- Gynaecological history. This is too often forgotten, and even in postmenopausal women it is important to exclude vaginal bleeding.
- Has the patient lost weight recently? This would clearly be a sinister symptom in this context.

Relevant past history

In particular you will want to know if the patient has had any previous gastrointestinal problems. Have they ever had any investigations of their bowel—barium meal, barium enema, endoscopy? Have they had any abdominal surgery—particularly Pólya's gastrectomy?

Examination

A full examination is required. The woman is likely to look pale and to have evidence of her rheumatoid arthritis, but look for the following:
- Does she look as though she has lost weight?
- Are there 'classic' signs of iron deficiency (e.g. koilonychia, glossitis)? But remember that these are more often absent than present.
- Is there lymphadenopathy?
- Is there aortic stenosis? This might require treatment in its own right, but is also associated with colonic angiodysplasia.
- Are there any abnormal signs on abdominal examination; in particular, are there any masses?

• Rectal examination with faecal occult blood testing and rigid sigmoidoscopy are mandatory.

Approach to investigations and management

Investigations

Blood tests

Check full blood count (microcytosis and hypochromia would suggest iron deficiency in this context, and an elevated platelet count might indicate active bleeding), electrolytes, renal and liver function tests, inflammatory markers, and serum ferritin, folate and B_{12}.

Clear interpretation of the results of blood tests (if possible) is important to distinguish iron deficiency from the anaemia of chronic disease in this context (see *Haematology*, Sections 1.1 and 1.3). A low serum ferritin is highly specific for iron deficiency but loses sensitivity in the context of any inflammatory process. Soluble transferrin receptor assay is available from some laboratories and is reported to remain sensitive for detection of iron deficiency in the context of inflammation.

> If there is doubt as to whether the patient has iron deficiency consider a bone marrow aspirate.

Examination of the bowel

> If iron deficiency is confirmed, then a gastrointestinal source of blood loss must be pursued in the absence of any other explanation.

UPPER GASTROINTESTINAL ENDOSCOPY

Any suspicious lesions should be biopsied, and duodenal biopsies should also be taken to exclude occult coeliac disease.

> Oesophagitis, gastritis or duodenitis should not be accepted as a cause for iron deficiency.

COLONOSCOPY/BARIUM ENEMA

The colon should be investigated unless a diagnosis of upper gastrointestinal malignancy, peptic ulcer or coeliac disease is made on gastroscopy. Colonoscopy has the advantages that biopsy and polypectomy (Fig. 27) can be performed, also that it is more likely to identify colonic angiodysplasia.

SMALL BOWEL ENEMA

In difficult cases where no cause for gastrointestinal blood loss is identified on the above investigations and there is

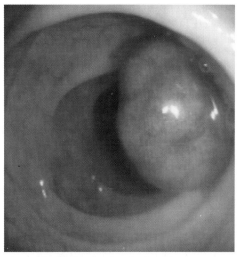
Fig. 27 A large colonic adenoma visualized at colonoscopy.

persistent severe iron-deficiency anaemia, then it can be necessary to consider small bowel imaging, but the yield is low.

Management

See the relevant sections of this module for information on management of specific conditions that may be diagnosed as the cause of iron-deficiency anaemia.

Iron replacement therapy

Along with treatment of any underlying condition, a 3–6 month course of iron replacement will be required. In cases where no cause for iron deficiency has been identified one approach is to prescribe such a course of iron replacement and consider repeating investigations if the patient were to become iron deficient again. Alternatively consider continuous oral iron therapy (i.e. 200 mg ferrous sulphate once daily as opposed to repeated 'courses' of higher dose iron) for those in whom repeated investigation is deemed inappropriate.

> See Sections 1.2, p. 8 and 1.5, p. 18.
> See *Haematology*, Sections 1.1 and 1.3.
> Goddard AF, McIntyre AS, Scott BB. Guidelines for the management of iron-deficiency anaemia. *Gut* 2000; 46 (Suppl. 4).

1.18 Abnormal liver function tests

Case history

A 40-year-old woman is referred for evaluation of abnormal liver function tests noticed when she volunteered to donate blood. She is obese and has a long history of non-insulin-dependent diabetes. She is on no medication.

Clinical approach

As the liver can be markedly damaged without any overt clinical manifestation, abnormal liver function tests may provide early warning of potentially serious pathology (Table 19). The detection of potential liver disease relies on careful clinical assessment, a variety of blood tests, radiological investigations, and ultimately on histological examination of a liver biopsy.

- Significant liver damage, including cirrhosis, may exist with little or no change in serum liver enzyme levels.
- Alkaline phosphatase can arise from liver, bone and intestine: isoenzymes can be determined to distinguish these sources.

- A normal GGT excludes the liver as a source of a raised alkaline phosphatase.
- Reduced serum albumin is part of the acute phase response, so levels may be reduced in severe infection even if hepatic function is otherwise normal.
- The prothrombin time may be elevated by vitamin K deficiency, which can result from prolonged cholestasis and malabsorption of fat-soluble vitamins.

History of the presenting problem

Since the presenting problem was detected at routine screening it is likely that there will be no symptoms to explore, but enquire about previously unnoticed symptoms suggestive of hepatic dysfunction. Ask specifically about general malaise, tiredness, weight loss, loss of libido and sexual potency (in men), and right hypochondrial pain or discomfort.

Relevant past history

Diabetes mellitus, obesity (both present in this woman) and hyperlipidaemia are all associated with hepatic steatosis, but are there any other reasons why the woman may have abnormal liver function tests? Ask about the following.

Previous liver disease or jaundice

Has the woman had any problem with her liver or with jaundice before? Chronic viral hepatitis may follow a poorly remembered episode of jaundice, and recurrent episodes of jaundice may signify cholelithiasis. If the only abnormality is mild hyperbilirubinaemia, consider Gilbert's syndrome. Common hepatic causes of abnormal tests are shown in Table 20.

Alcohol

This is the most common cause of liver disease in the Western world. Even moderate intake may cause liver damage in susceptible individuals. Be aware of a tendency to minimize drinking when the patient perceives it as morally or socially awkward to be accurate. Consider asking the CAGE questions (see Section 1.7, p. 23).

Table 19 Liver function tests and their significance.

Blood test	Significance of elevated level
Transaminases	Raised serum ALT and AST usually signify hepatocellular damage, but consider other source of AST (heart and skeletal muscle, kidney, and red cells)
	Extreme elevations of AST and ALT occur mainly with drug toxicity, acute viral hepatitis and ischaemic damage to the liver
	Moderate elevations of AST and ALT are seen in alcohol-related, autoimmune, chronic viral, and other acute and chronic liver disease
Alkaline phosphatase and γ-glutamyl transferase (GGT)	These 'biliary' enzymes usually indicate cholestatic liver disease or biliary tract disease
	The GGT levels are disproportionately raised in alcohol-related liver disease, or where an enzyme-inducing drug such as phenytoin or phenobarbitone is used
	Segmental, non-obstructive damage to the biliary tree, as in metastatic or infiltrative disease, often produces elevated biliary enzymes, mildly elevated transaminases and normal serum bilirubin
Bilirubin	Where hyperbilirubinaemia is due to excess haem breakdown serum bilirubin is predominantly unconjugated. Unconjugated bilirubinaemia also occurs with inherited disorders of bilirubin conjugation (Gilbert's and Crigler–Najjar syndromes)
	Conjugated bilirubinaemia can occur with any form of liver damage that interferes with hepatocyte function (intrahepatic cholestasis), but in chronic liver disease is typically a late feature, and usually signifies hepatic decompensation
	Primary diseases of bile canaliculi, ducts, and the gallbladder and large bile ducts (PBC, PSC, stones) produce hyperbilirubinaemia and elevated biliary enzymes
Albumin	Albumin is produced in the liver, and synthesis declines with worsening liver function. As the half-life of serum albumin is about 30 days, it is days before changes in synthesis are detectable
Prothrombin time	This is a sensitive test of hepatic synthetic capacity as the liver is responsible for the synthesis of factors II (prothrombin), V, VII and IX. The prothrombin time responds rapidly to changes in hepatic synthesis as the serum half-life of clotting factors is of the order of hours

ALT, alanine transaminase; AST, aspartate transaminase; GGT, γ-glutamyl transferase; PBC, primary biliary cirrhosis; PSC, primary sclerosing cholangitis.

Table 20 Hepatic causes of abnormal liver biochemistry.

Liver disease	Diagnostic blood tests
Alcohol related	Disproportionately elevated GGT and elevated mean MCV
	The AST is elevated greater than the ALT
Hepatic steatosis and non-alcoholic steatohepatitis	Associated with diabetes mellitus: therefore fasting glucose, glucose tolerance test (in patient without known diabetes)
	Associated with hypertriglyceridaemia and hypercholesterolaemia
	Associated with obesity (body mass index greater than 25)
	Associated with pregnancy (last trimester)
	May be idiopathic or associated with various drugs
	Diagnosis may require liver biopsy, although resolution of tests on correction of hyperglycaemia, hyperlipidaemia, obesity and pregnancy makes this unnecessary
Autoimmune hepatitis	(Table 21)
Primary biliary cirrhosis	Liver enzyme elevations usually show a biliary pattern
Chronic hepatitis C	The correct screening test is serum IgG to HCV
Chronic hepatitis B	The correct screening test is serum hepatitis B surface antigen
	Antibodies to hepatitis B antigens may reflect previous infection or immunization
Acute viral hepatitis	Serum IgM to hepatitis A, E, or B antigens may indicate acute infection, which in some patients may be subclinical
Genetic haemochromatosis	Consider the diagnosis in patients with a positive family history, diabetes mellitus, arthropathy, skin pigmentation or heart disease (Table 21)
Other causes	Primary sclerosing cholangitis (Table 21)
	Alpha 1-antitrypsin deficiency
	Wilson's disease
	Granulomatous hepatitis

ALT, alanine transaminase; AST, aspartate transaminase; GGT, γ-glutamyl transferase; HCV, hepatitis C virus; MCV, mean red cell volume.

Drugs and medications

Prescription drugs, the oral contraceptive pill, over-the-counter medications, herbal remedies, traditional medications and recreational drugs should all be considered. Also ask about surgery: recent exposure to anaesthetic agents may have provoked hepatitis, and gastro-intestinal surgery for obesity may provoke a steatohepatitis.

Pregnancy

Could the patient be pregnant? Pregnancy is associated with a number of hepatic disorders, including cholestasis of pregnancy and acute fatty liver of pregnancy.

Disease associations

Coeliac disease and Crohn's disease may be associated with abnormal liver function tests in the absence of primary liver pathology. Significant disease associations include:
• primary sclerosing cholangitis (PSC) and inflammatory bowel disease
• primary biliary cirrhosis (PBC) with coeliac disease
• PBC with other autoimmune diseases.
Autoimmune hepatitis is associated with thyroid disease. Multisystem disorders such as sarcoidosis and various vasculitides can all involve the liver, as may lymphoma and other neoplastic diseases.

Travel history

Enquire about travel to or residence in areas endemic for hydatid disease, amoebiasis, schistosomiasis and liver flukes.

Family history

Enquire particularly about a family history of liver disease, inflammatory bowel disease, coeliac disease, hyperlipidaemia and diabetes mellitus (which this woman has). Each of these can be familial and can be associated with liver abnormalities.

Examination

A full examination is required, paying particular attention to:
• measurement of the body mass index
• signs of chronic liver disease (see Sections 1.6, p. 20 and 1.7, p. 23)
• the abdomen. Is the liver enlarged and/or tender or shrunken and cirrhotic? Is the gall bladder palpable or tender, or the spleen enlarged? Typically none of these signs are present or helpful in cases of asymptomatic patients with abnormal liver function tests.

Alcohol-induced liver disease	May be a raised IgA level, relatively higher AST than ALT, and disproportionately raised GGT
Chronic viral hepatitis	HBsAg, HBeAg, HBV DNA
	Anti-HCV antibody, HCV RNA
Genetic haemochromatosis	Raised serum iron, transferrin saturation and ferritin levels
	Genetic testing for the common HFE mutation may be helpful (positive in 95% of affected individuals)
	Increased hepatocyte iron on liver biopsy
	Increased hepatic iron index
Autoimmune liver disease	Raised IgG levels, positive autoantibodies (antinuclear, antismooth muscle, antiliver and kidney microsomal antigens)
Primary biliary cirrhosis	Positive antimitochondrial antibody
Primary sclerosing cholangitis	Diagnostic ERCP findings
Alpha 1-antitrypsin deficiency	Reduced circulating α_1-antitrypsin, mutant form of protein on electrophoresis
Wilson's disease	Kayser–Fleischer copper deposits in iris on slit-lamp examination
	Raised serum copper, lowered serum caeruloplasmin level, increased urinary copper excretion basally and after oral penicillamine challenge
	Genetic testing may not identify all patients
	Increased liver copper content on biopsy

Table 21 Diagnostic tests for chronic liver disease.

ALT, alanine transaminase; AST, aspartate transaminase; GGT, γ-glutamyl transferase; HBsAg, Hepatitis B surface antigen; HBeAg, Hepatitis B envelope antigen; HBV, hepatitis B virus; HCV, hepatitis C virus; HFE, haemochromatosis iron; ERCP, endoscopic retrograde pancreaticocholangiography.

In this woman it will also be appropriate to look for evidence of diabetic complications.

Approach to investigations and management

 In an otherwise well person, a single isolated biochemical abnormality of liver function testing (particularly if marginal) is likely to represent the inherent variability of testing and the wide range of normality. Repeated testing at an interval is a reasonable first-line investigation.

Investigations

The clinical findings will determine the direction for further investigation, but the following investigations may be appropriate

Blood tests

Various diagnostic possibilities can be strengthened by serological and other tests (Table 21).

Abdominal ultrasound scan

This should be considered in most cases. Asymptomatic cholelithiasis and intrahepatic lesions such as abscesses, cysts and tumours should be sought. Cirrhosis can be hard to detect clinically, and altered hepatic texture coupled with splenomegaly is suggestive. Fatty infiltration of the liver is suggested by increased echogenicity ('bright liver') but is not diagnostic. Ultrasound scanning should be performed in all cases if liver biopsy is contemplated.

Liver biopsy

Liver biopsy may be required in many cases to make a precise diagnosis, stage disease, assess prognosis and guide therapy. A good core of tissue is required to diagnose macronodular cirrhosis: sampling error may result in false negative biopsy diagnosis.

- If haemochromatosis or Wilson's disease is suspected, unfixed samples should be set aside for quantitative iron and copper determination.
- If an infectious aetiology is suspected, unfixed material may be sent for viral, bacterial and mycobacterial culture. Electron microscopy may be useful in diagnosing viral inclusion bodies.

Figure 28 shows the microscopic appearance of hepatic steatosis (fatty liver), as present in this woman.

Management

See the relevant sections of this module for information on management of specific conditions that may cause abnormality of liver function tests.

In cases where a firm diagnosis is not established, patients should be followed at intervals of months, to determine if abnormalities resolve, or if there is any

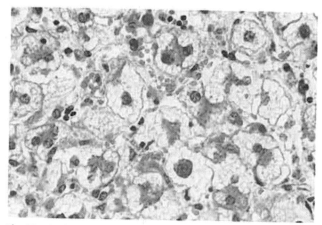

Fig. 28 Histological appearance of fatty liver. Fat droplets are seen filling most of the hepatocytes with the nucleus in the centre of the cells.

Table 22 Potential indications for nasogastric or percutaneous enterogastrostomy feeding.

Acute inability to swallow adequately
Acute cerebrovascular accident
Trauma and surgery to face, nose, throat area

Chronic inability to swallow adequately
Chronic neurological disease such as motor neurone disease
Oesophageal stricture, or dysmotility

Anorexia
With progressive neurological decline: e.g. Alzheimer's disease
Post-surgery; after severe, prolonged illness
Voluntary: hunger strike
Anorexia nervosa

deterioration in liver function, based on clinical features and measurement of bilirubin, albumin and prothrombin time. Referral to a specialist liver centre should be considered if there is ongoing damage with declining liver function. It seems sensible to advise patients to abstain from alcohol and avoid known hepatotoxins under such circumstances.

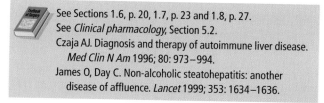

See Sections 1.6, p. 20, 1.7, p. 23 and 1.8, p. 27.
See *Clinical pharmacology*, Section 5.2.
Czaja AJ. Diagnosis and therapy of autoimmune liver disease. *Med Clin N Am* 1996; 80: 973–994.
James O, Day C. Non-alcoholic steatohepatitis: another disease of affluence. *Lancet* 1999; 353: 1634–1636.

1.19 Progressive decline

Case history

An 18-year-old man with severe neurological disability is difficult to feed, in particular because he cannot swallow properly, and he is losing weight.

Clinical approach

Enteral feeding, either by nasogastric tube (NGT) or by percutaneous enterogastrostomy (PEG), is often considered by physicians, nursing staff, dieticians, patients and patients' carers as a means of ensuring nutrition and avoiding the respiratory complications of aspiration. Medical indications are shown in Table 22, but logistical, legal and ethical aspects of these treatments should be considered carefully, whatever the medical indication.

The first issue in any case of swallowing difficulty is to ensure that carers have been given expert advice about how to attempt to feed the patient. Ensure that simple measures such as supervised feeding, modified diet and (when the problem is of anorexia) appetite-enhancing manoeuvres (e.g. steroids) have been explored: it may be that if this young man is propped up in bed and given thickened fluids he may be able to manage better than he has been doing. The next issue is to consider whether the problem is acute or chronic.

Acute and potentially reversible problem

If the problem is acute and potentially reversible and the patient cannot tolerate thickened fluids optimally administered, e.g. following stroke, then considerations are relatively straightforward. While immediate adequate hydration is essential for all patients, previously fit individuals are typically able to maintain homeostasis for at least 18 h, and potentially for a few days. Following this, NGT feeding may be adequate, but if longer-term nutritional support is necessary, then durable but resource-intensive PEG feeding is required.

However, if the main problem—as in many cases—is recurrent aspiration and respiratory infection, then it is important to remember that NGT and PEG feeding do not completely obviate the risk. Furthermore, if the patient, e.g. following stroke, does not improve, then the decision to continue feeding and other supportive measures may need to be reconsidered (see *Medicine for the elderly*, Section 1.4).

Chronic and probably irreversible problem

Many patients, such this young man, for whom the issue of artificial enteral feeding arises, have complicated medical histories. Specialist advice on the overall prognosis, e.g. from the neurological condition in this case, is absolutely essential. Consider whether the benefits of enteral feeding will have an impact on the patient's overall outcome, e.g. it is unlikely to benefit a moribund patient who has already suffered severe neurological damage and aspiration.

Approach to investigations and management

Ethical and communication issues

Any form of artificial feeding is a therapeutic intervention, and informed consent from the patient or carers with legal authority must be sought. The legal status of carers and interested parties may need to be established by a court of law.

Early consultation with interested parties rather than isolated decision-making is the key to finding a satisfactory outcome for the patient. When the patient can express views, these should be paramount, but when they cannot contribute to decision-making, as in this case, the views of relatives and carers become particularly important. They should be made to feel involved in the decision-making and management process, but not given the impression that they are being asked to make medical decisions that are rightly the doctors' responsibility (see *General clinical issues*, Section 3). Make an appointment to meet them, and talk in the presence of a nurse or other professional colleague who knows the patient well. Speak slowly, allowing time for silence and for the relatives or carers to interject at any point.

- Thanks for coming in. I wanted to speak with you about …
- As you know, he's getting worse, and now having difficulty swallowing …
- Even when he is sat up in bed and given thickened fluids, which are the easiest thing to take, he sometimes chokes …
- He isn't getting enough food, and he's losing weight …
- We have spoken with Dr Jones, the neurologist, who says that she is sure that he is not going to improve, and that he is likely to get gradually weaker and weaker …
- We have been thinking carefully about what we should do …
- The possibilities that we are considering are artificial feeding … (give brief details) …
- Or whether we should make sure that he is comfortable, by making sure that his mouth isn't dry and he isn't thirsty, and allow him to fade away …
- Did he ever speak with you about this sort of thing in the past?

An approach of this type allows plenty of opportunity for relatives or carers to say what they think the patient would want done in this situation, and to express any views of their own. Many will ask you to make the decision: 'We'll go along with whatever you think is best', but a few will express strong views that 'everything must be done'. Make thorough notes of the conversation.

If, after this discussion, and consultation with medical colleagues and other professionals involved in the patient's care, you decide that it would not be appropriate to institute artificial feeding, and the relatives and carers (on the basis of the discussion described above) will clearly accept such a medical decision, then speak with them along the following lines:

- As you know, his problem with feeding is getting worse …
- He isn't able to take enough food to sustain him …
- We have all thought hard about how we should handle this …
- And have come to the conclusion that the right thing to do is to make sure that he is comfortable …
- That we should keep his mouth moist and clean, so he doesn't feel thirsty …
- But we don't think that we should try to give him artificial feeding …
- Aside from the risks of doing this, we all know that he's deteriorating, and we think that it would prolong the misery, not make him better, and is something we wouldn't want to do …
- If we keep him comfortable in the way I've described, he is likely to fade away over the next few days or weeks …
- We will do everything we can to make sure that he does not suffer (the doctors and nurses will not abandon him because he is not being artificially fed).

Again, allow time for relatives or carers to interject, but if you have judged things correctly they will clearly agree with the sense of what you have said, and many will say 'thank you'. Make thorough notes of the conversation.

If, by contrast, the relatives and carers will clearly not accept a medical recommendation that it would be inappropriate (because futile) to institute artificial feeding, then the options are:

- To comply with the relatives'/carers' wishes to institute artificial feeding after explaining the risks and discomfort of placing an NGT (including the risk of feeding through a misplaced or displaced tube) and the risks of upper gastrointestinal endoscopy and placement of a PEG tube (Fig. 29).

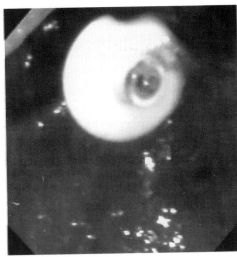

Fig. 29 View of a percutaneous enterogastrostomy feeding tube in the stomach at endoscopy.

• For the physician in charge of the case to discuss with the Trust responsible for the patient's care and with his or her personal medical defence society about how to obtain legal review, with the intention of not instituting artificial feeding against the express wishes of relatives/carers.

The option of 'doing nothing', i.e. hoping that the patient will fade away without anyone noticing, might seem tempting, but is not justifiable in the context of the proper discussions described above.

'Technical' issues

If the patient is to receive NGT or PEG feeding, then full dietary and nutritional assessment is necessary; see Section 2.14.1, p. 121.

The question of artificial nutrition in a patient in a persistent vegetative state was considered by the High Court in 1993, and four principles were established:
• The best interests of the patient is to be the guiding principle.
• Artificial nutrition is considered a medical intervention.
• Withholding and withdrawing artificial nutrition are equivalent acts.
• It was not unlawful to withhold or withdraw artificial nutrition.

Anorexia nervosa is considered a psychiatric condition and a patient may be detained and treated (e.g. artificially fed) under the terms of the Mental Health Act (see *Psychiatry*, Section 1.5).

See *General clinical issues*, Section 3.
See *Pain relief and palliative care*, Section 2.9.
See *Medicine for the elderly*, Section 1.4.
Lennard-Jones JE. Giving or withholding fluid and nutrients: ethical and legal aspects. *J Roy Col Phys Lond* 1999; 33: 39–45.

1.20 Factitious abdominal pain

Case history

A 34-year-old woman is referred by the casualty officer with a history of sudden onset of severe abdominal pain. The pain is intermittent and between episodes she appears well and unconcerned. She has just moved to the area and has not registered with a general practitioner.

Clinical approach

The patient's unconcern about her illness, often coupled with inconsistencies in the history, leads to suspicion that

Table 23 Causes of intermittent acute abdominal pain in young women.

Common	Less common	Rare
Functional bowel disease	Biliary colic	Pancreatitis
Pain related to ovulation (Mittelschmerz) or menstruation	Renal colic	Sickle cell crises
	Ileal Crohn's with a stricture	Acute intermittent porphyria
Cystitis		
Appendicitis ('grumbling')		

the condition is factitious. This is an unusual clinical problem, but everyone remembers a case. It is important to exclude organic pathology, but also to avoid overinvestigation: the balance can be very difficult to strike, particularly if the patient demands extensive tests.

When dealing with a patient who may have factitious symptoms:
• Remember that organic pathology often coexists with factitious symptoms (Table 23).
• Always try and corroborate the history with the general practitioner (if available) and with old hospital notes, also with relatives or friends (if available).

History of the presenting problem

Patients with factitious abdominal pain:
• may be health-care workers and so well informed about illness
• are often relatively unconcerned about their symptoms
• usually have inconsistencies within the history
• tend to be reluctant or evasive when corroborative information is requested
• are sometimes pathological liars.

The most important aspects of the history taking are to:
• Ask specifically about the pain. A full history is needed: When did it start? How often does it occur? See Sections 1.13, p. 39 and 1.14, p. 41. Does the pain seem characteristic of any of the conditions listed in Table 23, or is it atypical?
• Ask about associated symptoms that can be verified. Has there been any diarrhoea? Rectal bleeding?, etc.
• Ask her what she thinks is wrong, and what she expects from you in the form of treatment and investigation.

Relevant past history

Medical

This is particularly important, both to give information about previous organic illness, and also to reveal inconsistencies that would be typical of factitious disorder. Ask about the following:

- Previous episodes of pain.
- Previous investigations, and time spent in hospital. Be specific: When? Which hospital? Which ward? Which doctor? Which nursing sister? You will need this information to corroborate the story.
- Previous medications (particularly narcotic use for pain) and the doses she was taking.
- Who was the last GP you were registered with? Can you remember the address of the practice?
- Previous mental problems and treatment.

Social

Precisely how long have you lived in this area? Where are you staying? Do you have a job, and how long have you been doing it? Where did you live before moving to this area?

Examination

Examination of a patient with suspected factitious abdominal pain
- General impression: do they look well?
- Are there abdominal scars?
- Are the abdominal signs reproducible?

General appearance and vital signs

These are particularly important clinical observations. If she has genuine abdominal pain she is unlikely to look well and unconcerned between episodes. Vital signs will be normal in all but the most complex cases of factitious disorder: if using a thermometer to record the temperature, ensure that someone is in attendance whilst this is done.

Abdominal

Look particularly for the following:
- *Erythema ab igne.* Present with chronic pain due to hot water bottle so not factitious.
- *Abdominal scars.* May be due to abdominal surgery for pathology or repeated laparotomies for non-organic pain, usually performed in different hospitals.
- *Rebound tenderness.* Assess while the patient is distracted. More difficult to fake than guarding.
- *Bowel sounds.* Cannot be faked.
- *Other abnormalities*, e.g. organomegaly, are not expected.

Approach to investigations and management

When dealing with suspected factitious disorder, the immediate priority is to corroborate the history by:
- Speaking to the GP.
- Contacting family and friends.
- Contacting previous hospitals or GPs she claims to have visited and getting them to fax through operation notes, clinic and discharge letters.

Explain to the patient that you need to get more information:
- I am finding it difficult to work out what the cause of your pain is …
- I need to get all the information that I can about your medical history …
- Can I confirm the details of the GP/hospital that you mentioned?
- Ask the patient for permission to speak to relatives or friends:
- Who is your next of kin?
- I would like to explain to them that you are in hospital. Patients with factitious disorders (but also some with organic disorders) may be unwilling for you to do this, and will often say that none of them are contactable, or supply details that are incorrect.
- But won't they be worried about you?

Investigations

In all but the most obvious cases of factitious disorder, check the following:
- *Urinalysis.* A simple investigation that will exclude urinary tract infection. Make sure someone witnesses her producing the specimen so it is not tampered with.
- *Full blood count*, electrolytes, renal and liver function tests, inflammatory markers (CRP) and amylase.
- *Erect CXR and abdominal X-ray (AXR) kidneys, ureter, bladder (KUB).* Is there gas under the diaphragm? Is there bowel obstruction? Are there urinary stones? Are there any other abnormalities?

If these tests do not reveal any obvious leads then do not proceed to further investigation, e.g. abdominal ultrasound, unless there is clear clinical indication.

Management

If it is clear from the outset that the problem is factitious, then give simple non-addictive analgesics and avoid narcotics. Try to avoid hospital admission, and make early contact with the liaison psychiatric team.

In many cases, however, the situation in the Accident and Emergency Department is not clear; the patient has arrived at 3a.m., and appears to be in great pain. It is impossible to avoid admission, at least to an observation ward, and one or two doses of intramuscular pethidine are often required whilst the investigations described above are performed and the nature of the case becomes clear. However, within 24–48 h the diagnosis of factitious abdominal pain is usually apparent because of the continued unusual behaviour of the patient and unremarkable test results. How should you proceed from here? After discussion with senior medical colleagues, including the physician in charge of the case, a straightforward approach is to talk with the patient as follows:

- We have now had you in hospital for one/two days …
- I am pleased to say that we have not found anything terribly wrong in your abdomen …
- The tests give satisfactory results …
- I do not propose to organize any further tests …
- We should try to help the pain when you have it using simple pain killers …
- I would be happy for you to go home …
- I would suggest that you register with a GP, and I will give you a letter for them or for any other doctor that you meet … (this should as usual contain a simple statement of presentation, key test results, working clinical diagnosis and treatment given).
- I will also give you an appointment for the outpatient clinic, so that we can check how things are going in a few weeks' time … (patients with factitious disorder are unlikely to return, but should be offered the opportunity).

- If the pain were to get much worse or anything else were to happen, then the same rules apply to you as to me and everyone else—you should see your GP.

The patient may accept this, but they may not, and may request additional investigations or treatments or demand a diagnosis. These should be answered simply:
- Don't I need a CT scan?
- No, we don't think that a CT scan would help.
- I need pethidine.
- No, we don't think that the right way to manage your pain is with pethidine … the pain is unusual … if the treatment we are giving you is not satisfactory, then I think that we need to obtain specialist advice, and we should ask the doctors from the pain clinic to give us some help.
- What is wrong with me?
- I do not think that you have a serious problem in your abdomen … Pain in the belly can be caused by a number of things, including psychological factors …
- Are you saying that I'm mad?
- No, I'm not saying that … I'm saying that there can be psychological explanations for abdominal pain, and that if we want to improve things we need to consider these, and perhaps get some expert help.

1 Banerjee A. Factitious disorders presenting as acute emergencies. *Postgrad Med J* 1994; 70: 68–73.
2 Folks DG. Munchausen syndrome and other factitious disorders. *Neurol Clin* 1995; 13: 267–281.

2 Diseases and treatments

2.1 Inflammatory bowel disease

2.1.1 CROHN'S DISEASE

Aetiology/pathophysiology/pathology

The aetiology is unknown but:
• There is a presumed autoimmune process
• There is a measurable genetic component (genetic linkages and family studies)
• Candidate factors include various infectious agents, e.g. *Mycobacterium paratuberculosis*
• There is an increased incidence in cigarette smokers.
The characteristic histological features are (Fig. 30):
• Transmural inflammation with ulceration and granuloma formation
• May affect any part of the gastrointestinal tract (mouth to anus)
• May be restricted, e.g. terminal ileitis, Crohn's colitis or perianal Crohn's
• Often patchy distribution
• May cause strictures and fistulae to adjacent structures
• Usually accompanied by vigorous systemic response (raised CRP and ESR).

Epidemiology

Incidence is 6–8 per 100 000 and prevalence is 26–56 per 100 000 in Northern Europe, USA and Australia. Slightly more common in females. Bimodal age incidence: 15–40 is most common with second peak at around 70 years of age. Ten per cent of patients have a first-degree relative with the disease. The risk for siblings is 30-fold increased compared to the general population. Smoking gives a relative risk ×3. Other postulated causes are: highly refined diet, infective agents (atypical mycobacteria) and immunological factors.

Clinical presentation

Common

Diarrhoea, abdominal pain and weight loss are all common. Often associated general malaise, lassitude, fever and anorexia.

Rare

Occasionally mistaken for anorexia nervosa or irritable bowel syndrome.

Physical signs

Common

There may be few physical signs or the patient may be thin and unwell with clubbing, aphthous ulceration, abdominal tenderness or evident perianal skin tags, ulceration or fistulae.

Uncommon

Abdominal mass.

Rare

These include fistulae, seronegative arthritis, sacroiliitis, iritis and skin rashes (erythema nodosum, pyoderma gangrenosum: see *Dermatology*, Sections 2.10 and 2.18).

Investigations

The following tests are helpful:
• *Full blood count* often shows anaemia, which may be normochromic, normocytic (chronic disease) or result from iron, B_{12} or folate deficiency. Platelet count is often high in active disease (regard as an 'inflammatory marker').
• *Serum inflammatory markers* are raised (CRP≫ESR).
• *Serum albumin* is often low.
• *Vitamin B_{12} and folic acid* are often low due to terminal ileitis.

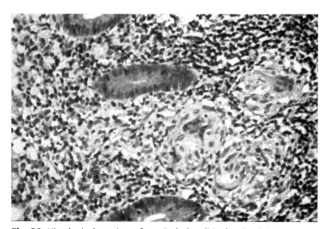

Fig. 30 Histological specimen from Crohn's colitis showing intense inflammation and granuloma.

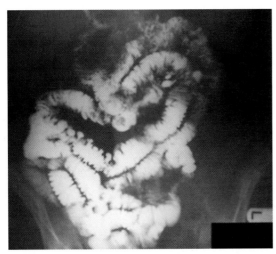

Fig. 31 Barium follow-through showing several tight strictures in the terminal ileum in a patient with Crohn's disease.

• *Sigmoidoscopy/colonoscopy* can show patchy inflammation, granulomas on biopsy, terminal ileitis.
• *Small bowel follow-through* can show segmental inflammation, strictures, fistulae. This should be the first investigation if pain and weight loss are predominant (Fig. 31).

> • MRI scanning is particularly useful for assessing complex perianal disease including fistulae.
> • Rectal biopsy in Crohn's may show granuloma even when macroscopically normal.

Differential diagnosis

• Ulcerative colitis—if colonic involvement
• Abdominal tuberculosis—particularly if terminal ileal disease and in 'at risk' group
• Malignancy/intestinal lymphoma.

Treatment

Emergency

Admit to hospital if ill (fever, tachycardia, tender abdomen, severe diarrhoea or pain), Nil by mouth initially [1]. (See Section 1.5, pp. 17–19.)

Short-term

Corticosteroids

If there is a response to i.v. hydrocortisone, or if the attack is less severe, commence oral prednisolone at 30–40 mg daily and taper down by approximately 5 mg per fortnight depending on response and inflammatory markers. Seventy per cent will be in remission in 3–4 months.

Budesonide, a new topically acting steroid with high potency and extensive first pass metabolism, is equivalent to prednisolone in inducing remission and has fewer side effects, but is much more expensive [2].

5-Aminosalicylic acids (5-ASAs)

These compounds have only marginal benefit in acute disease.

Dietary

Elemental diets, containing low molecular weight nutrients, seem to be as effective as steroids, but are unpalatable and often have to be given by nasogastric tube (for 6 weeks).

Other

No good data exist for the use of metronidazole or ciprofloxacin.

Long-term

Approximately 50% of Crohn's disease patients will have relapsed 1 year after initial treatment.

5-ASAs

5-ASAs have at best a modest effect in maintaining remission, with the postsurgical subgroup benefiting most.

Azathioprine

This immunosuppressant has been shown to induce remission in steroid-resistant and -dependent patients, to reduce relapse rates and to have steroid sparing effects. It takes 6–12 weeks to achieve its effects. All patients starting on this drug should be warned about possible bone marrow suppression effects, and have their full blood count checked at 8–10-week intervals.

Methotrexate

In those intolerant or failing to respond to azathioprine, methotrexate may be tried. In steroid-dependent patients it has been shown to achieve both remission and withdrawal of steroids in 39% vs 19% given placebo [3].

Tumour necrosis factor alpha (TNF-α) antibody

Early experience with Infliximab, a TNF-α antibody, shows promise for both refractory and fistulous Crohn's disease, although long-term side effects are unknown [4]. Cyclosporin has no role in either acute treatment or maintenance of remission.

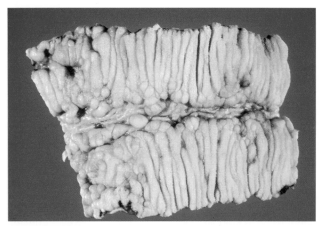

Fig. 32 Resected terminal ileum from a patient with Crohn's disease showing linear ulceration and pseudopolyps.

Surgery

Approximately three-quarters of patients require surgery at some point (Fig. 32). Failed medical therapy, abscesses, fistulae, intestinal obstruction and haemorrhage are indications. Between 50 and 80% will have relapsed within 10 years following surgery, but not all will require further surgery. Stricturoplasty may be performed, rather than resection, to preserve small intestinal length.

Complications

Common

Intestinal obstruction

This is usually subacute, and is very common. May be due to active disease causing oedema and narrowing, or by chronic fibrotic stricture. The former usually responds to steroids.

 Patients with small bowel strictures are advised to maintain a low-fibre diet to avoid food bolus obstruction.

Malabsorption

This is common. B_{12} deficiency and bile salt diarrhoea are caused by terminal ileal disease. Extensive involvement of the small bowel or surgical resections result in generalized malabsorption (short bowel syndrome). Bacterial overgrowth secondary to enteroenteric fistulae or strictures results in fat malabsorption.

Perforations

Contained perforations, resulting in abdominal, pelvic and ischiorectal abscesses, are fairly common and require drainage.

Uncommon

Massive rectal bleeding may occur, and is almost always secondary to colonic disease. Chronic blood loss is more usual, causing an iron-deficiency anaemia. Toxic megacolon can occur, but is less common than in ulcerative colitis. There is an increased risk of colonic carcinoma in patients with colonic Crohn's.

Rare

Free perforation is rare.

Prognosis

Morbidity

Some patients experience considerable morbidity from general ill health, pain, malnutrition, fistulous disease, abscess formation, repeated surgery or steroid side effects, but the majority are maintained relatively symptom free.

Mortality

Overall mortality is twice that for the general population. Those diagnosed with the disease before the age of 20 have >10× the standardized mortality ratio.

Prevention

Secondary

Cessation of smoking is of benefit in active disease, and reduces the risk of relapse.

Disease associations

Weak association with primary sclerosing cholangitis, arthralgia and arthritis; also with HLA B27.

 National Association for Colitis and Crohn's Disease provides information and support for patients.

 Further information on Crohn's disease from Doctors net: http://www.comedserv.com.crohns.htm.

1 McDonald J, Burroughs A, Feagan B (eds) *Evidence-based Gastroenterology and Hepatology.* London: BMJ Books, 1999.
2 Rutgeerts P, Lofberg R, Malchow H *et al.* A comparison of budesonide with prednisolone for active Crohn's disease. *N Engl J Med* 1994; 331: 842–845.
3 Feagan BG, Rochon J, Fedorak RN *et al.* Methotrexate for the treatment of Crohn's disease. *N Engl J Med* 1995; 332: 292–297.
4 Bell S, Kamm MA. Antibodies to tumour necrosis factor alpha as treatment for Crohn's disease. *Lancet* 2000; 355: 858–860.

2.1.2 ULCERATIVE COLITIS

Aetiology/pathophysiology/pathology

The aetiology is unknown but:
• There is a presumed autoimmune process
• There is a measurable genetic component (genetic linkages, and family studies)
• Enteric bacterial factors seem to be important
• There is a decreased incidence in cigarette smokers.
The histopathological features are (Fig. 33):
• Mucosal inflammation only (contrasting with Crohn's disease) with crypt distortion, crypt abscesses, and goblet cell depletion
• Rectal inflammation is almost universal; the extent of more proximal disease is variable
• Disease is usually continuous, i.e. extends from anus to wherever the proximal extent lies
• Does not cause fistulae or strictures, but may result in fibrotic narrowing of colon
• Not accompanied by vigorous systemic response unless the disease is severe.

Epidemiology

Incidence around 10 per 100 000. Affects any age group but typically youths and young adults [1].

Clinical presentation

Common

Bloody diarrhoea, general malaise.

Uncommon

Arthritis and arthralgia, uveitis, skin rashes.

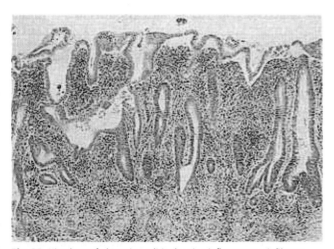

Fig. 33 Histology of ulcerative colitis showing inflammatory infiltrate within the mucosa.

Rare

Severe colitis and toxic megacolon.

Physical signs

Common

Few physical signs or thin, unwell patient with aphthous ulceration, abdominal tenderness, blood on rectal examination, mucopus on rigid sigmoidoscopy.

Uncommon

Tender, fibrotic, narrowed segment of colon on abdominal examination.

Rare

Toxic megacolon, arthritis, iritis, skin rashes (erythema nodosum, pyoderma gangrenosum).

Investigations/staging

Serum inflammatory markers

These are only raised in severe disease.

Plain abdominal radiograph

This may show segment of fibrotic colon, proximal faecal loading. In severe disease, dilated loop of inflamed colon. Mucosal oedema and ulcers may be detected.

Barium enema

This may confirm plain abdominal radiograph findings (Fig. 34).

Colonoscopy

This may show inflammation extending from rectum to proximal extent of disease (Fig. 35).

Differential diagnosis

Common differential diagnoses include:
• Crohn's colitis
• infectious colitis (bacterial, amoebic, viral, e.g. CMV in immunosuppressed patients)
• NSAID-induced colitis
• microscopic colitis, lymphocytic colitis, membranous colitis [2].

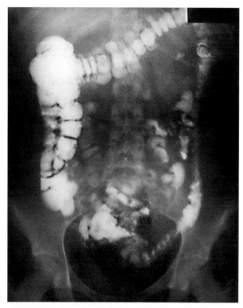

Fig. 34 Barium enema of ulcerative colitis extending to the splenic flexure.

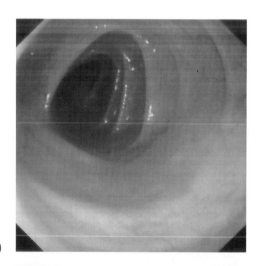

(a)

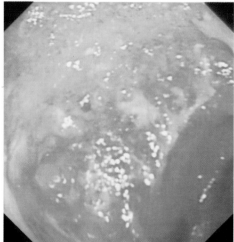

(b)

Fig. 35 Endoscopic appearance of (a) normal colon and (b) inflamed colon.

Treatment

Emergency

See Section 1.1, pp. 5–6.

Short-term

Steroids; immunosuppressants such as cyclosporin and azathioprine may have a role.

Long-term

5-aminosalicylic acid compounds can maintain remission in most patients. Panproctocolectomy is curative. Patients may opt for a permanent ileostomy or formation of a neorectum using a loop of ileum (pouch).

Complications

Common

These include malnutrition, steroid-induced side effects, arthralgias, arthritis, skin rash.

Uncommon

Uveitis, toxic megacolon and perforation or sepsis.

Rare

Malignancy (colorectal carcinoma).

Prognosis

Morbidity

About 25% of patients experience only one attack, 40% of patients are in remission in any one year, and a minority of patients have unremitting disease. About 30% of patients ultimately undergo colectomy. The longer a patient remains in remission, the better the chance of remaining in remission.

Mortality

The overall mortality is not increased compared to healthy controls, possibly due to a lower incidence of smoking.

Prevention

Secondary

5-Aminosalicylates, azathioprine.

Disease associations

Association with primary sclerosing cholangitis.

Stein RB, Hanauer SB. Medical therapy for inflammatory bowel disease. *Gastroenterol Clin N Am* 1999; 28: 297–321.
1 Andres PG, Friedman LS. Epidemiology and the natural course of inflammatory bowel disease. *Gastroenterol Clin N Am* 1999; 28: 225–281.
2 Giardiello FM, Lazenby AJ, Bayless TM. The new colitides, collagenous, lymphocytic, and diversion colitis. *Gastroenterol Clin N Am* 1995; 24: 717–729.

2.1.3 MICROSCOPIC COLITIS

Aetiology/pathophysiology/pathology

The aetiology of microscopic colitis (also known as lymphocytic colitis and membranous colitis) is not known [1]. Colonoscopy is normal, but histology shows lymphocytic infiltration and a thick subepithelial layer of collagen.

Persistent use of non-steroidal anti-inflammatories (NSAIDs) may produce a similar clinical and pathological picture, or may be associated with superficial mucosal ulceration.

Epidemiology

It occurs typically in middle-aged and elderly women. Incidence is uncertain.

Clinical presentation

Common

Persistent watery diarrhoea. NSAID enteropathy may produce abdominal pain and systemic symptoms.

Physical signs

Common

Few physical signs. Rigid sigmoidoscopy is typically normal.

Investigations/staging

Serum inflammatory markers, macroscopic appearance at colonoscopy and barium enema are usually normal.

Differential diagnosis

Common:
- ulcerative colitis
- infectious colitis.

Treatments

There is no satisfactory treatment. 5-Aminosalicylic acid compounds may be of benefit.

Prognosis

Morbidity

Most patients suffer repeated relapses.

Disease associations

Arthritis, thyroiditis, diabetes.

British Society of Gastroenterology Guidelines on Inflammatory Bowel Disease: http://www.bsg.org.uk.guidelines.
1 Kingham JGC. Microscopic colitis. *Gut* 1991; 32: 234–235.

2.2 Oesophagus

2.2.1 BARRETT'S OESOPHAGUS

Aetiology/pathophysiology/pathology

This condition is named after the surgeon Norman Barrett, who described ulceration in a tubular intrathoracic organ that appeared to be oesophagus except that its distal part was lined by a gastric type of columnar epithelium. It is defined as a replacement of the normal squamous epithelial lining of the oesophagus by metaplastic columnar epithelium.

It is strongly associated with gastro-oesophageal reflux of acid, which is thought to damage normal lining with replacement by columnar, acid-resistant lining.

Epidemiology

The true prevalence is unknown since many cases are silent and therefore not detected. Approximately 10% of patients undergoing upper GI endoscopy for reflux symptoms are found to have a columnar-lined oesophagus (Barrett's), and half will have specialized intestinal-type lining. Autopsy studies suggest a prevalence of around 1%.

Clinical presentation

Common

Gastro-oesophageal reflux symptoms or incidental finding at endoscopy. Most oesophageal adenocarcinomas have evidence of surrounding columnar epithelium.

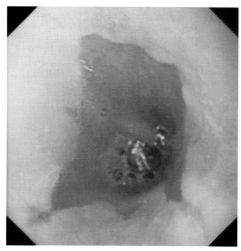

Fig. 36 Barrett's oesophagus. The squamous–columnar junction lies above the gastro-oesophageal junction.

Uncommon

Haematemesis or melaena may occur following bleeding from an oesophageal ulcer present in Barrett's oesophagus.

Physical signs

None.

Investigation/staging

Endoscopy

Characteristic, revealing red, velvety columnar epithelium extending proximally from the gastro-oesophageal junction (proximal end of gastric rugal folds) (Fig. 36). Biopsy confirms columnar metaplasia.

Differential diagnosis

It should be noted that biopsy from a point distal to the squamocolumnar junction (e.g. from the proximal end of a hiatus hernia) will lead to a false positive diagnosis of Barrett's oesophagus.

Treatment

Short-term

Proton pump inhibitor

Maintenance treatment with a proton pump inhibitor is used to treat reflux oesophagitis (symptomatic or endoscopic). This may also cause some regression of the Barrett's metaplasia, with the appearance of squamous mucosal islands, but does not effect a cure.

Anti-reflux surgery

May protect against the development of dysplasia and adenocarcinoma.

Endoscopic ablative therapy

The role of laser, photodynamic therapy or electrocoagulation is unclear, but may be considered for those who have high-grade dysplasia or carcinoma *in situ* and whose comorbidity prevents surgery.

Long-term

Endoscopic surveillance for adenocarcinoma

This involves yearly endoscopy, with multiple quadrantic biopsies, particularly if the segment of Barrett's is long (more than 3 cm) and shows intestinal-type metaplasia. Junctional and gastric type metaplasia probably have very low malignant potential and are not usually surveyed.

Oesophagectomy

This should be considered where there is high-grade dysplasia or carcinoma. The actual survival benefit gained by regular endoscopic surveillance is disputed.

Length of surveillance

Surveillance should only continue whilst the patient is fit enough (and willing) to undergo an oesophagectomy.

Complications

Common

As abnormal reflux is almost universally present in Barrett's patients, they are at risk of severe oesophagitis, oesophageal ulceration and stricture formation.

Uncommon

Oesophageal adenocarcinoma

There is a 40-fold increase in the risk of developing oesophageal adenocarcinoma in Barrett's oesophagus (intestinal metaplasia). Overall, approximately 1% of patients with Barrett's will develop oesophageal cancer per year.
 Risk factors are:
- increasing length of Barrett's
- male gender
- smoking
- presence of oesophageal ulceration.

Prognosis

Morbidity

Gastro-oesopagheal reflux is now usually well controlled following the advent of the powerful acid-suppressing proton pump inhibitors, with or without prokinetic agents such as cisapride and metoclopramide.

Mortality

Although Barrett's is a risk factor for oesophageal carcinoma, most patients die from other causes and have a normal life expectancy [1].

Prevention

Secondary

See above. Most are maintained on long-term proton pump inhibitors. Antireflux surgery is an alternative. Ablative therapies may cause regression, but none have been shown to prevent adenocarcinoma.

Daly JM, Karnell AH, Menck HR. National Cancer Data Base report on oesophageal carcinoma. *Cancer* 1996; 78: 1820–1828.
Spechler SJ. The columnar-lined oesphagus. *Gastroenterol Clin N Am* 1997; 26: 455–466.
1 van de Burgh A, Des J, Hop WCJ *et al*. Oesophageal cancer is an uncommon cause of death in patients with Barrett's oesophagus. *Gut* 1996; 39: 5–8.

2.2.2 OESOPHAGEAL REFLUX AND BENIGN STRICTURE

Aetiology/pathophysiology/pathology

Gastro-oesophageal reflux (GOR) of acid leads to mucosal injury (reflux oesophagitis), Barrett's oesophagus and peptic stricture formation [1]. It is caused primarily by dysfunction of the lower oesophageal sphincter which allows reflux of acid, compounded by ineffective oesophageal acid clearance. Gastric acid secretion is usually normal. Hiatal hernias, occurring in 10–15% of the general population, are more prevalent with increasing severity of reflux disease, and may contribute to abnormal reflux both by reducing basal lower oesophageal pressure and impairing effective oesophageal clearance of acid (Fig. 37).

Reflux may result in a spectrum of damage to the oesophagus, ranging from microscopic changes only through to circumferential oesophagitis with ulceration and stricture

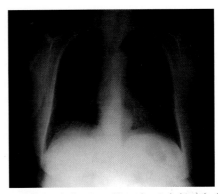
Fig. 37 Chest radiograph showing a hiatus hernia behind the heart.

formation. This can be graded using the Savary–Millar classification:
- grade I—one or more non-confluent erosions
- grade II—confluent but not circumferential erosions
- grade III—circumferential erosive oesophagitis
- grade IV—grade III plus ulceration, stricture formation or Barrett's oesophagus.

Epidemiology

Gastro-oesophageal reflux symptoms (retrosternal burning, acid regurgitation) are common and occur on a daily basis in up to 10% of the population. Only about one-third will have evidence of endoscopic oesophagitis. Peptic strictures occur in 7–23% of patients with untreated reflux oesophagitis.

Clinical presentation

Common

Burning retrosternal pain aggravated by lying down or bending forwards, and by spicy foods, citrus fruits and alcohol.

Regurgitation of acid, water brash, chest pain, odynophagia (painful swallowing) and dysphagia.

 Note that symptoms have a poor correlation with both the presence and severity of oesophagitis.

Uncommon

Haematemesis or iron-deficiency anaemia.

Physical signs

No physical signs. Weight loss if there has been a delayed presentation of an oesophageal stricture.

Investigation/staging

Upper gastrointestinal endoscopy

Indicated if troublesome or refractory reflux symptoms.

> • Gastroscopy is mandatory in those who have alarm symptoms (haematemesis, dysphasia, weight loss, anaemia), and desirable in middle-aged or elderly patients with new onset of symptoms.
> • Patients in their twenties or early thirties who require infrequent, intermittent courses of acid suppressing therapy probably don't warrant endoscopy, but those with persistent symptoms requiring long-term therapy should be examined to define the extent and severity of oesophagitis (or presence of Barrett's oesophagus) and therefore guide therapy.

Twenty-four hour ambulatory pH monitoring

This is useful in patients with atypical symptoms, in those who don't respond to acid suppressing therapy, and as part of the work-up for patients considered for antireflux surgery (along with oesophageal manometry).

Differential diagnosis

Common differential diagnoses include:
• cardiac pain
• oesophageal carcinoma—benign-looking peptic strictures must be brushed and biopsied to exclude malignancy
• infections with herpes simplex or *Candida*
• drugs (e.g. alendronate, NSAIDs, ferrous sulphate) that may cause heartburn
• radiotherapy-induced oesophagitis (e.g. treatment of bronchial carcinoma).

Treatment

Emergency

Patients with dysphagia need rapid assessment with either a barium swallow or endoscopy. Barium swallow is often performed first to define the position and extent of the stricture (and show pharyngeal pouches that may be perforated with the endoscope). Patients with a stricture demonstrated on barium swallow should proceed to endoscopy for biopsy and brushings to exclude malignancy. All patients with benign peptic oesophageal strictures should be commenced on proton pump inhibitors to prevent further acid reflux and damage. Concurrent oesophagitis *per se* may contribute to the dysphagia. If symptoms are significant, oesophageal dilatation should be performed. Initial improvement occurs in >80%, although one third require repeat dilatation within 12 months despite acid suppression therapy.

Short-term

Treatment of GOR should be directed at alleviating the symptoms. A graded approach is usual, starting with antacids and lifestyle measures (stopping smoking, avoiding precipitants), then H_2 antagonists with or without prokinetic agents (e.g. metoclopramide, cisapride), and finally proton pump inhibitors (PPIs) or antireflux surgery [2,3]. Healing of oesophagitis (grade II or more severe) is desirable to prevent complications of stricture formation or Barrett's metaplasia.

Long-term

Many patients with symptomatic GOR relapse following cessation of medical therapy. PPIs are the most effective agents in the initial healing of reflux oesophagitis (80–90% within 8 weeks with standard doses), and in subsequent maintenance therapy. Aggressive acid suppression therapy with PPIs has been shown to decrease the need for repeat dilatation of oesophageal peptic strictures.

Complications

Common

Most patients with GOR disease can be well controlled with acid suppression therapy. Relapse of symptoms is common on withdrawal of treatment. It is estimated that up to one quarter of patients with untreated reflux oesophagitis will develop strictures. Long-term acid reflux is important in the development of Barrett's oesophagus.

Prognosis

The advent of the powerful PPI agents means the vast majority of patients can be rendered asymptomatic. Antireflux surgery is an alternative where medical therapy fails, or if the patient is young and unkeen on long-term medication. Although reflux disease has little effect on life expectancy, it may predispose to the development of oesophageal adenocarcinoma [4].

Long-term severe reflux predisposes to Barrett's oesophagus with its malignant potential.

Oesophageal perforation occurs in <1% of procedures.

Prevention

Aggressive control of acid secretion is likely to be important in preventing peptic stricture formation in those with significant reflux oesophagitis. Once a stricture has formed long-term therapy with a PPI is indicated.

Disease associations

Scleroderma may result in severe oesophagitis and stricture formation.

1 Katz PO (ed.) Gastroesophageal Reflux Disease. *Gastroenterol Clin N Am* 1999; 28.
2 Smith PL, Kerr GD, Cockel R *et al.* A comparison of omeprazole and ranitidine in the prevention of recurrence of benign oesophageal stricture. The RESTORE Investigator Group. *Gastroenterol* 1994; 107: 1312–1318.
3 Vigneri S, Termini R, Leandro G *et al.* A comparison of five maintenance therapies for reflux oesophagitis. *N Engl J Med* 1995; 333: 1106–1110.
4 Lagergren J, Bergstrom R, Lindgren A, Nyren O. Symptomatic gastroesophageal reflux as a risk factor for oesophageal adenocarcinoma. *N Engl J Med* 1999; 340: 825–831.

2.2.3 OESOPHAGEAL TUMOURS

Aetiology/pathophysiology/pathology

The aetiology is shown in Table 24. Oesophageal carcinoma is microscopically squamous cell or adenocarcinoma. (See *Oncology*, Section 2.3.)

Epidemiology

There are geographical variations in the prevalence of the disease, with the highest rates (>100 per 100 000) in China, Iran and South Africa. In the Western world the incidence of adenocarcinoma of the oesophagus is rising rapidly for reasons that are unknown.

Clinical presentation

Common

Dysphagia with weight loss is the usual presentation. May be discovered as part of the work-up of iron-deficiency anaemia. Regurgitation common.

Table 24 Risk factors for carcinoma of oesophagus.

Squamous cell carcinoma	Adenocarcinoma
Smoking	Barrett's oesophagus
Alcohol	Gastro-oesphageal reflux
Malnutrition	
Achalasia	
Postcricoid web*	
Familial tylosis†	

* Brown–Kelly–Paterson/Plummer–Vinson syndrome; † Hyperkeratosis of palms of hands and soles of feet.

Uncommon

* Non-specific dyspepsia or heartburn
* Pain due to local invasion into the spine or intercostal nerves
* Hoarseness due to involvement of the recurrent laryngeal nerve by middle and upper third oesophageal carcinomas.

Rare

* Massive haemorrhage due to invasion into the aorta
* Oesophagobronchial fistulae.

Physical signs

Common

* Cachexia.
* Supraclavicular lymphadenopathy.

Uncommon

* Epigastric mass due to extension into gastric cardia.
* Ascites.

Rare

* Adenopathy in the thoracic inlet may cause venous congestion, including superior vena cava obstruction.

Investigation/staging

Barium swallow

This is the initial investigation of choice, although in practice endoscopy is often used first line with mild degrees of dysphagia ('difficulty with some solids') (Fig. 38).

Upper gastrointestinal endoscopy

To obtain multiple biopsies for histology and brushings for cytology for a tissue diagnosis.

CT of the thorax and abdomen

Undertaken to look for evidence of local invasion into mediastinal structures and for hepatic or pulmonary metastases [1].

Endoscopic ultrasound

If available this provides more accurate local staging of the tumour. Unfortunately most tumours are advanced at presentation (T3, invasion through the oesophageal

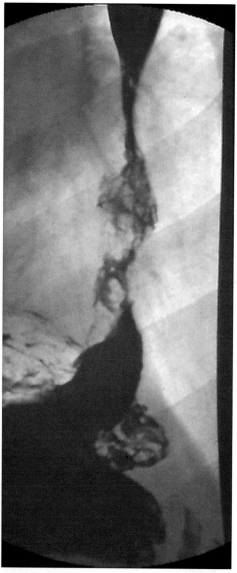

Fig. 38 Barium swallow showing an irregular malignant stricture in the distal oesophagus.

wall into the adventitia; or T4, into adjacent structures, e.g. aorta, pulmonary vessels).

Differential diagnosis

Benign oesophageal stricture. Usually obvious at endoscopy, confirmed with biopsy and brushings. If clinical suspicion but histology negative, repeat sampling.

Treatment

Emergency

Oesophageal dilatation

Presentation with complete or near-complete obstruction (liquids/liquidized food) not unusual. Dilatation may be needed at the time of diagnostic endoscopy.

 Risk of oesophageal perforation is higher with dilatation of malignant compared to benign strictures.

Short-term

Aim is rapid work-up to select appropriate candidates for curative surgery, usually with thoraco-abdominal CT and endoscopic ultrasound if available. Preoperative enteral or parenteral nutrition and physiotherapy important. Less than one third are suitable for surgery. Subtotal oesophagectomy with anastomosis to fashioned gastric 'tube' is often employed.

Long-term

Palliation indicated for the majority, with either endoscopic or radiological positioning of expandable metal stents, laser photocoagulation or radiotherapy (internal or external).

Complications

Oesophagectomy

Anastomosis may leak or dehisce (has less rich blood supply compared to rest of intestine).

Oesophageal stent

• Perforation during stent placement and laser photocoagulation.
• Stent migration.

Prognosis

Morbidity

Aim with the majority is palliation, i.e. ensuring reasonable swallowing.

Mortality

Overall median survival <1 year; 5-year survival rate 5%. Earlier stage and absence of lymph node involvement yields better results. There is 5–10% mortality with oesophagectomy.

Prevention

Primary

Endoscopic surveillance of Barrett's oesophagus for adenocarcinoma, but no evidence that this improves outcome.

Important information for patients

Most will need to mince food, since swallowing will not be normal even with stented, fully patent lumen.

 1 Tio TL, Cohen P, Coene PP *et al.* Endosonography and computed tomography of oesophageal carcinoma. *Gastroenterol* 1989; 96: 1478–1486.

2.2.4 ACHALASIA

Aetiology/pathophysiology/pathology

Achalasia is of unknown aetiology. It is characterized by a hypertensive lower oesophageal sphincter (LOS) with failure of LOS relaxation in response to swallowing. Peristalsis is absent in the body of the oesophagus. The oesophagus becomes progressively dilated. Histological examination reveals loss of myenteric plexus ganglia.

Epidemiology

Rare: approximate incidence 1 in 100 000 in the West.

Clinical presentation

Common

Dysphagia is universal and typically for both fluids and solids from the outset. Regurgitation is usual, causing nocturnal cough and respiratory complications.

Physical signs

Often absent. Weight loss may be evident.

Investigation/staging

Barium swallow

This shows food debris in the oesophagus with dilatation in later stages. Smooth, tapered 'bird's beak' at distal end (Fig. 39).

 Gastroscopy should always be performed to exclude malignancy at the gastro-oesophageal junction: this can mimic achalasia, particularly in elderly people.

Manometry

This confirms the diagnosis showing a hypertensive LOS that fails to relax on swallowing and diminished peristalsis.

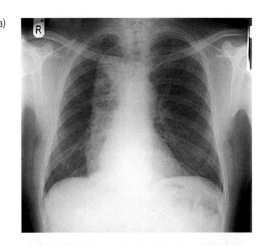
(a)

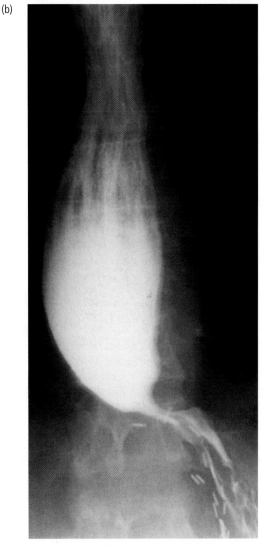
(b)

Fig. 39 (a) Chest radiograph and barium swallow of achalasia. Note the widened mediastinum on chest radiograph due to grossly distended oesophagus. (b) On the barium swallow the distal end of the dilated oesophagus has a characteristic 'beaked' appearance.

Differential diagnosis

Chagas' disease may present with identical clinical, endoscopic and radiological features.

Treatment

Pneumatic (balloon) dilatation or surgical myotomy (Heller's)

Results are comparable, with 75–85% having an excellent relief of their symptoms [1]. Perforation occurs in 1–5% after dilatation. Late stricture formation occurs in about 3% of surgically treated patients.

Intrasphincteric injection of botulinum toxin

This has recently been tried with similar results, although a second injection is often required after about 6 months [2,3].

Complications

Common

- Risk of oesophageal carcinoma is increased about 15-fold.
- Reflux oesophagitis and stricture formation (<1%) may occur after pneumatic dilatation.

Prognosis

Over 90% of patients are improved following pneumatic dilatation or surgical myotomy. Repeat dilatation is occasionally required.

1 Vantrappen G, Janssens J. To dilate or operate? That is the question. *Gut* 1983; 24: 1013–1019.
2 Annese V, Basciani M, Perri F *et al*. Controlled trial of botulinum toxin injection vs placebo and pneumatic dilation in achalasia. *Gastroenterol* 1996; 111: 1418–1424.
3 Pasricha PJ, Ravich WJ, Hendrix TR, Sostre S, Jones B, Kalloo AN. Intrasphincteric botulinum toxin for the treatment of achalasia. *N Engl J Med* 1995; 322: 774–778.

2.2.5 DIFFUSE OESOPHAGEAL SPASM

Aetiology/pathophysiology/pathology

Aetiology is unknown.

Clinical presentation

Intense, cramping chest pain often indistinguishable from cardiac pain. Dysphagia is variable and often precipitated by cold or carbonated drinks.

Physical signs

None.

Investigation/staging

Manometry

This shows simultaneous (i.e. aperistaltic) and repetitive contractions of high amplitude (pressure), which may be prolonged.

Barium swallow

This may demonstrate the classical 'corkscrew oeosphagus', segmental spasm or tertiary contractions (which are often asymptomatic and non-specific in elderly people).

Twenty-four hour pH measurements

This may show pathological reflux which is contributory to patients' symptoms.

Endoscopy

This rules out organic strictures and reflux oesophagitis.

Differential diagnosis

Cardiac chest pain.

Treatment

Reassurance is important. Calcium antagonists, e.g. nifedipine 10 mg t.d.s., or nitrates, e.g. isosorbide may be tried. Response is variable. Prokinetics may aggravate symptoms.

2.3 Gastric and duodenal disease

2.3.1 PEPTIC ULCERATION AND *HELICOBACTER PYLORI*

Aetiology/pathophysiology/pathology

Helicobacter pylori infection and non-steroidal anti-inflammatory drug (NSAID) use are important aetiological factors. It is unclear whether *H. pylori* infection increases the risk of NSAID-induced ulcers. There are different *H. pylori* strains: Cag-A is associated with more severe gastritis and intestinal metaplasia. *H. pylori* produces a urease which is made use of in the diagnostic tests.

Epidemiology

In the UK, serological testing for *H. pylori* shows that 50% of 50 yr olds and 20% of 20 yr olds have been infected.

Parameters	Score			
	0	1	2	3
Clinical				
Age (years)	<60	60–79	80+	
Shock				
Systolic BP (mmHg))	>100	>100	<100	
Pulse (min)	<100	>100		
Comorbidity	None	Other	Cardiac failure IHD	Renal failure Liver failure
Endoscopic				
Diagnosis	Mallory–Weiss No lesion	Other diagnoses	Malignancy	
Major SRH	None		Blood in upper GI tract Adherent clot Visible vessel	
Score	0	2	4	6	8+
Mortality (%)	0	0.2	5	17	41
Rebleeding (%)	5	5	14	32	41

Table 25 Combined clinical and endoscopic assessment of mortality and risk of rebleeding following an upper gastrointestinal haemorrhage.

BP, blood pressure; IHD, ischaemic heart disease; SRH, stigmata of recent haemorrhage; GI, gastrointestinal.

This is a cohort effect and does not mean that 1% acquire the infection each year. *H. pylori* causes 90% of duodenal ulcers and 60% of gastric ulcers.

The lifetime risk of duodenal ulcer is 4–10% and of gastric ulcer 3–4%, males more than females.

Clinical presentations

Common

- Epigastric pain or indigestion
- Lethargy from anaemia
- Melaena and/or haematemesis.

Uncommon

If present in the pylorus there may be pyloric obstruction with vomiting.

Rare

Perforation with abdominal pain and signs of an acute abdomen.

Physical signs

- Anaemia
- Epigastric tenderness.

Investigations/staging

Endoscopy

To establish the diagnosis and to take biopsies from a gastric ulcer to ensure it is benign. Antral and gastric body biopsies for *H. pylori*. Risk of rebleeding can also be assessed (Table 25).

H. pylori detection

This can be serological, looking for IgA and IgG antibodies to *H. pylori* if previously untreated or by histological examination of gastric tissue by CLO test or routine histology (silver stain) (Figs 40 and 41).

- Serology cannot be used to assess whether the infection has been successfully eradicated with treatment, as antibodies persist.

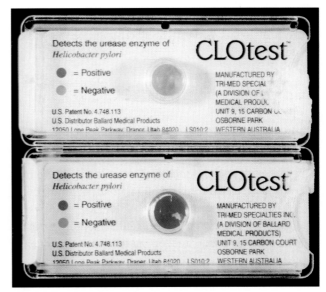

Fig. 40 CLO test. This relies on the fact that *Helicobacter pylori* produces a urease. A gastric biopsy is placed on the test card. If *H. pylori* is present the indicator turns from yellow to red. A result is obtained in an hour.

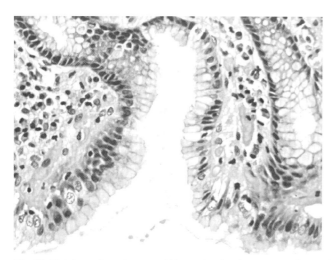

Fig. 41 Histology of gastric mucosal biopsy showing the presence of *Helicobacter pylori* on the epithelial surface.

^{13}C urea breath test

A non-invasive method of assessing whether *H. pylori* has been successfully eradicated.

Differential diagnosis

* If abdominal pain— see Section 1.9, p.30.
* If GI haemorrhage—see Section 1.3, p. 9.

Treatment

Emergency

See Section 1.3, p. 13.

Endoscopic therapy

Using either injection (adrenaline, saline, ethanolamine) or thermal contact devices (electrocoagulation) for bleeding peptic ulcer.

Short-term

Eradication of *H. pylori*

Triple drug regimes are effective in 80–95% of cases [1,2]. Effective regimes include 7 days of a proton pump inhibitor b.d., clarithromycin 500 mg b.d. or amoxycillin 1 g b.d., and metronidazole 500 mg b.d. Reinfection following eradication of *H. pylori* is rare in adults. Antibiotic resistance to metronidazole and/or clarithromycin occurs in 10–20%.

Ulcer healing

Six weeks of proton pump inhibitor to heal the ulcer.

Long-term

A patient who has had a complicated peptic ulcer (bleeding or perforation) should probably remain on long-term antisecretory therapy (proton pump inhibitor or H_2 blocker). If they require an NSAID following a GI bleed consider specific COX-2 inhibitors and a proton pump inhibitor [3]. If NSAID therapy is required after an uncomplicated peptic ulcer consider misoprostol or a proton pump inhibitor [4].

Complications

* Perforation and bleeding.
* Gastric carcinoma. Less than 3% of gastric ulcers are malignant.
* Oesophageal reflux. There is concern that eradication of *H. pylori* may be associated with an increased incidence of oesophageal reflux.

Prognosis

* Even if *H. pylori* infection is eradicated 20% will develop recurrent ulceration.
* The risk of rebleeding and mortality following a gastrointestinal haemorrhage is shown in Table 25.

Prevention

Primary

Avoidance of NSAIDs and smoking. Use of misoprostol with an NSAID or specific COX-2 inhibitors.

Disease associations

Gastrinoma—this is associated with multiple peptic ulcers. May occur in isolation or associated with multiple endocrine neoplasia (MEN) type 1.

1 Lee J, O'Morain C. Who should be treated for *Helicobacter pylori* infection? A review of consensus conferences and guidelines. *Gastroenterol* 1997; 113: S99–S106.
2 de Boer WA, Tytgat GNJ. Treatment of *Helicobacter pylori* infection. *BMJ* 2000; 320: 31–34.
3 Langamn MJ, Jensen DM, Watson DJ *et al.* Adverse upper gastrointestinal effects of rofecoxib compared with NSAIDs. *JAMA* 1999; 282: 1929–1933.
4 Hawkey CJ, Karrasch JA, Szczepanski L *et al.* Omeprazole compared with misoprostol for ulcers associated with non-steroidal anti-inflammatory drugs. Omeprazole vs misoprostol for NSAID-induced ulcer management group. *N Engl J Med* 1998; 328: 727–734.

2.3.2 GASTRIC CARCINOMA

Aetiology/pathophysiology/pathology

Histologically gastric carcinoma can be classified as diffuse or intestinal. It is associated with atrophic gastritis and intestinal metaplasia. By contrast there is no evidence that long-term drug-induced achlorhydria is associated with gastric cancer. However, distal gastrectomy is associated with a 12-fold increased risk of gastric cancer after 15–20 years. There is also increasing evidence of association between *H. pylori* and gastric cancer, with prospective serological studies showing a 3–6-fold increased risk mainly of distal tumours [1]. Countries with high rates of gastric cancer also have a high incidence of *H. pylori* infection (see *Oncology*, Section 2.3).

Epidemiology

The highest incidence is in Japan and China: it is 10 per 100 000 in the USA. Overall the incidence is falling, but adenocarcinoma affecting the cardia and gastroesophageal junction is becoming more common. It rarely occurs before the age of 40, peaking in the 70s [2].

Clinical presentations

Common

Small superficial tumours are often asymptomatic. Later symptoms are weight loss (61%), abdominal pain (51%), nausea (34%) and dysphagia (26%). Malaise due to iron-deficiency anaemia.

Rare

Vomiting from pyloric obstruction.

Physical signs

Common

Usually no clinical findings.

Uncommon

- Epigastric mass.
- Malignant ascites due to peritoneal seeding.

Rare

Enlarged supraclavicular lymph node (Virchow's).

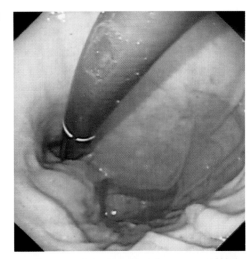
(a)

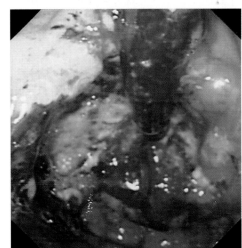
(b)

Fig. 42 Endoscopic appearance of (a) normal gastro-oesophageal junction and (b) gastric carcinoma.

Investigations

Full blood count

An iron-deficiency anaemia is present in 42%.

Tumour markers

Carcinoembryonic antigen (CEA) is not helpful diagnostically. It is elevated in 10–20% of patients with resectable tumour.

Endoscopy

For histological diagnosis and assessment of size and position of the tumour (Fig. 42).

Abdominal CT scan

Used for staging to assess whether surgically resectable. The tumour is staged from I to IV, dependent on tumour nodes metastases (TNM) classification.

Treatment

Surgery

Indicated if early tumour confined to stomach (i.e. stage I).

Chemotherapy

There is a role for neoadjuvant chemotherapy, which may reduce tumour bulk and invasion prior to surgery. Combined surgery and chemotherapy are better than chemotherapy alone.

Conservative

Indicated for linitus plasticus (involving whole of stomach) or those with locally-invasive as widespread metastatic disease.

Complications

Haemorrhage.

Prognosis

Five year-overall survival rates of 15%. Stage I (confined to stomach) with surgery: 50% 5-year survival in UK and 90% in Japan.

Prevention

Screening by endoscopy is advocated in Japan where 40–60% of early gastric cancers can be identified. Not the case in the UK, Europe and the USA.

Disease associations

Pernicious anaemia associated with 2–3-fold increased risk of carcinoma of stomach.

1 Huang JQ *et al.* Meta-analysis of the relationship between *Helicobacter pylori* seropositivity and gastric cancer. *Gastroenterol* 1998; 114: 1169–1179.
2 Fuchs CS, Mayer RJ. Gastric carcinoma. *N Engl J Med* 1995; 32–38.

2.3.3 RARE GASTRIC TUMOURS

Leiomyoma

This is a benign tumour of smooth muscle. Most tumours less than 2 cm are asymptomatic. By contrast, tumours greater than 2 cm may ulcerate and cause gastrointestinal haemorrhage. Submucosal endoscopic biopsy is often non-diagnostic but leiomyomas have a characteristic endoscopic appearance with central ulceration. Around 1% are malignant. If bleeding occurs then surgical resection is indicated.

Gastric and MALT lymphomas

Around 3–6% of gastric tumours are lymphomas, predominantly B cell. Low-grade lymphomas are associated with *H. pylori* infection in 72–98% of cases [1], *H. pylori* infection probably having resulted in the migration of B cells to gastric mucosa (mucosal-associated lymphoid tissue).

Most present over the age of 50 years, with non-specific dyspepsia, nausea and vomiting. There are usually no physical signs, and weight loss is rare. There may be no macroscopic abnormality or simply gastritis. Endoscopic biopsies are needed to make the diagnosis.

Eradication of *H. pylori* can cause resolution of low grade MALT lymphomas, confined to the mucosa, in the short term. Long-term follow-up studies are still awaited. Higher stage low-grade lymphomas and high-grade lymphomas are treated with gastrectomy and chemotherapy [2].

Gastrinoma

Gastrinoma causes multiple duodenal ulcers and is associated with watery diarrhoea. It may be sporadic or associated with MEN type 1. Sporadic tumours are usually single. They are found in the duodenal wall or pancreas; 50% are benign. There is a good 10-year prognosis. Treatment is by resection or with high-dose proton pump inhibitor.

1 Wotherspoon AC. *Helicobacter pylori* infection and gastric lymphoma. *Br Med Bull* 1998; 54: 79–85.
2 Steinbach G, Ford R, Glober G *et al.* Antibiotic treatment of gastric lymphoma of mucosal associated lymphoid tissue. An uncontrolled trial. *Ann Intern Med* 1999; 20: 131: 88–95.

2.3.4 RARE CAUSES OF GASTROINTESTINAL HAEMORRHAGE

Dieulafoy lesion

This is due to an artery in the submucosa with an overlying mucosal defect resulting in massive upper gastrointestinal haemorrhage. It is usually found within 6 cm of the gastrointestinal junction. The mean age at presentation is 50 years. The lesion may be missed at endoscopy when air inflates the stomach. The treatment of choice is surgical oversewing of the artery as the lesion rarely stops bleeding with injection therapy.

Vascular ectasia (angiodysplasia)

These are dilated distorted thin-walled vessels which are usually multiple. They occur anywhere along the gastrointestinal tract, but commonly in the caecum and descending colon. They usually present in middle age. Fifteen per cent are associated with massive bleeding. There is also an association with aortic stenosis. Treatments include oestrogens and surgical resection of the right colon.

Hereditary haemorrhagic telangiectasia

This is an autosomal dominant condition associated with skin and mucosal haemorrhage. The vascular lesions commonly occur in the stomach and small bowel and lead to recurrent gastrointestinal haemorrhage. Cutaneous manifestations include telangiectasia over the lips, fingers and oral mucosa. Treatment is with oestrogens.

Meckel's diverticulum

This congenital abnormality is present in 0.3–3% of the population. It is found on the antimesenteric border of the small bowel within 100 cm of the ileocaecal valve. Most are asymptomatic, but 80% contain gastric mucosa. Complications include haemorrhage (melaena or dark red blood per rectum), obstruction or intersussseption. The diagnosis is made by small bowel enema or technetium-99 scan (which detects parietal cells).

2.4 Pancreas

Diseases of the pancreas provide an enormous challenge to the clinician, and although patients with the more common forms of pancreatic disease (i.e. acute pancreatitis and pancreatic carcinoma) have historically been managed by surgical teams, there is a growing trend for non-surgical (i.e. medical) management.

2.4.1 ACUTE PANCREATITIS

Aetiology/pathophysiology/pathology

This is an acute inflammatory process of the pancreas with variable involvement of other regional tissues or remote organ systems [1]. Causes of acute pancreatitis include:
- gallstones 30–50%
- alcohol 10–40%—mechanism unclear
- idiopathic 15%
- trauma (ERCP, postoperative, blunt trauma) 5%.

Cause of acute pancreatitis

Other causes of acute pancreatitis are rare but should be considered in the absence of gallstones:
- *Drugs* e.g. azathioprine, sulphasalazine, frusemide
- *Pancreas divisum.* Congenital malfusion of the dorsal and ventral pancreatic buds
- *Sphincter of Oddi dysfunction*
- *Hypertriglyceridaemia.* May be associated with alcohol abuse or diabetes
- *Hypercalcaemia/hyperparathyroidism*
- *Viral.* Mumps, Coxsackie B, Epstein–Barr, cytomegalovirus
- *Hereditary pancreatitis.* Autosomal dominant inherited mutations in cationic trypsinogen gene (Ch7q). Increased lifetime risk of pancreatic carcinoma.

Once the process has started there is a variable degree of pancreatic necrosis in part related to proteolytic autodigestion of the gland.

Clinical presentation

Common

- Abdominal pain—usually epigastric and radiating through to the back
- Vomiting.

Uncommon

Jaundice—suggests the presence of an associated cholangitis and raises the probability of gallstones.

Rare

No pain.

Physical signs

Common

In mild acute pancreatitis there may be few physical signs:
- abdominal/epigastric tenderness
- infrequent or absent bowel sounds.

Uncommon

In patients with more severe disease there will be clinical evidence of hypovolaemia and systemic inflammation. Other features include:
- mental state—the patient may be agitated and delirious
- tachycardia
- hypotension
- fever
- peripheral cyanosis
- peritonism.

Rare

- Cullen's sign—periumbilical bruising
- Grey–Turner's sign—flank bruising.

Investigation/staging

Make the diagnosis

Serum amylase

This is diagnostic of pancreatitis if more than 3 times the upper limit of normal for the laboratory. Alternatives include serum lipase and possibly urinary trypsinogen.

Assess the severity

Assess the severity of the disease using the Glasgow/Ranson criteria [3]:

Glasgow/Ranson criteria

Three or more positive criteria, based on initial admission score and subsequent repeat tests over 48 h, constitutes severe disease.
- age >55 years
- white blood cell count >15 × 10⁹/L
- glucose >10 mmol/L
- urea >16 mmol/L
- Pao_2 <60 mmHg
- calcium <2 mmol/L
- albumin <32 g/L
- lactate dehydrogenase >600 units/L
- aspartate/alanine aminotransferase >100 units/L

APACHE II

The Acute Physiology and Chronic Health Evaluation scoring system is used in many intensive care units. An APACHE II score of 9 or more is considered to constitute a severe attack of acute pancreatitis.

C-reactive protein

A peak C-reactive protein level of >210 mg/L in the first four days of the attack (or >120 mg/L at the end of the first week) indicates severe disease.

Determine aetiology

Abdominal ultrasound

An ultrasound should be performed within 24 h of admission. This will determine whether there are gallstones present

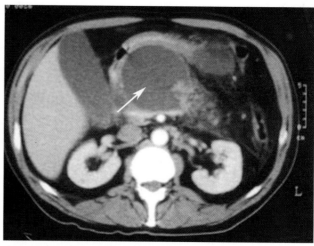

Fig. 43 Pancreatic pseudocysts complicating acute pancreatitis. The stomach is stretched over the large pseudocyst (arrow). (Courtesy of Dr ND Derbyshire, Royal Berks Hospital.)

and may demonstrate biliary dilatation, suggesting a common bile duct obstruction.

Identify local complications

Abdominal CT

A CT with contrast should be performed in cases of severe pancreatitis between 3 and 10 days after admission. In addition to identifying secondary complications such as pseudocyst formation (Fig. 43) the extent of pancreatic necrosis carries prognostic value (Table 26).

Differential diagnosis

This includes:
- perforated peptic ulcer
- intestinal ischaemia/infarction
- ectopic pregnancy
- aortic dissection
- myocardial infarction.

See Section 1.13, p.39.

Treatment

Emergency

Resuscitation

Intravenous fluids, CVP monitoring and oxygen. Patients with severe pancreatitis (as defined above) should be managed on an intensive care unit.

Nutrition

Although historically patients with acute pancreatitis were fasted, early nasojejunal feeding is now favoured.

Table 26 Contrast enhanced computed tomography (CT) grading of acute pancreatitis [2].

Grade	CT morphology
A	Normal
B	Focal or diffuse gland enlargement; small intrapancreatic fluid collection
C	Any of the above plus peripancreatic inflammatory changes and <30% gland necrosis
D	Any of the above plus single extrapancreatic fluid collection and 30–50% gland necrosis
E	Any of the above plus extensive extrapancreatic fluid collection, pancreatic abscess and >50% gland necrosis

Antibiotics

Use of 'blind' broad-spectrum antibiotics is controversial. Antibiotics should be used in cases of proven infection or organ failure.

Short-term

Cytokine antagonists

Antagonists of platelet activating factor (e.g. Lexipafant) have been used in acute pancreatitis although their use is not routine [2].

ERCP

If gallstones are present on the ultrasound or if the patient has clinical features of cholangitis (fever, jaundice) an early ERCP (i.e. within the first 24 h) should be considered on the principle that early relief of biliary obstruction will reduce complications. If this is not performed within 24–48 h oedema of the papilla makes ERCP technically difficult.

Other

The following interventions may also be needed:
- surgery—may be indicated in cases of infected necrosis
- CT drainage of pancreatic abscess.
- endoscopic cyst gastrostomy for internal drainage of pseudocyst (Fig. 44).

Long-term

Abstinence from alcohol. Early cholecystectomy is recommended if gallstones are confirmed to be the underlying cause of the pancreatitis.

Complications

Common

These include:
- pancreatic pseudocyst/abscess—persistent pain and/or fever suggests the development of a pancreatic pseudocyst or abscess

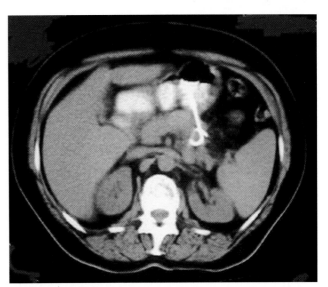

Fig. 44 Drainage of a pancreatic pseudocyst into the stomach. The internal transgastric drain is shown *in situ*. (Courtesy of Dr ND Derbyshire, Royal Berks Hospital.)

- paralytic ileus
- hypovolaemic shock
- renal failure
- hypocalcaemia
- hypoxia.

Uncommon

- Portal vein/mesenteric thrombosis
- Adult respiratory distress syndrome
- Ascites.

 In pancreatitis, ascites will have a high amylase content, differentiating it from other causes.

Rare

External pancreatic fistulae—may follow percutaneous drainage of pseudocyst.

Prognosis

Thirty per cent of patients have recurrent attacks. This is more likely in pancreatitis related to alcohol consumption. Overall prognosis may be worse in idiopathic pancreatitis.

Table 27 Prognosis from acute pancreatitis.

	Mortality (%)
Glasgow/Ranson's criteria*	
<2	5
3–5	10
>6	60
APACHE II†	
<9	'low'
>13	'high'

* Scored at 48 h from the onset of symptoms. Sensitivity 57–85%, Specificity 68–85%.
† Can be scored at any time. Sensitivity at admission 34–70%, at 48 h <50%; Specificity at admission 76–98%, at 48 h 100%.

Morbidity and mortality

This is dependant on the severity of the attack (Table 27).

Prevention

Primary

Other than a reduction in per capita alcohol consumption there is little scope for primary prevention of acute pancreatitis.

Secondary

- Cholecystectomy
- Abstinence from alcohol.

1 Balthazar EJ, Feeny PC, van Sonnenberg E. Imaging and intervention in acute pancreatitis. *Radiology* 1994; 193: 297–306.
2 Imrie CW, McKay CJ. The scientific basis of medical therapy of acute pancreatitis. Could it work and is there a role for lexipafant? *Gastroenterol Clin North Am* 1999; 28: 591–599.
3 United Kingdom guidelines for the management of acute pancreatitis: http://www.bsg.org.uk/guidelines/pancreatic.html.

2.4.2 CHRONIC PANCREATITIS

Aetiology/pathophysiology/pathology

Chronic pancreatitis is a chronic inflammatory condition of the pancreas characterized by fibrosis and eventual destruction of both exocrine and endocrine components of the gland [1]. Causes include:
- alcohol—the commonest underlying cause in the UK. Chronic pancreatitis appears to affect 5–15% of heavy drinkers
- hereditary pancreatitis [2]

- idiopathic 10–30%
- cystic fibrosis (see *Respiratory medicine*, Section 2.5).

Epidemiology

Rare. Estimated incidence in Western countries <4.0 per 100 000.

Clinical presentation

Common

- *Abdominal pain.* Typical pancreatic pain is epigastric radiating through to the back. It is often precipitated by eating fatty foods or drinking alcohol.

Uncommon

- *Exocrine pancreatic insufficiency.* Steatorrhoea and weight loss.
- *Endocrine pancreatic insufficiency.* Diabetes.

 Both exocrine and endocrine insufficiency may be absent in mild chronic pancreatitis their presence indicates substantial pancreatic damage.

Physical signs

Common

There are no specific physical signs until there has been sufficient destruction of the gland to cause pancreatic failure (either exocrine or endocrine).

Uncommon

Erythema ab igne may be evident on the anterior abdominal wall in patients with chronic pancreatic pain.

Investigation/staging

Serum amylase is often normal or at most only modestly elevated.

 Investigation of chronic pancreatitis
- Tests of pancreatic anatomy
- Tests of exocrine pancreatic function
- Tests of endocrine pancreatic function.

Tests of pancreatic anatomy

Plain abdominal radiograph

May show pancreatic calcification.

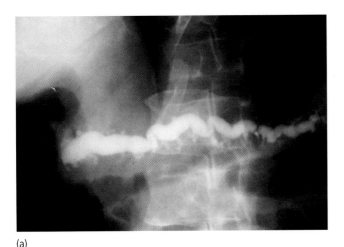

(a)

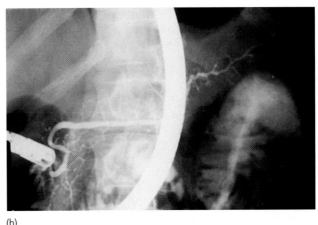

(b)

Fig. 45 Chronic pancreatitis shown on ERCP. (a) Dilated pancreatic duct with loss of side branches in severe disease, compared to (b) minimal duct changes.

Ultrasound

The pancreas may be obscured by overlying bowel gas.

Abdominal CT

The features of chronic pancreatitis include parenchymal calcification, duct irregularities and cysts.

ERCP

This may demonstrate both main duct and side branch irregularities (Fig. 45).

Tests of exocrine pancreatic function

These include:
• assessment of faecal fat either by Sudan staining of stool sample or microscopy
• faecal elastase
• measurement of pancreatic enzyme activity (e.g. pancreolauryl test).

Tests of endocrine pancreatic function

Glucose tolerance test.

Differential diagnosis

Of pain:
• peptic ulcer
• pancreatic cancer.
Of steatorrhoea and weight loss:
• coeliac disease
• small bowel bacterial overgrowth.

Treatment

Pancreatic enzyme replacement

Preparations such as Creon and Pancrex often improve both the pain and the malabsorption associated with chronic pancreatitis.

Analgesia

Where pain is the dominant feature opiate analgesia and local approaches such as coeliac axis block may be necessary.

Others

Treat diabetes—although hyperglycaemia may be relatively mild, early treatment with insulin is often useful. Ensure abstinence from alcohol.

Complications

Common

Malabsorption and diabetes [3].

Uncommon

Common bile duct obstruction.

Rare

Pancreatic carcinoma.

Prognosis

Morbidity

Although diabetes and malabsorption can be treated chronic

pain is a major source of morbidity with associated loss of employment, depression and opiate dependence.

Mortality

Survival may be reduced in alcoholic chronic pancreatitis, death in this group being due to many different causes.

Prevention

Secondary

Abstinence from alcohol along with medical management as outlined above will usually lead to clinical stabilization.

1 Naruse S, Kitagawa M, Ishiguro H, Nakae Y, Kondo T, Hayakawa T. Chronic pancreatitis: overview of medical aspects. *Pancreas* 1998; 16: 323–328.
2 Gates LK Jr, Urich CD 2nd, Whitcomb DC. Hereditary pancreatitis: gene defects and their implications. *Surg Clin N Am* 1999; 79: 711–722.
3 Apte MV, Keogh GW, Wilson JS. Chronic pancreatitis: complications and management. *J Clin Gastroenterol* 1999; 29: 225–240.

2.4.3 PANCREATIC CANCER

Aetiology/pathophysiology/pathology

The majority of primary malignant tumours of the pancreas are adenocarcinoma (see *Oncology*, Section 2.3). Risk factors include:
* age
* male sex
* smoking
* alcohol
* chronic pancreatitis
* diabetes
* hereditary pancreatitis.

Epidemiology

The incidence of carcinoma of the pancreas is increasing in the western world, in the range of 5–10 per 100 000. Male : female ratio is 1.3 : 1. It is rare at <45 years. It is a major cause of mortality.

Clinical presentation

Common

These include:
* painless cholestatic jaundice associated with varying degrees of pruritus, pale stools and dark urine due to common bile duct obstruction
* weight loss
* abdominal pain.

Uncommon

* Vomiting—from duodenal obstruction
* Malignant ascites.

Rare

* Venous thrombosis (thrombophlebitis migrans)
* Diabetes.

Physical signs

Common

Jaundice and cachexia.

Uncommon

* Palpable gall bladder (Courvoisier's sign)
* Palpable mass
* Ascites.

Investigation/staging

Blood tests

Routine blood tests show non-specific changes related to biliary obstruction. The pancreaticobiliary tumour marker CA19–9 may be elevated.

Non-invasive imaging

Abdominal ultrasound

May show a dilated biliary tree. A pancreatic mass may be demonstrated.

The absence of gallstones on ultrasound in a patient presenting with acute cholestasis and a dilated biliary tree suggests the presence of a common bile duct stricture due to a carcinoma of the pancreas or cholangiocarcinoma.

Abdominal CT or MRI

Useful for both diagnostic and prognostic features (i.e. demonstration of invasion into important local structures or evidence of distant metastases) (Fig. 46).

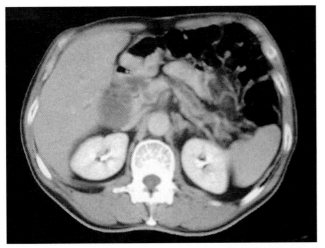

Fig. 46 Carcinoma of the head of the pancreas with distal pancreatic duct dilatation on a CT scan. (Courtesy of Dr ND Derbyshire, Royal Berks Hospital.)

Invasive imaging

ERCP

Very sensitive as diagnostic technique and allows palliation of biliary obstruction by the placement of an endobiliary stent if a bile duct stricture is demonstrated.

Percutaneous transhepatic cholangiography (PTC)

For cases where ERCP has failed (e.g. previous surgery such as Polya gastrectomy or roux-en-Y biliary reconstruction).

Endoscopic ultrasound

Increasingly available and may prove to be more sensitive than CT for both diagnosis of small lesions and preoperative staging [1].

CT-guided biopsy

In selected cases where the diagnosis remains obscure and where surgical resection might be considered if a positive diagnosis of adenocarcinoma is confirmed.

 Pancreatic tumours are very fibrotic and biopsy has a higher sensitivity than aspiration cytology.

Differential diagnosis

Of acute cholestasis:
• choledocolithiasis
• intrahepatic cholestasis (e.g. drug reaction).
Of pancreatic mass:
• ampullary carcinoma—tumour arising from the ampulla of Vater, which has a better prognosis.

Treatment

Short-term

ERCP and stenting—relief of biliary obstruction is the first priority in patients with obstructive jaundice [2].

Long-term or according to stage

Surgery

In a limited number of patients (<20%) pancreaticoduodenectomy (Whipple's procedure) offers the possibility of a surgical cure. Surgery may still be beneficial in patients with advanced disease by providing combined biliary and gastroduodenal bypass.

Chemotherapy/radiotherapy

Multimodal therapy (external beam irradiation combined with 5-flurouracil (5-FU) chemotherapy) may prove to be more efficacious than either approach alone.

Palliative measures

Relief of jaundice and pain control are the main objectives in patients with advanced disease and many require opiate analgesia. Anorexia and weight loss remain major problems.

Prognosis

Morbidity

The majority of patients with pancreatic cancer will have incurable disease at presentation and will experience pain in addition to progressive anorexia and weight loss [3].

Mortality

90% of individuals presenting with carcinoma of the pancreas are dead within a year.

1 Inui K, Nakazawa S, Yoshino J, Okushima K, Nakamura Y. Endoluminal ultrasonography for pancreatic diseases. *Gastroenterol Clin N Am* 1999; 28: 771–781.
2 Haycox A, Lombard M, Neoptlemos J, Walley T. Current treatment and optimal patient management in pancreatic cancer. *Aliment Pharmacol Ther* 1998; 12: 949–964.
3 Eskelinen MJ, Hayland UH. Prognosis of human pancreatic adenocarcinoma: review of clinical and histopathological variables and possible uses of new molecular methods. *Eur J Surg* 1999; 165: 292–306.

2.4.4 NEUROENDOCRINE TUMOURS

Aetiology/pathophysiology/pathology

Tumours arising from the specialized neuroendocrine tissue of the pancreas [1,2].

Epidemiology

All these conditions are rare.

Clinical presentation and physical signs

This depends on the tumour type:
• Gastrinoma (Zollinger–Ellison syndrome)—abdominal pain and diarrhoea
• Insulinoma—fasting hypoglycaemia
• VIPoma (Verner–Morrison syndrome)—watery diarrhoea, weight loss and flushing
• Glucagoma—dermatitis (necrolytic migratory erythema), diabetes, weight loss, diarrhoea
• Non-functioning tumours—incidental finding.

Investigation/staging

Stool weight

This is performed on a normal diet and then repeated fasting to distinguish secretory from osmotic diarrhoea.

 The diarrhoea associated with hormone excess is characteristically secretory rather than osmotic (i.e. not diminished by fasting).

Prolonged fast

Prolonged fast with measurement of glucose and C-peptide for insulinoma.

Fasting gut hormones

Most hormones can now be identified on a fasting serum sample. In the case of gastrin it is important that the patient is not taking acid-suppressing medication at the time of the test.

Pancreatic imaging

In most instances the clinical presentation of neuroendocrine tumours of the pancreas will be due to the systemic effect of the secreted hormone. Identification of the tumour is important as, with the exception of insulinomas, a significant proportion of these lesions are malignant. Spiral CT, MRI and increasingly endoscopic and intraoperative ultrasound are used.

Treatment

Long term or according to stage

Surgical resection

Probably the best treatment if a focal tumour can be identified.

Medical

Medical treatment depends on the secreted hormone:
• Gastrinoma—high-dose proton pump inhibitors improve both the pain and the diarrhoea
• Insulinoma—dietary advice, diazoxide, octreotide
• VIPoma—octreotide
• Glucagonoma—octreotide.

Prognosis

With the exception of insulinoma two thirds of the other tumour types will be histologically malignant. However with improved medical therapy (proton pump inhibitors and octreotide) these may still follow a relatively indolent course.

Disease associations

Multiple endocrine neoplasia (MEN) type 1 or Werner's syndrome comprises hyperparathyroidism associated with pancreatic endocrine tumours (usually non-functioning or gastrinomas).

1 Arnold R, Frank M. Gastrointestinal endocrine tumours: Medical management. *Baillière's Clin Gastroenterol* 1996; 10: 737–759.
2 Eriksson B, Oberg K. Neuroendocrine tumours of the pancreas. *Br J Surg* 2000; 87: 129–131.

2.5 Biliary tree

2.5.1 CHOLEDOCHOLITHIASIS

Aetiology/pathophysiology/pathology

There are three main types of stone: cholesterol, black pigment (occur in chronic haemolytic disease) and brown pigment stones (associated with infections in the biliary tree). They are almost always found in the gall bladder and are usually confined to the extrahepatic biliary tree. Intrahepatic biliary stones are rare, but seen more frequently in the Far East.

Epidemiology

Overall prevalence is 10%. Incidence increases with age and is twice as high in women as in men.

Clinical presentations

Common

- Indigestion, particularly exacerbated by fatty foods
- Biliary colic
- Acute cholecystitis (fever, right upper guadrant pain and tenderness, jaundice)
- Ascending cholangitis (high fever, rigors, jaundice, septicaemia)
- Acute pancreatitis.

Uncommon

In complete duct obstruction may cause cholestatic liver function tests (high ALP and GGT) without symptoms.

 Elderly patients commonly present with non-specific symptoms, e.g. 'off legs' due to cholangitis and secondary Gram-negative septicaemia.

Physical signs

Common

There may be no signs. Alternatively jaundice may be present with right upper quadrant tenderness.

Rare

The presence of splenomegaly suggests haemolytic anaemia with secondary pigmented common bile duct (CBD) stones.

Investigations

FBC and reticulocyte count

Elevated white cell count occurs with cholangitis. Macrocytic anaemia and elevated reticulocyte count suggests haemolysis.

Liver biochemistry

Classically elevated bilirubin and ALP/GGT. Rarely in acute biliary obstruction AST/ALT may be >1000 IU/L.

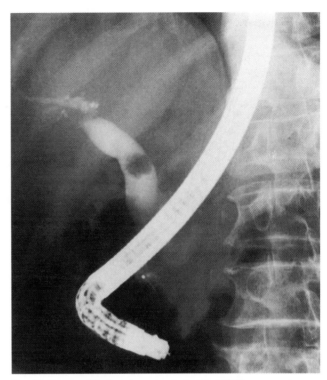

Fig. 47 Common bile duct stone demonstrated at ERCP.

Ultrasound

The preferred investigation to look for stones in the gall bladder. Sensitivity for CBD stones is only 70%.

 The common bile duct may not be dilated on an ultrasound in incomplete biliary obstruction.

ERCP

This is usually the investigation of choice to confirm that a stone is causing biliary obstruction (Fig. 47). It will also identify any distal common bile duct stricture, benign or malignant, that may have resulted in proximal stone formation.

Magnetic resonance cholangiopancreatography (MRCP)

This is a non-invasive method of imaging the CBD and pancreatic duct without the need for contrast. It can detect CBD stones and strictures [1].

Differential diagnosis

See Section 1.6, pp. 20–21.

Treatment

Emergency

Emergency early ERCP (within 72 h) with removal of CBD stones is indicated in patients with acute pancreatitis associated with obstructive jaundice. See Section 1.6, p. 22.

Short-term

Endoscopic removal of stones

A sphincterotomy or balloon sphincterplasty (cutting or dilating the sphincter of Oddi with a balloon) is performed to allow removal or passage of stones within the CBD. There is 8–12% risk of acute pancreatitis, bleeding or duodenal perforation with a 0.5–1% mortality. Stones are removed using a balloon, or basket to dredge the duct. Large stones can be crushed by lithotripsy inserted via the endoscope. A pigtail stent or nasobiliary drainage can provide temporary biliary decompression.

Long-term

Interval laparoscopic cholecystectomy in those for whom surgery is appropriate. In those who are not surgical candidates, and when it is not possible to remove large stones endoscopically, a CBD stent can be left in the bile duct providing adequate biliary drainage (Fig. 48). This may block within 3–12 months and need replacing at a further ERCP.

Complications

Common

Cholangitis and secondary septicaemia.

Rare

Prolonged asymptomatic biliary obstruction can lead to biliary cirrhosis.

Prognosis

Good if CBD stones removed.

Disease associations

• *Haemolytic anaemia*, e.g. sickle cell. Spherocytosis leading to pigmented large or intrahepatic stones.
• *Ileal disease/resection*. Interrupts enterohepatic circulation of bile acids.
• *Clonorchis infection*. Associated with intrahepatic stones. Rare in the UK.

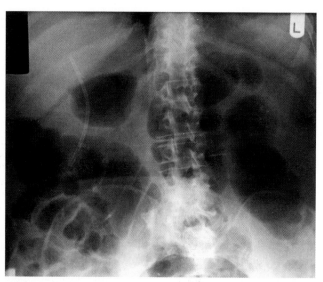

Fig. 48 A plastic stent within the common bile duct seen on a plain abdominal radiograph.

• *Total parenteral nutrition*. Associated with sludge and stones.

1 Zidi SH, Prat F, Le Guen O *et al*. Use of magnetic resonance cholangiography in the diagnosis of choledocholithiasis: a prospective comparison with a reference imaging method. *Gut* 1999; 44: 118–122.

2.5.2 CHOLANGIOCARCINOMA

Aetiology/pathophysiology/pathology

This is defined as adenocarcinoma of intrahepatic (peripheral), central (hilar) or extrahepatic bile ducts. Chronic inflammatory conditions and bile duct stasis are associated with tumours, e.g. primary sclerosing cholangitis, parasitic infections with liver flukes such as *Clonorchis* and *Opisthorchis* (south-east Asia), and recurrent bacterial cholangitis with hepatolithiasis. It is also associated with Thorotrast and choledochal cysts.

Epidemiology

Between 5 and 10% of malignant hepatic tumours are cholangiocarcinomas. Mean age is 50–70 years.

Clinical presentations

The patient is often asymptomatic until a late stage when symptoms include biliary obstruction, fever, weight loss and vague abdominal pain.

Physical signs

• Jaundice with or without hepatomegaly
• Weight loss.

Investigations

Liver biochemistry

Elevated bilirubin/ALP and GGT.

Tumour markers

CA19-9 rises but as this has low sensitivity and specificity it is not useful diagnostically, although it may be helpful in assessing response to therapy.

Ultrasound

To detect dilated ducts, mass in pancreatic head (carcinoma) and level of obstruction.

ERCP

This is both a diagnostic and a therapeutic procedure (Fig. 49). The sensitivity of cytology of brushing from the stricture is about 50–70% [1].

Percutaneous transhepatic cholangiogram (PTC)

In the presence of a lower CBD stricture it may not be possible to cannulate the papilla endoscopically and the biliary tree has to be accessed percutaneously (Fig. 50).

Differential diagnosis

Extrahepatic tumours must be differentiated from benign strictures, e.g. chronic pancreatitis, primary sclerosing cholangitis.

Treatment

Short-term

Relief of biliary obstruction with a stent placed percutaneously or endoscopically [2] (Fig. 51). Metal self-expanding stents have a longer patency time than cheaper plastic stents.

 Metal stents cannot be removed and can make subsequent surgery difficult. It is therefore important to have made the correct diagnosis before inserting one.

Long-term

Surgical resection

Appropriate in early disease if no evidence of spread. Roux-en-Y biliary anastomosis may relieve obstruction as a palliative procedure for low common bile duct cholangiocarcinomas.

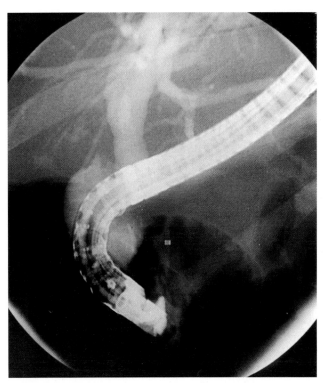

Fig. 49 A cholangiocarcinoma seen at ERCP. The common bile duct above the stricture is dilated.

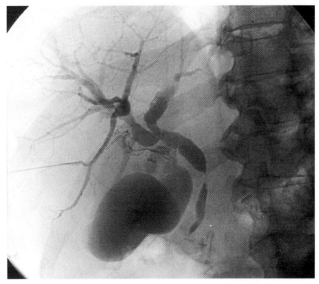

Fig. 50 A percutaneous transhepatic cholangiogram (PTC) showing a common bile duct stricture.

Liver transplantation

This is contraindicated in a patient with primary sclerosing cholangitis who develops a cholangiocarcinoma due to a high rate of tumour recurrence with immunosuppression.

Complications

Secondary bacterial cholangitis with or without a blocked stent.

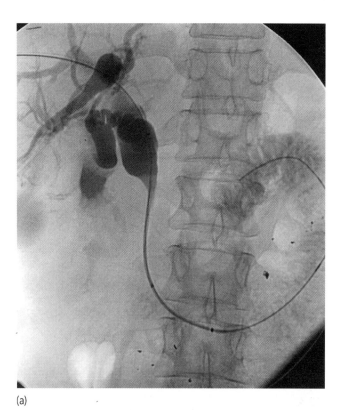

(a)

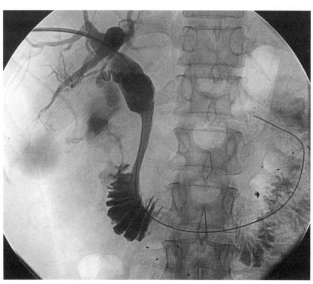

(b)

Fig. 51 (a) A high common bile duct stricture with dilated intrahepatic ducts above and a guidewire placed through the stricture percutaneously. (b) A metal stent has been placed through the stricture allowing contrast to pass through into the duodenum.

 The presence of cholangitis in the presence of a CBD stent usually indicates that the stent is blocked and is an indication for changing it, even if the liver biochemistry improves with treatment of the cholangitis.

Prognosis

This is poor with an overall survival rate of 40–53% at 1 year, and 10–19% at 2 years.

Disease associations

Primary sclerosing cholangitis.

 1 Mansfield JC, Griffin SM, Wadehra V, Matthewson K. A prospective evaluation of cytology from biliary strictures. *Gut* 1997; 40: 671–677.
2 Prat F, Chapat O, Ducot B *et al.* A randomised trial of endoscopic drainage methods for inoperable malignant strictures of the common bile duct. *Gastrointest Endosc* 1998; 47: 1–7.

2.5.3 PRIMARY SCLEROSING CHOLANGITIS

Aetiology/pathophysiology/pathology

There is diffuse inflammation and fibrosis involving the whole of the biliary tree, eventually leading to obliteration of bile ducts and a biliary cirrhosis with portal hypertension. The disease usually involves the intrahepatic ducts alone, but there may also be involvement of the extrahepatic duct and occasionally the disease is limited to the extrahepatic ducts. The aetiology is unknown, but the disease is probably immunologically mediated. There is an association with HLA DR3. Antibodies to perinuclear antineutrophil cytoplasmic antibody (ANCA) are non-specific but seen in 60–80% of cases [1].

Epidemiology

It has a prevalence of 6 per 100,000: 70% are male and the average age at diagnosis is 40 years.

Clinical presentations

These include:
* fatigue
* intermittent jaundice
* pruritus
* right upper quadrant pain
* no symptoms but abnormal liver biochemistry.

Physical signs

There are no signs in about 50% of symptomatic patients. Jaundice and hepatomegaly or splenomegaly may be present.

Investigations

Liver biochemistry

High ALP/GGT. Mild elevations in serum transaminases (AST/ALT). Bilirubin may be raised. A low

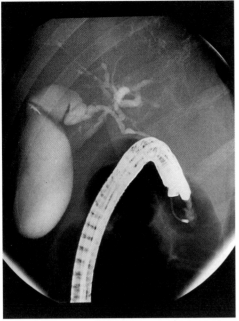

Fig. 52 ERCP showing the classical beading of the intrahepatic bile ducts seen in primary sclerosing cholangitis.

albumin and raised PT are only found in late stage disease (biliary cirrhosis).

Cholangiography (PTC or ERCP)

Multiple irregular stricturing and dilatation (beading) of intrahepatic ducts (Fig. 52), with or without extrahepatic stricture.

Liver biopsy

May be normal. Periductal onion skin fibrosis and inflammation with expansion of portal tracts, bile duct proliferation and portal oedema. Late progressive fibrosis with loss of bile ducts (Fig. 53).

Differential diagnosis

Secondary sclerosing cholangitis due to cytomegalovirus or cryptosporidium infection in AIDS, previous bile duct surgery, bile duct stones causing cholangitis.

Treatment

Short-term

There is no curative therapy.

Management of complications

Antibiotics (e.g. oral ciprofloxacin, which is excreted in bile) for cholangitis. Well defined extrahepatic biliary strictures can be stented or balloon dilated at ERCP.

Ursodeoxycholoic acid

Improves liver biochemistry but has no effect on histology or survival. Neither steroids, azathioprine, methotrexate nor cyclosporin have affected disease outcome.

Long-term

Liver transplantation

Indicated for end-stage biliary cirrhosis. Cholangiocarcinoma is a contraindication.

Complications

These include:
- cholangitis
- common bile duct or intrahepatic stones
- extrahepatic biliary strictures

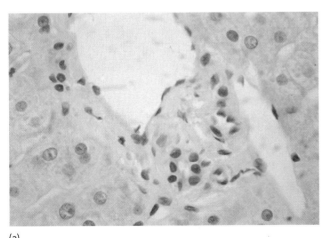
(a)

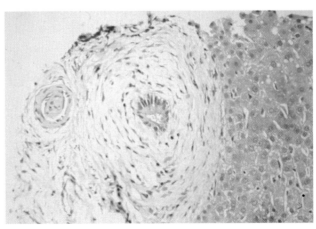
(b)

Fig. 53 A liver biopsy showing (a) normal portal tract (bile duct, hepatic artery and portal vein) and (b) periductal sclerosis, 'onion skin fibrosis' typical of primary sclerosing cholangitis.

- biliary cirrhosis with portal hypertension
- cholangiocarcinoma occurs in 10–30%; more commonly if the patient has ulcerative colitis.

Most of these complications present as increasing jaundice.

 It can be difficult to differentiate a benign biliary stricture from a cholangiocarcinoma, even after cholangiography and cytology of brushings from the stricture.

Prognosis

This is variable. In symptomatic patients the median survival from presentation to death or transplantation is 12 years; 75% of asymptomatic patients are alive at 15 years [2].

Disease associations

Five to ten per cent of patients with ulcerative colitis and 1% of those with Crohn's disease develop primary sclerosing cholangitis (PSC). Up to 70% of patients with PSC will have clinical or histological evidence of ulcerative colitis. The colitis may predate the diagnosis of PSC or present many years later.

 1 Mitchell SA, Chapman RW. Review article: the management of primary sclerosing cholangitis. *Aliment Pharmaocol Ther* 1997; 11: 33–43.
2 Broome U, Olsson R, Loof L *et al.* Natural history and prognostic factors in 305 Swedish patients with primary sclerosing cholangitis. *Gut* 1996; 38: 610–615.

2.5.4 PRIMARY BILIARY CIRRHOSIS

Aetiology/pathophysiology/pathology

There is progressive destruction of small intrahepatic bile ducts (smaller ducts than involved in PSC). This is thought to be immune mediated as there is a predominantly T-cell infiltration in the liver. Possible aetiological factors include failure of immune regulation, loss of tolerance, immune complex bile duct damage, and mitochondrial antibodies cross reacting with bacteria [1].

Epidemiology

Females account for 90% of cases and most present between the ages of 40 and 60. Prevalence is 25 per 100 000 in women >18 years.

Clinical presentations

Common

- Asymptomatic (diagnosed as a result of biochemical screening)
- Itching
- Lethargy.

Uncommon

- Jaundice
- Haematemesis (from varices)
- Abdominal distension (ascites)
- Confusion (hepatic encephalopathy).

Physical signs

Common

Initially none. Subsequently pigmentation, xanthelasma, hepatomegaly, scratch marks.

Uncommon

Late signs of portal hypertension (ascites and hepatic encephalopathy).

Investigations

Liver biochemistry

High ALP and mild increase in ALT. Rising bilirubin is a poor prognostic marker. Falling albumin and rising PT only occur at a very late stage in the disease as it is a biliary cirrhosis.

 The level of the alkaline phosphatase does not correlate with the extent of liver disease. Insidious progression to cirrhosis may occur without significant changes in liver blood tests.

Antimitochondrial antibody (AMA)

This is present in 95% of cases and is specific for PBC. Individuals with AMA and normal liver histology will eventually develop PBC. The antibody is specifically directed against E2 which is part of the pyruvate dehydrogenase complex that lies on the inner mitochondrial membrane.

Immunoglobulins

The IgM is often high.

Liver biopsy

The histology is of lymphoid aggregates and granuloma in portal tracts. There is bile duct damage and eventually bile duct loss. Progressive fibrosis results in a biliary cirrhosis (Fig. 54).

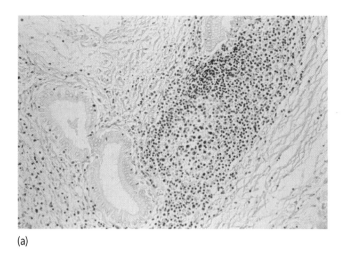

(a)

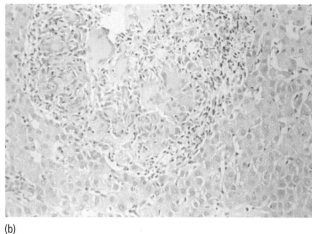

(b)

(c)

Fig. 54 Liver biopsy of a patient with primary biliary cirrhosis showing (a) portal tract with lymphocytic infiltration and loss of bile ducts, (b) granuloma and (c) progression to a biliary cirrhosis.

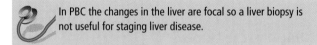

In PBC the changes in the liver are focal so a liver biopsy is not useful for staging liver disease.

Differential diagnosis

Large bile duct obstruction. Sclerosing cholangitis. Other causes of intrahepatic cholestasis (drugs, sepsis, total parenteral nutrition).

Treatment

Short-term

Ursodeoxycholic acid

Its role is controversial but it appears to delay time to transplantation and death in late stage disease [2]. It may improve itching. Treatment should be directed to symptomatic patients.

Other immunosuppressives

Steroids, azathiaprine and methotrexate have not been shown to be effective.

Itching

Responds to cholestyramine. If persistent other drugs which are worth trying include rifampicin, benzodiazepines and naltraxone (opiate antagonist).

Long-term

Liver transplantation

There is a 90–95% survival rate for end-stage liver disease. Recurrence in hepatic grafts occurs but this does not have an adverse effect on outcome in the first 5–10 years.

Complications

Common

Osteoporosis and portal hypertension in late disease.

Rare

Osteomalacia is rarely seen now.

Prognosis

Variable and unpredictable. Some asymptomatic patients may have a normal life expectancy. Symptoms generally develop within 2–7 years. Subsequent life expectancy varies from 2 to 10 years.

Disease associations

Other autoimmune conditions: rheumatoid arthritis, Calcinosis, Raynauds, Esophagus (hypomotility), Sclero-dactyly, Telangiectasia (CREST), hypothyroidism. Sicca syndrome (dry mouth and eyes). Coeliac disease.

1 Neuberger J. Primary biliary cirrhosis. *Lancet* 1997; 350: 875–879.
2 Poupon RE, Lindor KD, Cauch-Dudek K, Dickinson ER, Poupon R, Heathcote EJ. Combined analysis of randomised controlled trials of ursodeoxycholic acid in primary biliary cirrhosis. *Gastroenterol* 1997; 113: 884–890.

2.5.5 INTRAHEPATIC CHOLESTASIS

Intrahepatic cholestasis from sepsis

Jaundice associated with cholestatic liver biochemistry (elevated ALP and GGT) is common in patients with extrabiliary bacterial infections, particularly on the intensive care unit. Treatment is of the underlying condition and must be differentiated from cholestasis due to total parenteral nutrition, gallstones and drugs (e.g. flucloxacillin).

Trauner M, Meier PJ, Boyer JL. Molecular pathogenesis of cholestasis. *N Engl J Med* 1998; 339: 1217–1227.

2.6 Small bowel

2.6.1 COELIAC DISEASE

Aetiology/pathophysiology/pathology

Coeliac disease (gluten-sensitive enteropathy) is characterized by total or subtotal villous atrophy of the small intestinal mucosa due to an intolerance to gluten, a group of proteins present in wheat, barley and rye [1,2]. The aetiology of coeliac disease is unknown, but probably requires both environmental and genetic factors:
• Ten per cent of first-degree relatives of an affected individual have the disease.
• There is an association with the MHC class II markers HLA DR3 and HLA DQW2 that are present in 80–90% of Caucasians with the disease (but less than 0.1% of individuals with this haplotype actually develop coeliac disease).
• Tissue transglutaminase has recently been identified as the possible autoantigen [3].

The condition results in patchy damage to the small intestinal mucosa, with the proximal small bowel more severely affected. On stereomicroscopy, the villi are either absent (total villous atrophy) or blunted (subtotal or partial villous atrophy), with preservation of the crypts. Light microscopy demonstrates shortened or absent villi, but lengthened crypts (overall hypertrophied mucosa), with a plasma cell infiltrate in the lamina propria and the presence of intraepithelial lymphocytes.

Epidemiology

Its prevalence worldwide ranges from 1 : 300 (Galway, Ireland) to 1 : 12 800 (Greece), and is quoted as being approximately 1 : 2000 in the UK. Recent evidence, however, suggests that this is likely to be an underestimate, with the true prevalence in the UK probably as high as 1 : 200 [4]. It is extremely rare in Africa, and has not been described in China or the Caribbean. It occurs more commonly in females (2 : 1). In adults, diagnosis peaks in the fourth and fifth decades in women, and the fifth and sixth decades in men.

Coeliac disease may present for the first time in the seventh or eighth decade of life.

Clinical presentation

Symptoms and signs are as shown in Table 28.

The diagnosis of coeliac disease should be seriously considered in any patient with diarrhoea/steatorrhoea, and iron or folate deficiency anaemia.

Investigation

Histological

Histological examination of small bowel biopsies remains the gold standard for diagnosing coeliac disease, and must be performed if the condition is suspected. Previously jejunal material was obtained via a Crosby capsule, but now the standard technique is to obtain four (because of the patchy nature) duodenal biopsies.

Histological appearances of the duodenal biopsies are usually characteristic, but if the patient's symptoms and/or repeat duodenal biopsies fail to improve on a gluten-free diet (assuming compliance), other conditions should be considered.

Table 28 Symptoms and signs of coeliac disease (*denotes commonest signs and symptoms in infancy).

Common	Less common	Rare
Anaemia* (iron, folate or mixed deficiency, often found by chance)	Infertility/amenorrhoea	Neurological (peripheral neuropathy, cerebellar ataxia, etc.)
Diarrhoea* (typically pale, bulky, offensive and difficult to flush)	Bone pain (osteomalacia, osteoporosis)	Tetany (hypocalcaemia)
Weight loss*/failure to thrive*/short stature	Dermatitis herpetiformis	Rickets
Abdominal distension/abdominal pain*/bloating/borborygmi		Bruising and night-blindness (deficiencies of fat-soluble vitamins A and K)
Anorexia, nausea, vomiting*		Constipation
Aphthous oral ulceration, glossitis, stomatis		
General malaise, lethargy		
Mood change*, anxiety, depression		
Clubbing		

Blood tests

A full blood count may show anaemia (iron and/or folate deficiency) and the film a dimorphic population of red blood cells with Howell–Jolly bodies (associated hyposplenism). Liver function tests are often mildly abnormal, but correct after treatment.

Serology

Antigliaden antibodies are commonly present and the antiendomysial antibody test has a sensitivity and specificity of around 95%.

 Persistence of antiendomysial antibodies 6 weeks after starting dietary therapy suggests non-compliance.

Barium follow-through

This is often abnormal but is not normally needed to make the diagnosis. The normal fine feathery appearance of the mucosa is replaced by a coarser pattern (transverse barring) or a tubular, featureless appearance in severe disease.

Differential diagnosis

- If diarrhoea—giardiasis, infection, inflammatory bowel disease
- If abdominal pain and/or weight loss—Crohn's disease and thyrotoxicosis
- If steatorrhoea—exocrine pancreatic failure
- Iron-deficiency anaemia (see Section 1.17, pp. 48–49).

Other causes of villous atrophy:
- giardiasis
- hypogammaglobulinaemia
- bacterial overgrowth
- tropical sprue
- cow's milk sensitivity

- Whipple's disease
- lymphoma
- non-steroidal anti-inflammatory drugs.

Treatment

Gluten-free diet

Strict withdrawal of gluten from the diet is advocated. Physicians and dieticians should be involved in educating the patient about the condition, and membership of the Coeliac Society encouraged. Eighty-five per cent of cases respond to withdrawal of gluten from the diet, and relapse on its reintroduction.

Dietary supplementation

Iron, folate, vitamin D and calcium supplementation may be required at diagnosis depending on the degree of abnormality and symptoms.

 A small proportion of patients do not respond to a gluten-free diet (symptomatically and/or histologically). In these instances ask yourself:
- Is the patient truly compliant with the diet?
- Are there alternative diagnoses that also result in villous atrophy?
- Is there another or associated condition present (e.g. lactose intolerance, exocrine pancreatic insufficiency)?
- Has the patient developed small bowel lymphoma?

Immunosuppression

In those coeliacs who do not respond to dietary treatment, steroids and other immunosuppressants may induce remission.

Complications

These include:
- bone disease (osteoporosis and osteomalacia)

• increased risk of gastrointestinal malignancy (T-cell small bowel lymphoma, squamous cell carcinoma of the pharynx and oesophagus, and small intestinal adenocarcinoma)
• hyposplenism is common and related to duration and severity of disease, but rarely causes problems
• ulcerative enteritis, a rare complication that may be an early manifestation of malignant lymphoma.

 Osteopenia and osteoporosis are relatively common at diagnosis, but malignant complications are rare.

Prognosis

Mortality

Mortality is increased in coeliac disease, chiefly due to an excess of malignant disease [5]. Adoption of a gluten-free diet appears to protect against this complication, and results in a normal life-span.

Disease associations

Associated diseases include:
• type 1 diabetes mellitus
• primary biliary cirrhosis
• rheumatoid arthritis
• thyroid disease
• inflammatory bowel disease
• IgA deficiency
• IgA mesangial nephropathy
• epilepsy with cerebral calcification
• sarcoidosis
• Down's syndrome.

Important information for patients

Condition and complications usually 'cured' by permanent adoption of strict gluten-free diet. Advise to join Coeliac society.

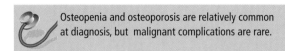 British Society for Gastroenterology Guidelines for Management of Coeliac Disease: http://www.bsg.org.uk/guidelines.

1 Howdle PD (ed.) Coeliac disease. *Baillière's Clin Gastroenterol* 1995; 9 (no. 2).
2 Hadjivassiliou M, Grunewald RA, Davies-Jones GAB. Gluten sensitivity: a many headed hydra. *BMJ* 1999; 318: 1710–1711.
3 Dieterich W, Ehnis T, Bauer M *et al.* Identification of tissue transglutaminase as the autoantigen of celiac disease. *Nat Med* 1997; 3: 797–801.
4 Hin H, Bird G, Fisher P, Mahy N, Jewell D. Coeliac disease in primary care: case finding study. *BMJ* 1999; 318: 164–167.
5 Logan RFA, Rifkind EA, Rutner ID, Ferguson A. Mortality in coeliac disease. *Gastroenterol* 1989; 97: 265–271.

2.6.2 BACTERIAL OVERGROWTH

Aetiology/pathophysiology/pathology

Akin to fresh water in a free flowing river, and stagnant water in a pond, bacterial overgrowth is promoted by any condition that impedes the normal flow of intestinal contents and therefore promotes stagnation.

The normal small intestine is not sterile, but houses $<10^4$ organisms/mL. In bacterial overgrowth the figure rises to 10^4–10^9 organisms/mL. The mechanisms by which bacterial overgrowth produce diarrhoea (usually steatorrhoea) are not completely clear. Deconjugation of bile salts by bacteria may interfere with fat micelle formation and thus impair fat absorption. Other mechanisms may include direct damage to the enterocytes or brush border enzymes, or indirect damage by the deconjugated bile salts. Bacteria also metabolize B_{12}.

Epidemiology

Incidence and prevalence are unknown but may be decreasing as a result of reduced surgical intervention for peptic ulcer disease.

Clinical presentation

Common

Diarrhoea (usually steatorrhoea).

Uncommon

Neurological disorder, e.g. peripheral neuropathy, subacute combined degeneration of the spinal cord (secondary to B_{12} deficiency).

Physical signs

None due to bacterial overgrowth *per se*. Look for neuropathy and associated diseases, e.g. Crohn's, previous peptic ulcer disease surgery.

Investigation

 Bacterial overgrowth

Be alert to the diagnosis in patients developing diarrhoea who have a predisposition for this problem, e.g. those with structural abnormalities of the small bowel.

Jejunal aspiration and culture

Although this is the gold standard for diagnosis, it is an invasive and rarely used test.

Glucose or lactulose hydrogen breath test

This is used in preference to an aspirate to make the diagnosis. Glucose is absorbed completely in the upper small bowel; if bacteria are present they will metabolize glucose to H_2 and cause a rise in breath H_2. Lactulose is a non-absorbable synthetic dissacharide that is metabolized by colonic bacteria. Bacterial overgrowth of the small bowel causes an early rise, but false positives may occur with rapid small intestinal transit.

Small bowel follow-through

In those patients who do not have a known underlying structural small bowel abnormality, small bowel radiology is indicated to look for diverticula.

Differential diagnosis

Other causes of diarrhoea and steatorrhoea.

Treatment

Cyclical rotating courses of antibiotics, e.g. tetracycline and metronidazole. B_{12} injections may be required. (See Section 1.11, p. 34.)

Complications

Malnutrition, neuropathy, deficiencies of fat-soluble vitamins.

Prognosis

Often a chronic recurring condition unless cyclical antibiotics are employed because most of the predisposing conditions are not correctable. Morbidity probably mostly due to lack of diagnosis. Unlikely to have any effect on mortality.

Disease associations

See Table 29.

Table 29 Causes of bacterial overgrowth.

Anatomical	Functional	Immune deficiency
Surgical blind loops	Autonomic neuropathy	Hypogammaglobulinaemia
Bilroth II	Amyloid	Achlorhydria
Roux-en-Y	Diabetes	
Jejunal diverticulae	mellitus	
Strictures	Systemic sclerosis	
Crohn's disease		
Radiation		
Enterocolic fistulae		

1 Farthing MJG. Bacterial overgrowth of the small intestine. In: Misiewicz JJ, Pounder RE, Venables CW, eds. *Diseases of the Gut and Pancreas*, 2nd edn. Oxford: Blackwell Scientific Publications, 1993.

2.6.3 OTHER CAUSES OF MALABSORPTION

Chronic pancreatitis

May occur following repeated acute attacks of pancreatitis, or without any identifiable cause. Alcohol is the most common culprit cystic fibrosis and α_1-antitrypsin deficiency other causes. Steatorrhoea develops when less than 10% of pancreatic exocrine function remains. ERCP is the gold standard for diagnosis. Pancreatic function tests may be helpful (Pancrealauryl). Pancreatic enzyme supplements are titrated against response.

Whipple's disease

A rare disease caused by *Tropheryma whippelli* that usually occurs in white middle-aged or elderly males. It is characterized by malabsorption, migratory polyarthritis, anaemia and weight loss. Neurological and cardiac involvement may occur, as well as pigmentation and clubbing. Jejunal biopsy shows large 'foamy' macrophages in lamina propria that contain positive periodic acid–Schiff staining material. Treatment is for 1 year with sulphamethoxazole and trimethoprim. Prognosis is good.

Tropical sprue

Occurs in residents of the tropics—India, Asia, Central America—but is rare in Africa. It usually follows an acute diarrhoeal illness. There is persistent bacterial overgrowth in the small bowel, resulting typically in steatorrhoea, weight loss, anaemia, hypoproteinaemia and glossitis. Small bowel biopsy (jejunal) shows partial villous atrophy and round cell infiltration of the lamina propria. Untreated, the mortality is 10–20% within months. It responds readily to tetracycline 250 mg q.d.s. and folic acid 5 mg t.d.s.

Giardiasis

Caused by the flagellated protozoan *Giardia lambia*. It is usually contracted abroad, though it can occur in UK. It has faecal—oral transmission and is characterized by persistent diarrhoea after an acute diarrhoeal episode. Malabsorption is unusual but can occur. Diagnosis is made by finding trophozoites in jejunal aspiration and biopsy (stool culture is less sensitive). Tinidazole 2 g as a single dose or metronidazole 800 mg t.d.s. for 3 days is very effective.

Hypolactasia

Primary hypolactasia is common in most races apart from North Europeans. Lactase, a brush border enzyme that breaks lactose into glucose and galactose, disappears after weaning. Subsequent lactose ingestion (milk) causes an osmotic diarrhoea. It is diagnosed on clinical grounds, or by lactose H_2 breath test.

Secondary hypolactasia is caused by anything that damages the small bowel mucosa (e.g. viral gastroenteritis, coeliac disease, Crohn's disease), and reverses on treatment of the underlying disorder.

Short bowel syndrome

Malabsorption occurs when the effective small intestinal length is reduced to less than 100 cm by surgical resection, mesenteric infarction, severe Crohn's disease or radiation injury. The absorptive capacity is overwhelmed and diarrhoea and malabsorption ensues. Adaptation occurs, with improvement for up to 2 years. The colon contributes to energy supplies via fermentation of non-absorbed dietary fibre to short-chain fatty acids which are then absorbed.

Post gastric surgery

Frank malabsorption following gastric surgery is rare. Iron deficiency is common. The cause is multifactoral and includes hypoacidity, chronic bleeding from friable anastomosis and decreased intake. B_{12} deficiency may also occur due to lack of intrinsic factor, or bacterial overgrowth. Frank malabsorption is due to steatorrhoea, which is attributed to an impaired pancreatic response (due either to bypassing the duodenum in a Bilroth II gastrectomy, vagal denervation, or rapid gastric emptying preventing optimal mixing with pancreatic juices).

2.7 Large bowel

 Colorectal cancer remains a major cause of death worldwide. It commonly presents at an advanced stage with complications such as colonic obstruction or perforation.
A recognition that the majority of colorectal cancers arise within adenomatous polyps of the colon (Fig. 55) has led to a greater emphasis on early diagnosis (see Section 2.16, pp. 127–128).

2.7.1 ADENOMATOUS POLYPS OF THE COLON

Aetiology/pathophysiology/pathology

Benign neoplastic polyps. The risk of subsequent carcinoma is increased in polyps greater than 1 cm in diameter, and those with villous architecture or severe dysplasia.

Clinical presentation

Common

Incidental finding at colonoscopy.

Uncommon/rare

Iron-deficiency anaemia. Rectal bleeding.

Differential diagnosis

Not all colonic polyps are neoplastic or carry a significantly increased risk of colorectal cancer.

Hyperplastic polyps

These are diminutive polyps, usually less than 5 mm in diameter found in the distal colon and rectum. They are not neoplastic and carry no significant risk of colorectal cancer.

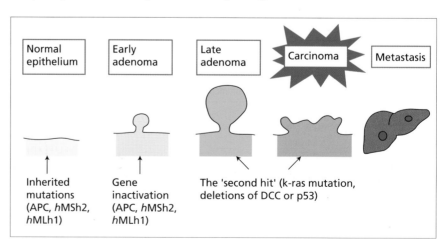

Fig. 55 The colonic adenoma carcinoma sequence. DCC, deleted in colon cancer; APC, *h*MLH1, *h*MSH2 are genes.

Hamartomatous polyps

These are associated with Peutz–Jeghers syndrome. Hamartomatous polyps are not themselves neoplastic, although there is an increased risk of gastrointestinal tumours in these patients.

Inflammatory pseudopolyps

These are seen in longstanding colitis (Crohn's disease, ulcerative colitis) and are not neoplastic.

Treatment

Colonoscopic polypectomy is recommended for all adenomatous polyps.

Complications

Colorectal carcinoma.

2.7.2 COLORECTAL CARCINOMA

 Colorectal cancer is a major public health problem in the developed world. Increasing efforts are being directed towards identifying the condition early in individuals considered to be at risk.

Aetiology/pathophysiology/pathology

There are several conditions that are recognized to predispose to colorectal cancer. (See *Oncology*, Section 2.3.)

Adenomatous polyps of the colon

Tubulovillous adenomas carry an increased risk of colorectal cancer. It is generally felt that colorectal cancer usually develops in pre-existing adenomatous polyps in the colon (Fig. 55, p. 94).

Ulcerative colitis

Longstanding total ulcerative colitis predisposes to colorectal cancer and patients with a 10-year history of total colitis should be offered 2-yearly surveillance colonoscopy with random colonic biopsies taken to detect histological dysplasia.

Family history

There is a family history in 14% of new cases of colorectal cancer. A greater understanding of the genetic predisposition to colorectal cancer is resulting in an increasing number of individuals referred for colonoscopic screening/surveillance (Table 30).

Table 30 Family history and lifetime risk of colorectal cancer. There is benefit of surveillance colonoscopy at risk of 1 : 12 or greater.

Family history of CRC	Lifetime risk
None	1 : 40
One first-degree relative >45 years	1 : 17
One first-degree and one second-degree relative	1 : 12
One first-degree relative <45 years	1 : 10
Two first-degree relatives (any age)	1 : 6
Dominant inheritance (e.g. HNPCC)	1 : 2

CRC, colorectal cancer; HNPCC, hereditary non-polyposis colon cancer syndromes.

Familial cancer syndromes

There are some rare but important hereditary cancer syndromes [1,2]:
• *Familial adenomatous polyposis (FAP)*. Autosomal dominant. Hundreds of adenomatous polyps are seen throughout the colon and evident from an early age. The risk of neoplasia is such that prophylactic colectomy is performed before the age of 20.
• *Hereditary non-polyposis colon cancer (HNPCC)*. This is inherited in an autosomal dominant fashion and is due to mutations in DNA mismatch repair genes. Individuals at risk are offered colonoscopic screening.

Epidemiology

The incidence of colorectal cancer increases with age and overall this has increased over the last 50 years. Colorectal cancer now accounts for 20 000 deaths per year in the UK.

Clinical presentation

Common

• Change in bowel habit—new-onset constipation or 'spurious' diarrhoea
• Large bowel obstruction—constipation, pain and vomiting
• Iron deficiency
• Rectal bleeding.

Uncommon

Evidence of metastatic disease (ascites).

Rare

Anorexia and weight loss.

Physical signs

Common

In most cases there will be no diagnostic physical signs.

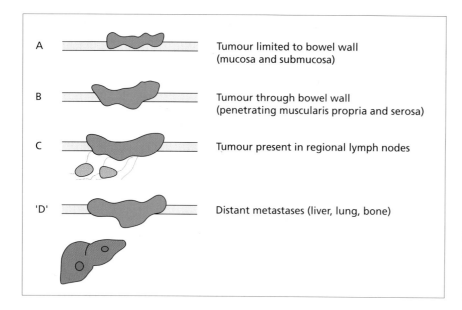

A   Tumour limited to bowel wall (mucosa and submucosa)

B   Tumour through bowel wall (penetrating muscularis propria and serosa)

C   Tumour present in regional lymph nodes

'D'   Distant metastases (liver, lung, bone)

Fig. 56 Dukes staging for colorectal carcinoma. Originally used for the staging of rectal cancer but now widely adopted for colorectal cancer in general. Stage D was not originally described by Dukes.

Uncommon

- Palpable abdominal mass
- Signs of iron deficiency—pallor, koilonychia, glossitis
- Signs of metastatic disease—hepatomegaly, ascites.

Investigation/staging

Dukes staging of colonic carcinoma (Fig. 56).

Blood tests

Blood count, iron indices—may demonstrate iron-deficiency anaemia.

 Liver blood tests may be normal or there may be an isolated elevation in alkaline phosphatase (may be >1000 IU/L) in the presence of liver metastases.

Tumour markers

Carcinoembryonic antigen (CEA). This tumour marker is not useful for diagnosis but may be useful in monitoring the patient's response to treatment and for the identification of disease relapse.

Colonoscopy

Total examination of the colon should be undertaken, even in instances of proven distal tumours, to exclude the presence of synchronous tumours or polyps. If this has not been performed prior to resection it ought to be done subsequently.

Barium enema

This remains a common investigation in patients presenting with a symptomatic change in bowel habit (Fig. 57).

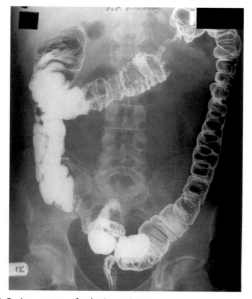

Fig. 57 Barium enema of colonic carcinoma.

If the appearances are unequivocal and there are signs of impending bowel obstruction a tissue diagnosis before laparotomy is unnecessary.

Liver ultrasound, abdominal CT

To identify metastatic disease. Although surgery is required in most cases it is often useful to identify whether or not the patient has metastatic disease prior to laparotomy.

Differential diagnosis

Of change in bowel habit:
- diverticular change
- irritable bowel syndrome.

Of iron deficiency:
- peptic ulceration
- coeliac disease

- upper gastrointestinal neoplasia
- colonic angiodysplasia.

Of rectal bleeding:
- haemorrhoids—usually cause fresh red blood visible on the toilet paper and the surface of the stool
- diverticular disease—usually produces heavy, acute colonic bleeding rather than chronic persistent blood loss
- distal colitis.

Treatment

Emergency

Acute large intestinal obstruction is a surgical emergency with a high risk of caecal perforation (see Section 1.9, p. 30).

Short-term

Surgery

This is required in most cases of colorectal cancer. The extent of bowel resection depends on the site of the tumour. Attempts are made to resect at least 5 cm of normal bowel either side of the tumour.

Palliative approaches

Although surgery is the usual treatment for patients with impending colonic obstruction, stenting of tumours with self-expanding metal stents offers an alternative approach for the palliative relief of obstruction.

Long-term or according to stage

Chemotherapy

Treatment with 5-fluorouracil (5-FU) improves survival for Dukes B and C cancers.

Radiotherapy

Pre-operative radiotherapy to 'down-stage' rectal tumours reduces local recurrence but has limited effect on survival.

Complications

Common

Large bowel obstruction and metastatic disease.

Prognosis

Mortality

Prognosis following surgery depends on the histological

Table 31 Five-year survival after resection of colorectal cancer.

Duke's stage	5-year survival
A	95–100%
B	65–75%
C	30–40%
Distant metastases	<1%

grade of the tumour and the Dukes stage (Fig. 56 and Table 31).

Prevention

See Section 2.16, pp. 127–128.

1 Terdiman JP, Conrad PG, Sleisenger MH. Genetic testing in hereditary colorectal cancer: indications and procedures. *Am J Gastroenterol* 1999; 94: 2344–2356.
2 Lynch HT, Watson P, Shaw TG *et al*. Clinical impact of molecular genetic diagnosis, genetic counselling and management of hereditary cancer. Part II hereditary non-polyposis colorectal carcinoma as a model. *Cancer* 1999; 86: 2457–2463.

2.7.3 DIVERTICULAR DISEASE

Aetiology/pathophysiology/pathology

Although there are suspicions that there may be an underlying genetic predisposition to diverticular disease, it is best considered as an acquired condition. Diverticula form as herniations of colonic mucosa through the muscularis. This process tends to occur more commonly in the distal colon and usually occurs at the point of entry of penetrating blood vessels through the muscle layers (hence the presentation with acute haemorrhage) [1,2].

Epidemiology

The prevalence of diverticular disease of the colon increases with age: it is present in 50% of the population over the age of 50.

Clinical presentation

Common

Diverticula are common in elderly people and often asymptomatic. Presentation is usually in the form of one of the common complications:
- *Diverticulitis.* An associated inflammation of the colon, often related to infection which is thought to result from impaction of faeces within a diverticulum.
- *Colonic bleeding.* This is a frequent presentation of diverticular disease. This is thought to result from the fact that diverticula form at the point of maximal weakness in the colon, i.e. at the point where blood vessels penetrate the muscle coat.

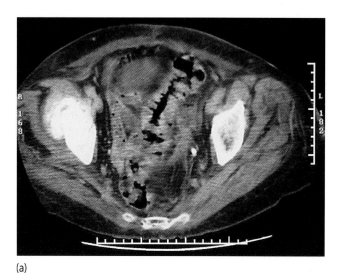

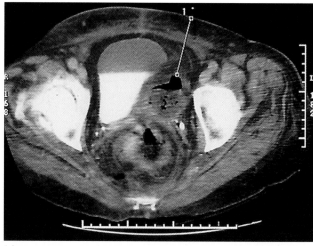

(a)   (b)

Fig. 58 Diverticular disease: (a) CT scan showing a loop of bowel (lumen in black) with diverticula; (b) adjacent collection (identified by tip of white marker line) due to a perforated diverticulum adjacent to the bladder.

Uncommon

This includes:

- diverticular abscess
- colovesical fistula
- colonic stricture—after repeated episodes of inflammation the colon may become strictured, resulting in subacute colonic obstruction.

Physical signs

There are no specific external physical signs of diverticular change itself.

Investigation

Barium enema/colonoscopy

Asymptomatic diverticular change may be demonstrated by either barium enema or colonoscopy.

Abdominal CT

Computerized tomography (CT) is the best way to demonstrate abscess formation (Fig. 58). Colovesical fistulae require a high index of suspicion (recurrent urinary tract infections, pneumaturia, etc.) but may be identified on barium contrast radiology (Fig. 59).

Differential diagnosis

This includes:

- colonic carcinoma
- colonic ischaemia
- inflammatory bowel disease.

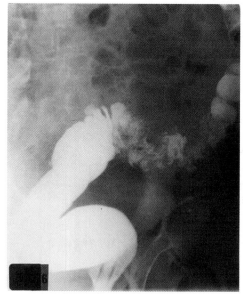

Fig. 59 Fistulae complicating diverticular disease.

Treatment

Short-term

The management of diverticular disease is often conservative. Treatment of complications:

- Acute diverticulitis requires intravenous fluids, antibiotics and analgesics.
- Diverticular abscess may require drainage in addition to the above.
- Bleeding will usually settle with supportive treatment.

Long-term

- A high-fibre diet is recommended in the belief that this may reduce the risk of complications.

- Surgery is usually reserved for complicated diverticular disease (i.e. bleeding, abscess, stricture).

Prognosis

Morbidity

Many patients experience recurrent diverticulitis or bleeding.

Mortality

Diverticular change is not a progressive pathology and there is no increased risk of colonic neoplasia.

1 Stollman NH, Raskin JB. Diverticular disease of the colon. *J Clin Gastroenterol* 1999; 29: 241–251.
2 Stollman NH, Raskin JB. Diagnosis and management of diverticular disease of the colon in adults. Ad hoc practice parameters committee of the American College of Gastroenterology. *Am J Gastroenterol* 1999; 94: 3110–3121.

2.7.4 INTESTINAL ISCHAEMIA

Aetiology/pathophysiology/pathology

As with vascular disease elsewhere in the body, the gut is prone to ischaemia from either progressive atheromatous narrowing of the mesenteric arteries or thromboembolism from intracardiac or proximal vascular sources [1,2].

Epidemiology

Vascular disease in general is increasing in most developed countries.
  Risk factors include:
- age
- male sex
- family history
- smoking
- diabetes
- hypertension
- hyperlipidaemia.

Clinical presentation

Common

Ischaemic colitis

Bloody diarrhoea, usually of sudden onset and associated with abdominal pain.

Ischaemia usually affects the splenic flexure of the colon. This represents the 'watershed' between areas supplied by the superior and inferior mesenteric arteries.

Small bowel infarction

This is usually due to arterial embolism and presents as an acute abdomen, often with severe systemic disturbance (hypotension, acidosis).

Uncommon

Mesenteric angina—recurrent postprandial abdominal pain.

Physical signs

These include:
- other features of atheroma—arcus, xanthelasma
- potential sources of arterial embolism—atrial fibrillation, heart valve disease
- abdominal bruits and other evidence of vascular disease.

Investigation

Helpful tests include:
- Plain abdominal radiograph, which may show aortic calcification and colonic mucosal oedema, often with thumb-printing. This may be of relatively limited distribution compared to other forms of colitis (e.g. the distal transverse colon and splenic flexure).
- Flexible sigmoidoscopy/colonoscopy.
- Mesenteric angiography.

Differential diagnosis

This includes:
- colorectal carcinoma
- diverticular change
- inflammatory bowel disease.

Treatment

Acute intestinal infarction often requires emergency surgery and resection. Lesser degrees of ischaemia (e.g. ischaemic colitis) are usually managed conservatively.

Complications

Intestinal strictures and obstruction.

Prognosis

Excess mortality is associated with other features of vascular disease (ischaemic heart disease, stroke, renal failure, etc.).

1 Gandhi SK, Hanson MM, Vernava AM, Kaminsk DL, Longo WE. Ischaemic colitis. *Dis Colon Rectum* 1996; 39: 88–100.
2 Toursarkissian B, Thompson RW. Ischaemic colitis. *Surg Clin N Am* 1997; 77: 461–470.

2.7.5 ANORECTAL DISEASE

Aetiology/pathophysiology/pathology

Haemorrhoids (piles)

'Varicose' perianal veins. Associated with chronic constipation and straining at stool.

Anal fissure

Tear in anal mucosa associated with straining and passage of a very hard constipated stool.

Fistula-in-ano

A fistulous tract originating in the rectum and opening onto the perineum or into other pelvic organs (most commonly the vagina).

Solitary rectal ulcer

Ulceration of the anterior rectal wall due to excessive straining.

Clinical presentation

Haemorrhoids

Common findings are:
• *Rectal bleeding*. Usually bright red blood seen on the toilet paper. Sometimes dramatic bleeding.
• *Perianal irritation*. Itching.
• *Pain*. Usually associated with thrombosis.

Anal fissure

• *Anal pain on defaecation*.
• *Constipation* which is sometimes secondary to the pain associated with defaecation.

Fistula-in-ano

• *Discharge*. Pus, mucus and blood may discharge spontaneously onto the perineum.
• *Pain*. Persistent pain usually represents a complicating abscess.

Solitary rectal ulcer

• *Tenesmus and rectal bleeding*.

Investigation

Haemorrhoids

Proctoscopy

This is the investigation of choice.

Sigmoidoscopy

Sigmoidoscopy (rigid or flexible) is necessary to exclude other causes of rectal bleeding (proctitis, rectal cancer, polyps, etc.). In some circumstances investigation of the more proximal colon by barium enema or colonoscopy may be necessary.

Anal fissure

Sigmoidoscopy and examination under anaesthetic.

Fistula-in-ano

Sigmoidoscopy

This may be very uncomfortable for the patient and may provide only limited information.

Examination under anaesthetic (EUA)

This allows thorough sigmoidoscopy and the probing of any identified tracts.

MRI

This is of increasing utility in delineating the course of fistulae and identifying associated abscess cavities.

Solitary rectal ulcer

Sigmoidoscopy and rectal biopsy.

Treatment

Haemorrhoids

Therapeutic options include:
• *Conservative*. Simple advice on diet, use of aperients and toilet habits.
• *Injection sclerotherapy*. With phenol.
• *Banding*. Now replacing injection therapy.
• *Surgery*. Haemorrhoidectomy is reserved for very troublesome haemorrhoids.

Anal fissure

Conservative

Give advice on diet and hydration to avoid constipation.

Glyceryl trinitrate (GTN) paste

When applied to the anus this leads to reduction in anal sphincter tone and healing of fissures.

Surgery

Lateral sphincterotomy performed for resistant cases.

Fistula-in-ano

Conservative

Give advice on diet and hydration to avoid constipation.

Seton drain

A plastic seton drain placed through a fistula will keep the tract open and prevent the recurrent formation of abscess.

Fistulotomy

Superficial fistulae may be laid open.

Defunctioning stoma

In very severe cases it may be necessary to perform either a sigmoid colostomy or a split ileostomy.

Solitary rectal ulcer

Conservative—advice on diet and hydration to avoid constipation.

Complications

Fistula-in-ano

Incontinence—fistulae that pass through the anal sphincter may result in long-term faecal incontinence.

Disease associations

Fistula-in-ano

Crohn's disease—should always be considered in patients with recurrent or complex perianal fistulae.

2.8 Irritable bowel

 The term irritable bowel syndrome is widely (and often loosely) used but has relatively limited clinical value. It represents one of many functional syndromes of gut sensitivity and/or motility that may affect any part of the gastrointestinal tract (Table 32). In practice the common link between these conditions is that they have a combination of characteristic symptom complexes and in any one patient there are no features (either clinical or biochemical) to suggest any progressive intestinal pathology.

Aetiology/pathophysiology/pathology

The hallmark of the functional gastrointestinal disorders is altered (usually increased) visceral sensitivity. Some evidence suggests that this may be associated with increased release of 5HT from enterochromaffin cells in the gut, whilst other studies have identified central (psychosocial, neurohumoral) factors.

Epidemiology

The prevalence of the functional bowel disorders depends entirely on definition. It is estimated that only 10–50% of patients with functional gut symptoms consult medical practitioners, yet this represents as much as 5% of all general practice consultations in the UK. Within the group that do consult their doctor there is an excess of individuals that harbour fear of serious disease.

Table 32 The functional gastrointestinal disorders.

Classification	Examples
Oesophageal disorders	Globus Functional heartburn Functional dysphagia
Gastroduodenal disorders	Functional dyspepsia Functional vomiting
Bowel disorders	Irritable bowel syndrome Functional constipation Functional diarrhoea
Functional abdominal pain	
Biliary disorders	Sphincter of Oddi dysfunction
Anorectal disorders	Functional faecal incontinence Proctalgia fugax
Functional paediatric disorders	

Clinical presentation

Common

The agreed definition of the irritable bowel syndrome comprises [1]: 'At least 12 weeks, which need not be consecutive, in the preceding 12 months of abdominal discomfort or pain that has two of the following three features:
• relieved with defaecation; and/or
• onset associated with a change in frequency of stool; and/or
• onset associated with a change in form (appearance) of stool.'
This rather rigid definition does not take into account other symptoms which are commonly reported:
• bloating
• marked gastrocolic reflex (i.e. the need to defaecate shortly after eating)
• identifiable dietary precipitants.

There are some clinical features that should not be put down to a functional cause without careful further investigation. These include:
• dysphagia
• anorexia and/or weight loss
• mouth ulcers
• nocturnal diarrhoea
• rectal bleeding.

Physical signs

There are no characteristic physical signs.

Investigation

The extent of clinical investigation to exclude a progressive intestinal pathology must be tailored to each individual patient. A detailed history (including a good dietary history) is central to both the correct clinical diagnosis and the subsequent management. Investigations depend largely on the patient's particular symptom complex. At the very least a full blood count and ESR should be performed.

Differential diagnosis

The following should always be considered:
• coeliac disease
• hypolactasia
• inflammatory bowel disease
• giardiasis
• depressive illness
• gastrointestinal malignancy.

Treatment

A thorough history and physical examination—the most important part of the management is to listen to the patient. Often the 'qualified reassurance' of being told that there is no objective evidence of physical disease is sufficient to lead to an improvement in symptoms (or at least the resulting concern).

Antispasmodic drugs

Mebeverine or alverine are useful in patients with colicky abdominal pain.

Peppermint oil preparations

Colpermin may benefit those with bloating.

Sedative antidepressants

Low doses of tricyclic drugs such as amytriptyline may help those with depressive features (low mood, anhedonia, rumination, poor sleep, etc.).

Dietary measures

Patients resistant to the above measures, or those with clearly identifiable dietary intolerances, may benefit from dietary intervention (low lactose diet, exclusion diet). Many patients with an irritable bowel find that their symptoms worsen with a high-fibre diet [2].

New agents

Early trials of 5-HT3 receptor antagonists (e.g. Alosetron) suggested that these may be beneficial in some patients [3]. However, concerns about ischaemic colitis as a side effect has led to withdrawal of this compound.

Prognosis

Most patients will continue to have intermittent gastrointestinal symptoms and some may develop more overt psychiatric problems. There is no excess mortality associated with the diagnosis.

1 Rome II: A Multinational Consensus Document on Functional Gastrointestinal Disorders. *Gut* 1999; 45 (Suppl. II).
2 King TS, Elia M, Hunter JO. Abnormal colonic fermentation in irritable bowel syndrome. *Lancet* 1998; 352: 1187–1189.
3 Camilleri M, Mayer E A, Drossmond A *et al.* Improvement in pain and bowel function in female irritable bowel patients with alosetron, a 5-HT3 receptor antagonist. *Aliment Pharmacol Ther* 1999; 13: 1149–1159.

2.9 Acute liver disease

2.9.1 HEPATITIS A

Aetiology/pathology

Hepatitis A is an RNA virus that can cause acute hepatitis and is spread by the faecal–oral route. Figure 60 shows the histological picture of acute viral hepatitis.

Epidemiology

Hepatitis A is the commonest cause of viral hepatitis in the UK, with an incidence of symptomatic disease of about 6 per 100 000, most commonly between the ages of 20 and 45. The incubation period is between 15 and 45 days. Most cases are sporadic. Asymptomatic disease is common in childhood. Five per cent of the population will be immune by 5 years of age and 74% of people over the age of 50 are immune in the UK. Better sanitation means age of first exposure is increasing.

Clinical presentation

Common

Most cases are asymptomatic, with symptoms and severe disease more common with increasing age. If symptomatic the presentation is of an acute hepatitis with non-specific symptoms of lethargy, arthralgia, anorexia, nausea and mild upper quadrant discomfort (prodrome) followed by jaundice. The latter is associated with pale stools and dark urine. Itching can occur in the cholestatic phase of illness.

Physical signs

Common

Those of an acute hepatitis: tender mild hepatomegaly, jaundice.

Uncommon

Splenomegaly in 15%.

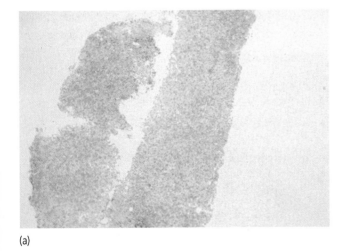

(a)

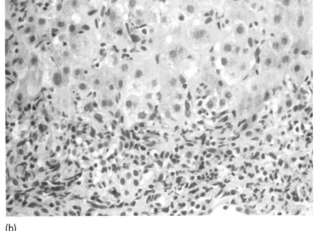

(b)

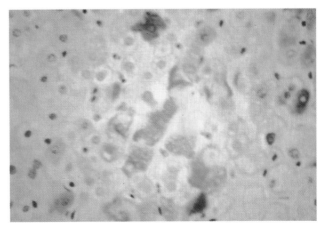

(c)

Fig. 60 Histology of acute viral hepatitis. (a) Unlike cirrhosis the normal hepatic architecture is preserved. (b) Higher power showing mixed (neutrophil and polymorphonucleocyte) portal tract inflammation and infiltration of the lobule. Other findings are hepatocyte necrosis and ballooning of hepatocytes (c) Hepatitis B infection with positive immunohistochemical staining for HBsAg in hepatocytes.

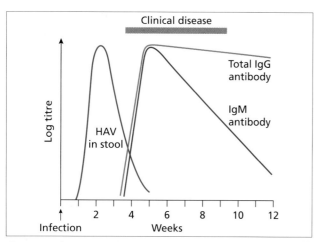

Fig. 61 Serology in acute hepatitis A. HAV, hepatitis A virus.

Table 33 Differential diagnosis of acute liver disease.

Common	Uncommon
Viral hepatitis	Halothane
Hepatitis A	Liver infiltration (adenocarcinoma/
Hepatitis B	lymphoma)
Non-A non-B non-C	Venous hepatic outflow obstruction
Drugs	Pregnancy-associated liver disease
Paracetamol	
NSAIDs	
Flucloxacillin/augmentin	
Dextropropoxyphene	
Alcoholic hepatitis	
Autoimmune chronic	
active hepatitis	

Investigations

Liver biochemistry

High serum transaminases (peak usually >1000 IU/L) with or without raised serum bilirubin. Alkaline phosphatase raised in cholestatic phase. Normal albumin.

Serology

The presence of Hepatitis A IgM indicates a recent infection (Fig. 61).

Differential diagnosis

See Table 33.

Treatment

This is supportive, with intravenous fluids if vomiting. Rare cases of acute liver failure need special management.

Complications

A cholestatic phase is common, can last between 12 and 18 weeks, and is associated with rising bilirubin level (i.e. 400–500 μmol/L) and alkaline phosphatase level and falling serum transaminases.
Relapsing disease is rare, occurring in 6%.

Prognosis

Morbidity

Hepatitis A is self-limiting with no residual liver damage. Symptoms and signs usually resolve within 3 weeks. Acute liver failure occurs in 0.14–0.35% [1].

Mortality

Death occurs in 0.04% of patients with symptomatic disease.

Prevention

Passive immunization

Pooled serum immunoglobulin can be given to close contacts of a case of hepatitis A within 2 weeks of exposure.

Active immunization

Formalin inactivated vaccine is indicated for travellers to high-risk areas, homosexuals and intravenous drug users. It lasts 5–10 years.

See *Infectious diseases*, Section 2.10.8.
1 Willner IR, Uhl MD, Howard SC, Williams EQ, Riely CA, Waters B. Serious hepatitis A: an analysis of patients hospitalized during an urban epidemic in the United States. *Ann Intern Med* 1998; 128: 111–114.

2.9.2 HEPATITIS B

Aetiology/pathophysiology/pathology

Hepatitis B is a double-stranded DNA virus. The e antigen is a protein subunit of the core of the virus that is excreted by hepatocytes. Excess surface antigen is also found free in serum.

The histological picture is of an acute hepatitis with liver damage due to immune clearance of the virus.

Epidemiology

Horizontal transmission is via parenteral transmission and sexual contact, and probably by close contact in young

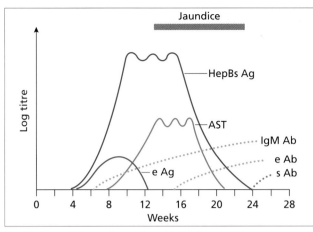

Fig. 62 Natural history of acute hepatitis B infection. AST, aspartate transaminases.

Table 34 Serological markers of hepatitis B infection.

	HBsAg	HBeAg	HBsAb	HBcAb (IgG)
Acute hepatitis B	+	+		
Resolved acute infection	–	–	+	+/–
Vaccination			+	–

children. Vertical transmission accounts for the high rates of infection worldwide. The prevalence is falling, although worldwide there are still 350 million chronic carriers.

Clinical presentations

Common

Most infected individuals are asymptomatic. Up to 4 months after exposure there may be self-limiting jaundice, which rarely lasts more than 1 month (Fig. 62).

Rare

Unlike hepatitis A, a cholestatic phase and relapses are uncommon. There are extrahepatic associations due to the presence of immune complexes containing hepatitis B, e.g. polyarteritis, glomerulonephritis and myocarditis.

Physical signs

These are of an acute hepatitis.

Investigations

Liver biochemistry

High serum transaminases and an elevated bilirubin.

Serology

See Table 34.

 Hepatitis B core IgM is often the only marker of infection in acute liver failure as the virus will have been eradicated by the immune system by the time liver failure occurs.

HBV DNA

This can be detected by molecular techniques of variable sensitivity. Hybridization techniques have a sensitivity of 10^5–10^7 copies/mL. Polymerase chain reaction (PCR) is more sensitive. Low viral replication with undetectable e Ag is usually associated with levels of less than 10^5 copies/mL. Rarely mutations in the gene encoding the e Ag mean undetectable e Ag but still high levels of viral replication (precore mutants).

Treatment

There is none. Antiviral therapy is not indicated in acute hepatitis B infection. Liver transplantation for acute liver failure.

Complications

Chronicity

Persistence of HBsAg in serum for longer than 6 months suggests chronicity. Overall 10% of adults and 90% of neonates or those who become infected in infancy will become chronic carriers. The carrier rate in the UK is 0.1% compared to 10–15% in Africa. Chronicity is less common if the acute attack is more severe, i.e. jaundice.

Acute liver failure

Due to enhanced immune response with rapid clearance of the virus.

Others

Polyarteritis and glomerulonephritis are rare.

Prognosis

Good unless acute liver failure.

Prevention

Children and adults

Recombinant vaccine is given intramuscularly. Give a booster every 5–7 years to maintain HBsAb levels >100 IU/L.

105

Table 35 Indications for vaccination for hepatitis B.

Universal
Selected
Surgical and dental staff
Hospital staff in contact with blood products
Mental abnormality
Close family and sexual contact of HBsAg
Drug abusers
Homosexually active men
Travellers to high risk areas

HBsAg, hepatitis B surface antigen.

After three injections 94% will become immune. Low responders may need a further booster; this is commoner in elderly people and the immunosuppressed. There is an argument for universal vaccination in childhood to eradicate HBV worldwide [1] (Table 35).

Neonates

If the mother has hepatitis B give hepatitis B immunoglobulin at birth as passive immunization together with hepatitis B vaccination. See *Infectious diseases*, Section 2.10.8.

Remember to tell the patient to avoid unprotected sexual intercourse unless their partner is immune to hepatitis B.

1 Chang M-H, Chen C-J, Lai M-S *et al.* Universal hepatitis B vaccination in Taiwan and the incidence of hepatocellular carcinoma in children. *N Engl J Med* 1997; 336: 1855–1859.

2.9.3 OTHER VIRAL HEPATITIS

Hepatitis E

This is an RNA virus transmitted by the faecal–oral route. It accounts for sporadic and major epidemics of viral hepatitis in developing countries, e.g. 50% of non-A non-B (NANB) hepatitis in Hong Kong. It is rare in the UK with only about 2% of adults being immune. There is low viral faecal excretion so low secondary spread.

Hepatitis E is seen in young adults and resembles hepatitis A. The incubation period is 34–46 days. Jaundice is often of sudden onset and liver biochemistry is cholestatic. Acute liver failure is rare. It is diagnosed by IgG and IgM antibodies to recombinant HEV proteins. Alternatively HEV RNA can be detected by PCR.

The disease is self-limiting. Acute haemorrhagic syndrome with encephalopathy and renal failure is a complication seen classically in women in the last trimester of pregnancy and is associated with a 20% mortality.

Cytomegalovirus

Cytomegalovirus (CMV) can cause an acute hepatitis, most commonly in those who are immunosuppressed. Patients may be asymptomatic, with hepatitis recognized solely from elevation of serum transaminases, but symptoms can range from fever and malaise through to a devastating illness with jaundice and other features of CMV infection including pharyngitis, oesophagitis, gastroenteritis, pneumonitis, retinitis and bone marrow suppression. Diagnosis is by demonstrating CMV on tissue biopsy, detection of CMV by PCR in blood or urine, or by finding IgM to CMV. Treatment is with intravenous ganciclovir.

Epstein–Barr virus

Primary infection in children is asymptomatic. In young adults it can mimic viral hepatitis with fever and right upper quadrant pain together with elevated bilirubin (in 50%) and transaminases (up to 20x normal). Diagnosis is made by a positive Monospot or raised IgM to EBV capsid antigens. The disease is self limiting.

Other

Other rare causes of viral hepatitis include herpes simplex, adenovirus and rubella in the immunosuppressed. Parvovirus also rarely causes hepatitis in association with pancytopenia. Note that hepatitis C is not a cause of acute liver disease, but is the commonest cause of chronic hepatitis in the world.

2.9.4 ALCOHOL AND ALCOHOLIC HEPATITIS

Aetiology/pathophysiology/pathology

Ethanol is primarily oxidized in the liver (Fig. 63). The recommended safe limits for drinking are 21 units/week for women and 28 units for men. Men who drink more than 52 units (420 g) per week and women who drink more than 35 units (280 g) per week are at increased risk of alcohol-related liver disease. About 20% of those misusing alcohol will develop cirrhosis. The histology of alcoholic liver diseases is shown in Fig. 64.

Epidemiology

Alcohol intake is directly related to death from chronic liver disease.

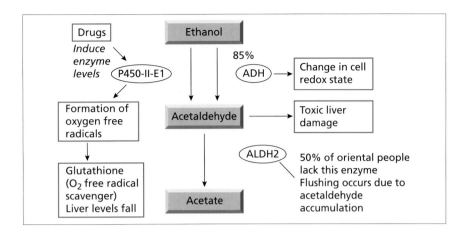

Fig. 63 Metabolic pathways involved in alcohol metabolism; 85% of alcohol is metabolized via the ADH pathway. ADH, alcohol dehydrogenase; ALDH2, acetaldehyde dehydrogenase 2; P450-II-E1, cytochrome P450-II-E1.

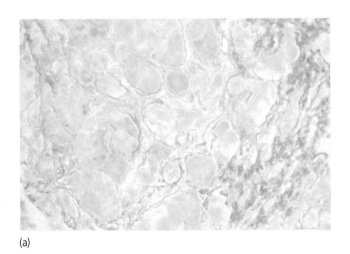

(a)

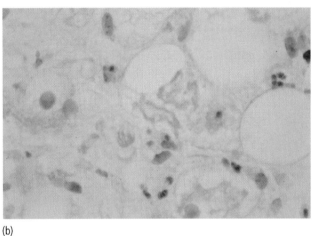

(b)

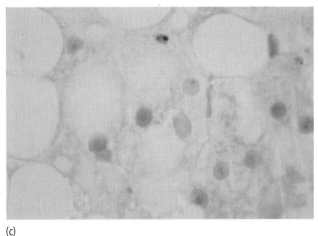

(c)

Fig. 64 Acute alcoholic hepatitis. (a) Pericellular fibrosis, fibrosis around individual hepatocytes giving a 'chicken wire' appearance. (b) Mallory's hyaline within hepatocyte. (c) Megamitochondria and fat within hepatocytes. Other features are predominantly neutrophil infiltration around portal tracts and fibrosis around hepatic vein. More extensive fibrosis or an established cirrhosis may also be present.

Clinical presentations

Minor alcoholic hepatitis may be asymptomatic with elevated serum transaminases as the only abnormality.

Physical signs

Common

This depends on the severity:

- *Mild/moderate alcoholic hepatitis.* Tender hepatomegaly, and jaundice in 10–15%.
- *Severe alcoholic hepatitis.* Jaundice, ascites, hepatic encephalopathy and rarely a hepatic bruit.

Uncommon

Parotid gland enlargement and testicular atrophy.

Investigations

Assessment of severity

Full blood count

There is often a leucocytosis (more common with viral hepatitis) and a macrocytosis. An initial low platelet count is seen with acute alcohol use in the absence of portal hypertension. Low-grade haemolysis is also common.

Prothrombin time

This is an important prognostic marker.

Liver function tests

Aspartate transaminase (AST) is greater than the alanine transaminase (ALT) in alcoholic liver disease. Usually AST <300 IU/L.

Transaminase levels >1000 IU/L are seen if there is associated paracetamol toxicity, which can occur with doses of as little as 4–6 g [1].

The alkaline phosphatase is often elevated, with levels up to 3–4 times normal in the absence of pancreatic disease (i.e. lower common bile duct stricture from chronic pancreatitis).

Chronic liver disease screen

Alcoholic hepatitis can coexist with other chronic liver diseases, e.g. haemochromatosis, hepatitis C, hepatitis B.

Abdominal ultrasound

This is needed to exclude biliary obstruction and signs of portal hypertension suggestive of cirrhosis.

Liver biopsy

This is needed to establish the extent of hepatic fibrosis.

Differential diagnosis

Drugs, viral hepatitis and autoimmune liver disease.

Treatment

Emergency

See Section 1.6, p. 22.

Short-term

Corticosteroids should be considered in severe alcoholic hepatitis as long as there is no evidence of infection or renal failure.

Long-term

Abstinence

Psychological input and counselling both reduce readmission rates.

Drugs

Acamprosate and naltrexone (12 months) may reduce alcohol dependence [2]. Antabuse should probably be avoided because of the side effects.

Complications

Ascites, hepatic encephalopathy, septicaemia, hepatorenal failure and chronic liver disease.

Prognosis

In mild/moderate alcoholic hepatitis, 30-day mortality is 2–17%; it is 42% in severe alcoholic hepatitis (i.e. PT >4 s prolonged). Overall survival at 5 years is 60% if the patient remains abstinent, falling to 40% if the patient continues to drink. If cirrhosis coexists at presentation the overall 5-year survival is 50%.

Prevention

Psychological input and counselling (including referral to Alcoholics Anonymous) is indicated when there is alcohol misuse.

Disease associations

These include:
- alcoholic cardiomyopathy
- chronic pancreatitis
- duodenal ulceration
- peripheral sensory neuropathy
- cerebellar atrophy
- cerebral atrophy
- Wernicke's encephalopathy
- Korsakoff's dementia.

1 Zimmerman HJ, Maddrey WC. Acetaminophen (paracetamol) hepatotoxicity with regular intake of alcohol: analysis of instances of therapeutic misadventure. *Hepatol* 1995; 22: 767.
2 Whitworth AB, Fischer F, Lesch OM *et al.* Comparison of acamprosate and placebo in long-term treatment of alcohol dependence. *Lancet* 1996; 25: 1438–1442.

2.9.5 ACUTE LIVER FAILURE

Aetiology/pathophysiology/pathology

Acute liver failure is distinguished from chronic liver disease by the absence of pre-existing clinical liver disease.
• Hyperacute liver failure is encephalopathy occurring within 7 days of onset of jaundice, e.g. caused by paracetamol overdose.
• Acute liver failure is encephalopathy occurring within 8–28 days of jaundice.
• Subacute liver failure (previously known as late onset hepatic failure) is defined by encephalopathy that occurs between 5 and 12 weeks from onset of jaundice [1].

The conditions are characterized by acute hepatocellular necrosis. Table 36 shows the causes.

Clinical presentations

Common

Increasing jaundice and confusion, i.e. encephalopathy, after a known paracetamol overdose.

Physical signs

Common

Jaundice, mild tender hepatomegaly. Small amounts of ascites may develop later. In hepatic venous outflow obstruction (Budd–Chiari) there is sudden onset of tender hepatomegaly and tense ascites.

Investigations

Blood tests

These should include:
• *Full blood count.* Haemolysis suggests Wilson's disease.
• *Prothrombin time or INR.* This is an indicator of the severity of acute liver injury.
• *Liver function tests.* A hepatitis (high serum transaminase) occurs in a viral hepatitis.

Table 36 Aetiology of acute liver failure.

	USA	UK
Paracetamol	20%	73%
Cryptogenic/NANBNC	15%	8%
Idiosyncratic drug toxicity	12%	2%
Hepatitis B	10%	2%
Hepatitis A	7%	2%

NANBNC, non-A non-B non-C hepatitis.

• *Urea and electrolytes.* In hepatorenal failure urea and creatinine rise.

Ultrasound

The liver is usually small or of normal size. It is important to exclude chronic liver disease (splenomegaly or varices). Hepatic vein patency must be assessed to exclude Budd–Chiari [2].

Liver disease screen

This should include:
• hepatitis A IgM
• hepatitis B core IgM
• smooth muscle antibody
• tests for Wilson's disease in patients <40 years old, i.e. serum copper and caeruloplasmin and 24 h urinary copper
• ophthalmological assessment if <40 years for Kayser–Fleischer rings seen in Wilson's disease.

Differential diagnosis

See Table 33, p. 104.

Treatment

Emergency

See Section 1.16, pp. 45–48.

Short-term

In the majority of cases treatment is supportive until liver function recovers. Criteria have been developed by King's College Hospital to help to decide when to consider liver transplantation in appropriate cases. (See Section 2.15, p. 126.)

 Patients should be discussed with or referred to a liver transplant centre sooner rather than later. Central venous access helps in managing haemodynamic changes and giving drugs in a concentrated form.

Supportive of complications

These include [3]:
• *Hypoglycaemia.* Give boluses of 50% dextrose.
• *Hypovolaemia.* Keep CVP at 10 mmHg with colloid (such as 4.5% human albumin solution).
• *N-acetyl cysteine.* This is of benefit in all patients, with both paracetamol- and non-paracetamol-induced acute liver failure. It can be given as an infusion at a dose of 100 mg/kg/24 h and has been shown to improve tissue oxygen delivery.

Complications

Common complications include:

- *Cerebral oedema.* Occurs in between 40 and 70% of patients who develop grade III/IV hepatic encephalopathy.
- *Infection.* Bacterial occurs in about 82% and fungal in 34% (often occult).
- *Acidosis.*
- *Coagulopathy.* Bleeding, however, is rare.
- *Renal failure.* Hepatorenal failure and/or acute tubular necrosis from paracetamol.
- *Acute pancreatitis.* Seen particularly in paracetamol-induced toxicity.

Prognosis

The overall mortality from subacute hepatic failure is 81%.

Prevention

Treatment of paracetamol overdose within 16 h of overdose with *N*-acetyl cysteine.

1 O'Grady J. Acute liver failure. *J Roy Col Phys Lond* 1997; 31: 603–607.
2 Rowbotham D, Endon J, Williams R. Acute liver failure secondary to hepatic infiltration: a single centre experience of 18 cases. *Gut* 1998; 42: 576–580.
3 Raham TM, Hodgson HJ. Review articles: liver support systems in acute hepatic failure. *Aliment Pharmacol Ther* 1999; 13: 1255–1272.

2.10 Chronic liver disease

Aetiology/pathophysiology/pathology

Chronic liver disease is liver damage occurring for more than 6 months. It results in progressive fibrosis and eventually cirrhosis (Fig. 65). Cirrhosis comprises fibrotic liver damage with regenerative nodule formation, and consequent portal venous hypertension (Fig. 66).

Fatty infiltration of the liver, which is a common cause of abnormal liver tests (about 90% of cases where no other cause is found), rarely progresses to cirrhosis, although as it is a recently recognized entity, this clinical impression may change in time. Common causes of chronic progressive liver disease are shown in Table 37.

Autoimmune hepatitis (relatively common) and Wilson's disease (very rare) may progress rapidly to cirrhosis. Rapid progression to cirrhosis due to recurrent disease in the liver graft can also occur after liver transplantation, e.g. in recurrent hepatitis C or recidivist alcohol use.

Epidemiology

Incidence varies with geographic region, age and sex. The commonest cause of chronic hepatitis in the world is hepatitis C. In the UK the commonest cause of cirrhosis is alcohol, followed by hepatitis C.

Hepatitis C

Hepatitis C is an RNA virus that is parenterally transmitted. The majority of those infected develop hepatitis 14–160 days after exposure. Prodromal symptoms are fever and malaise, jaundice is rare, and the vast majority are asymptomatic. Fifty per cent recover completely, but 50% go on to develop persistent viraemia and slowly progressive chronic liver disease, passing in the course of 20–40 years from acute to chronic persistent hepatitis, to chronic active hepatitis, to cirrhosis (in 10%) and eventually hepatocellular carcinoma. In the UK, 0.1–0.5% of the population have been infected.
For further information, see *Infectious diseases*, Section 2.10.8.

Clinical presentation

Common

Non-specific malaise, loss of libido, mental changes. Hepatic

(a)

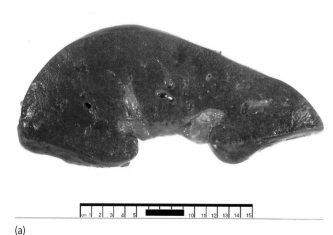

(b)

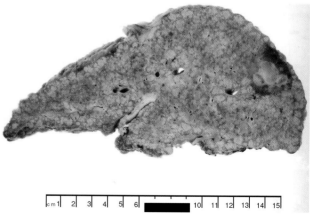

Fig. 65 (a) Normal liver; (b) cirrhotic liver containing a benign cyst.

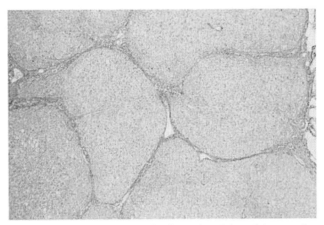

Fig. 66 Histological appearance of cirrhosis. There is loss of the normal architecture which is replaced by nodules.

decompensation: jaundice, ascites, hepatic encephalopathy, variceal haemorrhage.

 Most patients with chronic liver disease are asymptomatic until cirrhosis develops. It is also possible to be asymptomatic in the presence of cirrhosis if portal hypertension has not developed.

Physical signs

Common

Wasting, tiredness, loss of body hair, jaundice, encephalopathy, spider naevi, leuconychia, Dupuytren's contracture, testicular atrophy, ascites, firm, smooth or nodular hepatomegaly, splenomegaly.

Uncommon

Skin pigmentation in haemochromatosis (see *Endocrinology*,

Sections 1.5 and 2.5.3; *Rheumatology and clinical immunology*, Section 1.18).

Investigations/staging

Causes

Blood tests

Finding the cause of chronic liver dysfunction is an essential guide to treatment. Common causes and diagnostic tests are shown in Table 21, p. 52.

Liver biopsy

This is often used to confirm the diagnosis, especially as more than one aetiology may coexist, and establish the degree of hepatic fibrosis.

Extent of damage

Synthetic function

A low serum albumin and elevated prothrombin time are an indicator of the severity of liver damage.

Excretory function

An elevated serum bilirubin is an indicator of severe liver disease in patients with viral hepatitis.

Portal venous hypertension

An abdominal ultrasound may show splenomegaly and portosystemic collaterals (varices). An endoscopy may show oesophageal varices.

Table 37 Important causes of chronic liver disease and cirrhosis.

Alcohol-induced liver disease	See Sections 1.7, p. 23 and 2.9.4, p. 106
Chronic viral hepatitis	Lobular lymphocytic infiltration, variable hepatocyte necrosis and fibrosis progresses to cirrhosis. The damage is most likely due to immune mediated mechanisms rather than a viral cytopathic effect
Genetic haemochromatosis	Excess iron absorption from the intestine results in accumulation in hepatocytes, hepatocyte necrosis and cirrhosis
Autoimmune liver disease	Immune cell infiltration and hepatocyte damage leads to rapidly progressing fibrosis and cirrhosis
Primary biliary cirrhosis	See Section 2.5.4, p. 88
Primary sclerosing cholangitis	See Section 2.5.3, p. 86
Alpha 1-antitrypsin deficiency	Abnormal protein cannot be adequately exported from hepatocytes, where it accumulates causing hepatocyte damage
Wilson's disease	Abnormalities in the biliary copper transporter results in excess copper accumulation in the liver and brain, with hepatocyte damage and basal ganglia disease. The disease is genetically heterogeneous and this is reflected in variable clinical presentations (e.g. rapid neurological deterioration, early onset fulminant liver failure, or chronic liver disease presenting with cirrhosis)

Alcohol-induced liver disease	Abstinence
Chronic viral hepatitis [1,2]	Hepatitis C is cleared in 40% by a combination of interferon alpha and ribavirin (a nucleoside analogue) given for 6–12 months
	Hepatitis B responds to interferon alpha in 30% who are HBeAg positive with elevated transaminases. Other antivirals including lamivudine may be useful in the future
Genetic haemochromatosis [3]	Venesection to reduce iron load and return serum iron indices to normal reduces the rate of progression of liver disease
Autoimmune liver disease	Systemic steroid treatment, with or without azathioprine maintains long-term remission
Alpha 1-antitrypsin deficiency	No effective treatment exists
Wilson's disease	Penicillamine to increase urinary copper excretion and prevent hepatic and neurological disease progression
	Oral zinc may also promote copper excretion

Table 38 Specific treatment options for various causes of chronic liver disease.

HBeAg, Hepotitis B e antigen.

Looking for complications

Abdominal ultrasound and/or CT scanning and α-fetoprotein level to detect hepatocellular carcinoma.

Treatments

Emergency

Attention to supportive measures, including nutrition is the main priority. Serious complications such as variceal haemorrhage and bacterial peritonitis require emergency treatment.

Short-term

Progressive liver disease can sometimes be arrested where the cause is known. The appropriate interventions are shown in Table 38.

Wilson's disease

Wilson's disease may present as asymptomatic liver disease with predominant neurological abnormalities, as chronic liver disease with cholestatic features in early adulthood, or as fulminant liver failure in younger patients. A clue to Wilson's disease in these patients is the presence of significant red cell haemolysis. The diagnosis should be considered as prompt treatment can be life saving.

Long-term

Apart from specific treatments (Table 38), therapy is aimed at managing and preventing complications, e.g. diuretics to reduce ascites, non-selective β-blocker (propanolol) to reduce portal hypertension, and adequate nutrition to maintain general health.

Refer patients with chronic liver disease for consideration of liver transplantation, particularly if complications develop or there is a deterioration in markers of liver function (albumin and prothrombin time).

Complications

Common

Coagulopathy

This is caused by decreased synthesis of coagulation factors II, V, VII and IX with worsening liver function, or as a result of chronic cholestasis and reduced vitamin K levels. It is aggravated by thrombocytopenia caused by hyper-splenism due to portal hypertension.

Encephalopathy

The cause is multifactorial, and ill-understood. Abnormal amino acid synthesis and increased ammonia production may play a role, as may abnormal enteric bacterial metabolism and reduced hepatic clearance of neurotoxic substances due to portal hypertension and shunting. Resting EEG shows slowed α-wave frequency.

Ascites

This results from a combination of portal hypertension, increased sodium and water retention, and hypoalbuminaemia. Spontaneous bacterial peritonitis (SBP) in cirrhotic patients with ascites is common and potentially fatal.

Hepatorenal failure

See *Nephrology*, Section 2.7.10.

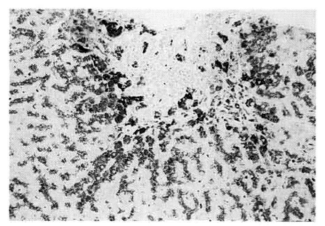

Fig. 67 Haemochromatosis. Iron deposition in hepatocytes shown as blue staining with Perl's stain.

Variceal haemorrhage

The most common site is oesophageal and gastric varices, but varices can form at any site of contact between the portal and systemic circulation (see Section 1.4, p. 13).

Cachexia

As the liver is the primary regulator of glucose, lipid and protein metabolism, profound abnormalities occur with advanced liver disease, and patients eventually become profoundly wasted. This is aggravated by haemorrhage, ascites, infection and anorexia.

Hepatocellular carcinoma (HCC)

This develops almost exclusively in cirrhotic livers, and patients with chronic viral hepatitis are most at risk, followed by those with haemochromatosis (Fig. 67). HCC is less common in females of reproductive age. Development of HCC can precipitate ascites, encephalopathy and rapid hepatic failure.

Prognosis

Morbidity

There is significant morbidity from malaise, malnutrition, sepsis and bleeding. Figure 68 shows the natural history of hepatitis C infection.

Mortality

Life expectancy is severely reduced, but varies depending on the cause and whether specific treatment is available. Most patients die from sepsis, bleeding or progressive liver failure. Successful liver transplantation much improves the prognosis.

1 Poynard T, Marcellin P, Lee SS *et al.* Randomised trial of interferon alpha 2b plus ribavirin for 48 weeks or for 24 weeks vs interferon alpha 2b plus placebo for 48 weeks for treatment of chronic infection with hepatitis C virus. *Lancet* 1998; 352: 1426–1432.
2 Malik AH, Lee WM. Chronic hepatitis B virus infection: treatment strategies for the next millennium. *Ann Intern Med* 2000; 132: 723–731.
3 Meeting Report. Hereditary Haemochromatosis. *Gastroenterol* 1999; 116: 193–207.

2.11 Focal liver lesions

Aetiology/pathophysiology/pathology

The common causes are (Table 39):
• *Infective lesions.* Pyogenic hepatic abscess is often related to colonic disease or appendicitis, amoebic abscess requires environmental exposure to *Entamoeba histolytica*, while hydatid cysts and abscesses are associated with exposure to dogs and sheep.

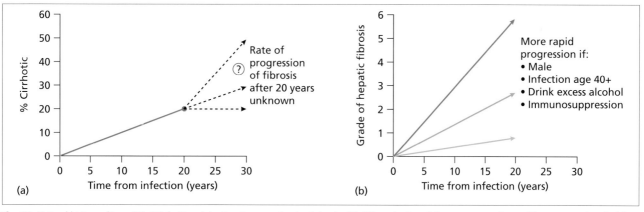

Fig. 68 Natural history of hepatitis C infection: (a) rate of progression to cirrhosis; (b) different rates of disease progression and factors associated with rapid progression.

Table 39 Differential diagnosis of focal liver lesions.

Infectious
Pyogenic abscess
Amoebic abscess
Hydatid cyst

Benign tumours
Haemangioma
Hepatic adenoma
Focal nodular hyperplasia, focal regenerative hyperplasia

Secondary deposits
Colorectal cancer
Gastrointestinal tract cancer including pancreatic and carcinoid tumours
Breast, cervix, ovary, prostate, lung, skin cancer

Primary liver cancer
HCC related to cirrhosis
Cholangiocarcinoma in patient with PSC
HCC developing in hepatic adenoma (rare, except in inherited glycogen diseases)

HCC, hepatocellular carcinoma; PSC, primary sclerosing cholangitis.

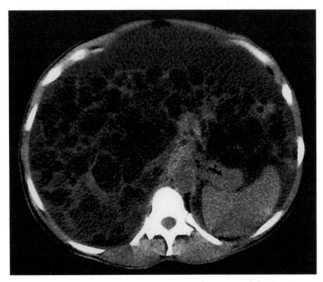

Fig. 69 Multiple hepatic cysts in a patient with autosomal dominant polycystic kidney disease. The CT scan also shows ascites and absence of kidneys following a bilateral nephrectomy.

• *Neoplastic benign lesions*. Simple cysts, haemangiomas or hyperplastic lesions (focal nodular hyperplasia) (Fig. 69).
• *Benign adenomas*. Occur almost exclusively in women on the oral contraceptive pill, and in this group are the commonest significant focal liver lesions.
• *Secondary deposits*. From colorectal carcinoma, other gastrointestinal tract tumours, breast, lung, prostate and other tumours (Fig. 70) (see *Oncology*, Section 2.10).
• *Primary liver cell cancer* (hepatocellular carcinoma, hepatoma or HCC). Occurs mainly in patients with cirrhosis. Cell proliferation in regenerating cirrhotic nodules may favour malignant change, as may the effects of chronic viral infection on the host genome (Fig. 19, p. 29) (see *Oncology*, Section 2.10).
• *Cholangiocarcinoma*. See Section 2.5.2, p. 84.

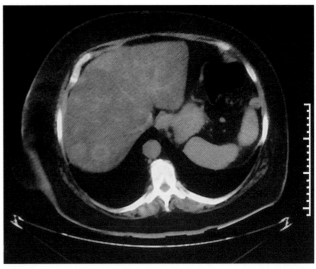

Fig. 70 Multiple liver metastases from adenocarcinoma of the pancreas on a CT scan.

Epidemiology

• *Hydatid disease*. Found mainly in patients from agricultural regions.
• *Haemangiomas*. Extremely common, occurring in up to 20% of people, and detected usually as an incidental finding.
• *Hepatic adenomas*. Occur in 3–4 per 100 000 of women on oestrogen-containing contraceptives, and may occur in men on androgen treatment.
• *Benign liver lesions*. Commoner in women than in men.
• *HCC*. Found in about 20–30% of patients dying with cirrhosis, and is commoner in men than in premenopausal women. HCC is particularly common in cirrhosis associated with chronic viral hepatitis and haemochromatosis.
• *Cholangiocarcinoma*. Occurs in up to 15% of patients with primary sclerosing cholangitis (PSC).

Clinical presentations

Common

These include:
• abscess—fever, pain and tenderness
• incidental finding on ultrasound scanning
• during investigation of abnormal liver tests
• detected on screening ultrasound in at-risk patients
• clinical deterioration or decompensation in cirrhotic patients
• onset of jaundice in patient with PSC.

Uncommon

• Weight loss
• Abdominal pain
• Increased ascites secondary to portal vein thrombosis.

Rare

Bleeding or tumour rupture.

Physical signs

Common

There are often few signs but there may be:
- HCC—signs of chronic liver disease
- hepatomegaly—tender in the case of liver abscess
- jaundice.

Uncommon

Hepatic bruit with hepatocellular carcinoma.

Investigations/staging

- Ultrasound scanning is most useful, but vascular tumours may have a diagnostic appearance on CT and MRI scanning and angiography, obviating the need for biopsy.
- Endoscopic retrograde cholangiopancreatography (ERCP) is useful for evaluating if jaundice in a patient with PSC is caused by cholangiocarcinoma, and allows collection of bile and brushings for cytological examination.
- Certain blood tests (Table 40) may help to confirm or refute a diagnostic possibility.
- Histological diagnosis may be established by liver biopsy, but beware of vascular lesions that may bleed catastrophically on biopsy.
- If the patient has ascites, cytological examination may provide a diagnosis, particularly if the lesion is a secondary malignant deposit.

 Beware of haemangiomas and hydatid cysts, where biopsy may result in catastrophic bleeding or disseminated infection.

Differential diagnosis

Common causes of focal liver lesions are considered in Table 39.

Table 40 Tumour markers.

Tumour marker	Disease
Alpha-fetoprotein level (AFP)	Hepatocellular carcinoma (also acute hepatitis, and germ cell tumours)
CA 19-9 tumour antigen level	Cholangiocarcinoma (also other pancreatic and biliary diseases)
Carcinoembryonic antigen (CEA)	Colorectal carcinoma
Amoebic and hydatid serology	Past infection with amoeba or *Echinococcus* species

Treatments

Emergency

- Liver abscess requires prompt antimicrobial treatment, and may require diagnostic or therapeutic aspiration or drainage.
- Ruptured liver abscess or haemangioma require surgical intervention.

Short-term

- Biliary obstruction can be relieved endoscopically or radiologically.
- Small hepatocellular carcinomas can be treated locally (e.g. by percutaneous alcohol injection), reducing tumour load and prolonging patient survival.
- Local resection of secondary deposits may be feasible in some cases.

Long-term

- Pyogenic and amoebic liver abscess may be cured by antimicrobial treatment alone or with percutaneous drainage.
- Hydatid cysts usually require careful excisional surgery under antimicrobial cover.
- Benign neoplastic liver lesions may require surgical removal (partial hepatectomy or liver transplant) if there is a risk of major complications (usually impending rupture or haemorrhage).
- Cessation of oral contraceptive use is associated with regression of adenomas.
- Early hepatocellular carcinoma may be cured by resection or liver transplantation.

Complications

Common

- Septicaemia in patients with pyogenic abscess.
- Decompensated liver failure in patients with cirrhosis or PSC.

Uncommon

- Vascular thrombosis, particularly portal vein thrombosis or inferior vena cava thrombosis, can occur.

Rare

- Haemorrhage or rupture of haemangioma and large adenoma.
- Malignant transformation of adenoma.

Prognosis

Morbidity

- Incidental liver lesions rarely cause morbidity.
- Fever, pain or vague right upper quadrant discomfort are common.

Mortality

Without curative resection hepatic secondaries and hepatocellular carcinoma usually have a dire prognosis.

Prevention

Primary

- Low-dose oestrogen formulations reduce the risk of hepatic adenoma in patients using the oral contraceptive pill.
- The risk of HCC is reduced in patients with cirrhosis who abstain from alcohol and in patients with chronic viral hepatitis in whom viral replication is suppressed by antiviral therapies.

Disease associations

- *Pyogenic liver abscess.* Cholangitis, diverticular disease, inflammatory bowel disease, appendicitis, colorectal neoplasia.
- *Amoebic liver abscess.* Amoebic colitis.
- *Adenoma.* Glycogen storage disease.
- *HCC.* Liver cirrhosis.
- *Cholangiocarcinoma.* PSC.

Reddy KR, Schiff ER. Approach to a liver mass. *Semin Liver Dis* 1993; 13: 423–435.
Rubin RA, Mitchell DG. Evaluation of the solid hepatic mass. *Med Clin N Am* 1996; 80: 907–928.
Vukmir RB. Pyogenic hepatic abscess. *Am Family Phys* 1993; 47: 1435–1441.

2.12 Drugs and the liver

2.12.1 HEPATIC DRUG TOXICITY

Aetiology/pathophysiology/pathology

Over 10 000 drugs are implicated [1]. Damage occurs to hepatocytes, bile ducts and hepatic veins (Table 41). The effect may be predictable and dose dependent, e.g. paracetamol, but is more commonly idiosyncratic. Mechanisms of drug toxicity include:

- direct toxicity
- indirect damage via the formation of reactive metabolites. Reactive metabolites may deplete essential enzymes, e.g. glutathione (paracetamol), or bind to liver proteins forming adducts. Adducts can subsequently mediate an immuno-allergic response. Autoantibodies to halothane and nitrofurantoin have been identified. Genetic factors are also important. Thus deficiency in certain cytochrome P450 enzymes is associated with hepatotoxicity. Histological features depend on the type of drug but may be differentiated from other causes of acute liver injury by the presence of large numbers of eosinophils (Table 41 and Fig. 71).

	Bilirubin	ALP/GGT	ALT/AST	Drug causes
Acute hepatitis	++	+	+++	Paracetamol NSAID Isoniazid Halothane
Acute cholestasis	+++	+++	+	Oestrogens Flucloxacillin Chlorpromazine Dextropropoxyphene
Fatty liver			++	Tetracycline
Steatohepatitis		++	++	Amioderone
Granuloma	+	++		Carbamezepine Allopurinol
Hepatic fibrosis	N	N	N	Methotrexate
No liver disease (enzyme induction)		–/+		Rifampicin

Table 41 Clinical presentations of drug hepatoxicity.

ALP, alkaline phosphatase; ALT, alanine transaminase; AST, aspartate transaminase; GGT, γ-glutamyl transferase; N, normal liver biochemistry; NSAID, non-steroidal anti-inflammatory drug.

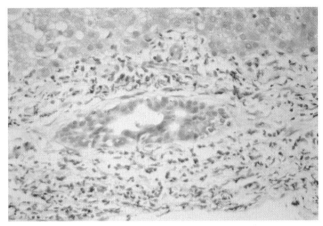

Fig. 71 Bile duct damage due to clavulinic acid–amoxycillin. The bile duct epithelium is irregular and infiltrated with lymphocytes.

Epidemiology

The incidence of hepatic drug toxicity is under-reported; it has been estimated to occur in 1 in 10 000–100 000 persons. Prevalence increases with age, with drugs being responsible for 40% of acute hepatitis in those aged >50 years.

Drugs most commonly implicated in causing drug toxicity have changed over the last 40 years. In the 1960s toxicity was primarily due to:
- chlorpromazine
- halothane
- high oestrogen containing oral contraceptives
- intravenous tetracyclines
- methotrexate [2].

Now the commonest causes are:
- non-steroidal anti-inflammatory drugs (NSAIDs)
- dextropropoxyphene
- clavulanic acid–amoxycillin
- flucloxacillin
- herbal remedies [3].

Clinical presentations/physical signs

 Always consider drug toxicity in the presence of jaundice or abnormal liver biochemistry. This often means obtaining the drug history directly from the general practitioner. Always ask about herbal remedies.

The clinical presentation depends on the type of liver injury:
- *Jaundice.* More likely if bile duct damage or cholestasis, but also occurs in severe hepatitis.
- *Symptoms of hypersensitivity, fever, arthralgia,* but these may be absent.
- *Acute hepatitis.* Nausea and upper abdominal discomfort.
- *Acute cholestasis.* Jaundice and itching.
- *Fatty liver.* Usually asymptomatic.

 There is usually a temporal association between starting the drug and the occurrence of hepatotoxicity, although liver biochemistry may become abnormal before symptoms develop. However, halothane and clavulanic acid–amoxycillin hepatotoxicity occurs up to 3 weeks after cessation of drug exposure.

Investigations

Eosinophilia

A peripheral eosinophilia may be present.

Liver biochemistry

The pattern of liver biochemistry is shown in Table 41.

Differential diagnosis

This depends on the type of liver injury caused by the drug as indicated below.

Acute hepatitis

Viral hepatitis. Autoimmune chronic active hepatitis. Alcoholic hepatitis.

Steatohepatitis

This has to be differentiated from alcoholic hepatitis.

Acute cholestasis

Biliary disease, extrahepatic obstruction and intrahepatic disease including PSC, PBC and intrahepatic cholestasis of sepsis.

Treatment

Stop the drug. Supportive care.

Complications

Acute liver failure

This is more likely in elderly people. It has been frequently reported with antituberculous medication [4]. It occurs in about 20% who are jaundiced. Overall 15–20% of acute liver failure is due to drugs.

Chronic cholestasis

Loss of bile ducts (ductopenia) has been reported.

117

Prognosis

- In the absence of liver failure most reactions are self-limiting with no chronic liver damage.
- If acute liver failure develops outcome is not as good as that of viral hepatitis.

Disease associations

In severe reactions—erythroderma, bone marrow suppression.

See *Clinical pharmacology,* Sections 4 and 5.
1 Farrell GC. *Drug Induced Liver Disease.* London: Churchill Livingstone, 1994.
2 Kremer JM, Alarcon GSS, Lightfoot RW *et al.* Methotrexate for rheumatoid arthritis. Suggested guidelines for monitoring liver toxicity. *Am Coll Rheumatol* 1994; 37: 316–328.
3 Schuppan D, Jia J-D, Brinkhaus B, Hahn EG. Herbal products for liver diseases: a therapeutic challenge for the new millennium. *Hepatol* 1999; 30: 1099–1104.
4 Thompson NP, Caplin ME, Hamilton MI *et al.* Anti-tuberculosis medication and the liver: dangers and recommendations in management. *Eur Respir J* 1995; 8: 1384–1388.

2.12.2 DRUGS AND CHRONIC LIVER DISEASE

Clinical presentations

The following drugs should be avoided or used cautiously:
- *Narcotics/anxiolytics.* Accumulation results in hepatic encephalopathy.
- *Codeine.* Causes constipation and secondary hepatic encephalopathy.
- *NSAIDs.* May initiate an oesophageal variceal haemorrhage and precipitate hepatorenal failure.

2.13 Gastrointestinal infections

- Gastrointestinal infections can be caused by viruses (most commonly), bacteria (or their toxins), or protozoa.
- They present abruptly with diarrhoea and/or vomiting and colicky abdominal pain.
- They are usually self-limiting.
- Stool cultures often fail to grow an organism.
- The commonest causes in the UK are *Campylobacter, Salmonella, Shigella* and *Clostridium difficile.*
- All cases of 'food poisoning' are notifiable by law.

Sigmoidoscopic and histological examinations may be indistinguishable in gastrointestinal infections from idiopathic inflammatory bowel disease. The two conditions may also coexist.

2.13.1 CAMPYLOBACTER

Aetiology/pathophysiology/pathology

This infection is contracted mainly from infected food, particularly poultry.

Epidemiology

This is probably the most common cause of bacterial gastroenteritis in the UK.

Clinical presentation

The incubation period is 3–5 days. Remission usually occurs over 1–2 weeks, but bacterial excretion in stool often lasts longer. It typically causes severe, crampy abdominal pain and diarrhoea, which may be bloody, and affects small and large bowel. There is often associated malaise, headache and myalgia.

Complications

It may rarely cause Reiter's syndrome, erythema nodosum, toxic dilatation, Guillain–Barré syndrome.

Treatment

Antibiotics are rarely required; erythromycin or ciprofloxacin may be used.

2.13.2 SALMONELLA

Aetiology/pathophysiology/pathology

- *Salmonella* causes a spectrum of disease ranging from asymptomatic carriage to acute gastroenteritis to typhoid (enteric) fever.
- Salmonella gastroenteritis is usually caused by *S. typhimurium* and *S. enteritidis.* The organism is present in chickens and eggs.
- The gall bladder (gallstone nidus) may account for asymptomatic carriage.
- Enteric fever caused by *S. typhi* and *S. typhimurium* is a systemic illness and caused by contamination in food or water primarily in the tropics or subtropics.

Clinical presentation

Acute gastroenteritis. Headache, abdominal pain, fever and diarrhoea (blood rare) with an incubation period of 8–48 h.
Enteric fever. Presents usually as pyrexia of unknown origin (PUO). Constipation is an initial GI symptom followed by diarrhoea. The incubation period is usually 10–14 days.

Physical signs

Enteric fever. There is often a relative bradycardia and a rash (rose spots) develops over the trunk after about 1 week.

Investigations

The highest yield of positive culture results is from blood and bone marrow culture in the first week, faecal and urine culture in the second week. Leucopenia with relative lymphocytosis is common.

Complications

Enteric fever. Severe toxaemia, haemorrhage, perforation (small bowel), coma and death may occur in the third week in untreated cases of enteric fever; relapse may occur.

Treatment

Acute gastroenteritis. If antibiotic treatment is required, ciprofloxacin is the drug of choice. Antibiotics are only indicated in the severely ill, or bacteraemic, since they lead to prolonged stool carriage.

Enteric fever. Chloramphenicol, ciprofloxacin, trimethoprim and amoxycillin may all be used.

Prevention

Three negative stool samples are advised in certain occupations (e.g. food handlers, nurses) before allowing return to work.

2.13.3 SHIGELLA

Aetiology/pathophysiology/pathology

Shigella multiplies in the small intestine causing water and electrolyte secretion, and invades the colonic wall resulting in bloody diarrhoea.

Clinical presentation

The incubation period is 2–3 days. Bloody diarrhoea, fever, headache and myalgia are common.

Complications

Aseptic meningitis, febrile convulsions, Reiter's syndrome, respiratory symptoms and haemolytic uraemic syndrome may all rarely complicate shigellosis.

Treatment

The infection is usually self-limiting and treatment is not needed. Amoxycillin is the antibiotic of choice if required.

Prevention

As with *Salmonella* infections, negative stool cultures are required for certain occupations before it is possible to return to work.

Shigella sp. and some species of *Escherichia coli* cause 'bacillary dysentery', characterized by bloody diarrhoea.

2.13.4 CLOSTRIDIUM DIFFICILE

Aetiology/pathophysiology/pathology

This is associated with antibiotic usage, particularly clindamycin, but widespread use of cephalosporins are responsible for most cases [1].

Clinical presentation

It may be present in asymptomatic individuals, or cause mild diarrhoea or severe bloody diarrhoea (pseudomembranous colitis).

Investigations

Diagnosed by culture and detection of toxin in stool (in pseudomembranous colitis, sigmoidoscopy reveals punctate yellow-white plaques adhering to inflamed mucosa).

Treatment

Effectively cleared by metronidazole 400 mg t.d.s. for 1 week. Relapse is common (up to 30%) and can be treated by vancomycin 125 mg qds.

1 Kelly CP, Pothoulakis C, LaMont JT. *Clostridium difficile* colitis. *N Engl J Med* 1994; 330: 257–262.

2.13.5 GIARDIA LAMBLIA

Aetiology/pathophysiology/pathology

Small intestinal protozoan parasite occurring worldwide. Infection usually by contaminated drinking water.

Clinical presentation

Presents as acute diarrhoea with excessive flatus after an incubation period of 1–4 weeks. Malabsorption may occur, with pale, bulky, offensive stools and weight loss. Symptoms may persist for months.

Investigations

Diagnosed by presence of trophozoites in jejunal aspirate or biopsy taken at endoscopy, or cysts in the stool.

Treatment

Metronidazole or tinidazole are highly effective.

2.13.6 YERSINIA ENTEROCOLITICA

Aetiology/pathophysiology/pathology

Infection via contaminated food, milk, animal excreta and raw pork.

Clinical presentation

Incubation period of 24–36 h.

Invades intestinal mucosa and multiplies within Peyer's patches, causing mesenteric adenitis and terminal ileitis, which can mimic Crohn's disease.

Investigations

Diagnosed by stool or blood cultures, or rising antibody titre.

Complications

May cause a reactive arthritis (or Reiter's syndrome) and erythema nodosum.

Treatment

Tetracycline or ciprofloxacin may be used.

2.13.7 ESCHERICHIA COLI

Most *E. coli* strains are normal commensals in humans. Pathogenic strains are divided into four groups:
- enteropathogenic
- enterotoxigenic
- enteroinvasive
- enterohaemorrhagic.

The incubation period is 12–72 h. Enterohaemorrhagic strains are responsible for haemorrhagic colitis and haemolytic uraemic syndrome. Treatment is with co-trimoxazole, ciprofloxaxin or gentamicin.

Mead PS, Griffin PM. *Escherichia coli* 0157:H7. *Lancet* 1998; 352: 1207–1212.

2.13.8 ENTAMOEBA HISTOLYTICA

Aetiology/pathophysiology/pathology

It is responsible for amoebic dysentery and is spread via person-to-person contact and ingestion of infected water or food.

Clinical presentation

Incubation period is 1–4 weeks. Symptoms range from mild diarrhoea to severe bloody diarrhoea (colonic ulceration).

Investigations

Diagnosed by stool culture, rectal biopsy or serology.

Complications

Liver abscesses occur in 1–3% of cases.

Treatment

Metronidazole is effective.

2.13.9 TRAVELLER'S DIARRHOEA

This describes diarrhoea occurring during or after a journey. Enteropathogens responsible include: enterotoxigenic *E. coli* (most common), viruses, enterohaemorrhagic *E. coli*, *Campylobacter*, *Shigella* sp., *Salmonella* sp., protozoa.

The illness is usually short-lived and self-limiting. Ciprofloxacin or doxycycline afford reasonable prophylaxis.

Persistent diarrhoea in a patient with traveller's diarrhoea should alert the physician to the possibility of giardiasis, cryptosporidiosis or strongyloidiasis.

2.13.10 HUMAN IMMUNODEFICIENCY VIRUS (HIV)

HIV may cause an enteropathy which histologically has the appearance of partial villous atrophy with crypt hyperplasia and polymorph infiltration. This results in diarrhoea, malabsorption and weight loss.

Diarrhoea can also be caused by simple opportunistic infections such as cryptosporidium and cytomegalovirus which rarely cause gastroenteritis in immunocompromised individuals.

Immunodeficiency leads to increased severity of infection.

HIV infection is also associated with oral candidiasis, herpes simplex oesophagitis and proctitis.

2.14 Nutrition

2.14.1 DEFINING NUTRITION

Nutritional requirements in health

A balanced diet supplies energy (fat and carbohydrate), nitrogen (protein), electrolytes, and vitamins/trace elements. Fat is the most efficient storage form of energy, yielding approximately 10 kcal/g, compared to glucose and protein (both 4 kcal/g).

Nutritional requirements vary depending on:
* age
* weight
* degree of activity
* growth
* pregnancy
* illness (catabolic states, e.g. sepsis, trauma, surgery).

In health, approximately 2000–2500 kcal of energy are required daily, as well as 14–20 g nitrogen (a minimum of 40–50 g protein). There are eight or nine essential amino acids (i.e. cannot be synthesized by humans) and one essential fatty acid (linoleic acid). Vitamins and trace elements are also required (Table 42).

Assessment of nutritional status

The term malnutrition strictly includes both energy undernutrition and overnutrition (e.g. obesity), also specific deficiencies or excesses of vitamins or trace elements. However, malnutrition is often used synonymously with undernutrition.

Nutritional assessment of hospitalized patients is vital, since almost half may be malnourished and this predicts a poorer outcome. There is no single adequate parameter of nutritional status. Assessment is mainly made by a combination of history and examination (Tables 42–44).

History

The following features from the history are important in assessing the nutritional state:
* altered intake and pattern of intake
* recent weight loss (>10% significant)
* ability to chew or swallow, presence of dysphagia
* anorexia, early satiety
* recent vomiting
* altered bowel habit suggesting malabsorption
* vitamin deficiency—angular stomatitis, glossitis, night blindness.

Examination

The following findings suggest impaired nutrition:
* *General muscle and fat mass.* Hollow cheeks, wasting of temporalis, squaring of shoulders (loss of deltoid), wasting of quadriceps.
* *Oedema.* May indicate hypoalbuminaemia.
* *Petechial or subcutaneous haemorrhage.* Vitamin C/K deficiencies.
* *Wrinkling, dryness of conjunctiva.* Vitamin A deficiency.
* *Ophthalmoplegia.* Thiamine deficiency; may be other signs of Wernicke's encephalopathy.
* *Chelosis, angular stomatitis, glossitis.* Vitamin B complex deficiency.
* *Myelopathy, ataxia, retinopathy, blindness.* Vitamin E deficiency.

Table 42 List of vitamin requirements. (Vitamin B is covered separately in Table 43.)

Vitamin	Requirement	Effect of deficiency	Notes
A	1000 IU/day	Night blindness, Bitot's spots, hyperkeratosis and keratomalacia of skin	Found in dairy products, liver, fish. Plasma retinol levels can be measured
C	60–100 mg/day	Scurvy	Necessary for collagen synthesis (hydroxylation of proline to hydroxyproline). Seen in elderly or people who don't eat vegetables. Signs are perifollicular haemorrhages, 'corkscrew hair', bleeding gums, loose teeth, spontaneous bruising/haemorrhage, anaemia, poor wound healing
D	200 IU/day	Osteomalacia, rickets, bone pain, proximal myopathy, Looser's zones	Normal or low Ca^{2+}, low PO_4, high ALP, high PTH. Main source is from action of sunlight on skin photoactivating 7-dehydrocholesterol
E	10–20 mg/day	Neurological disorders	Found in vegetable oils and fish
K	1 μg/kg/day	Bleeding diathesis	Found in leafy vegetables. Deficiency most commonly seen in biliary obstruction

ALP, alkaline phosphatase; PTH, parathyroid hormone.

Table 43 List of vitamin B requirements.

Vitamin	Requirement	Effect of deficiency	Notes
B$_1$ (thiamine)	0.5–1 mg/1000 kcal intake	Neuropathy, cardiac failure (beri-beri), ophthalmoplegia (Wernicke's) encephalopathy, severe acidosis	Suspect in alcoholics, i.v. feeding with high glucose intake. Red cell transketolase levels can be measured
B$_2$ (riboflavin)	0.6 mg/1000 kcal intake	Angular stomatitis, chelosis, glossitis, conjunctival injection	Suspect in alcoholics. Can measure blood and urine levels
B$_6$ (pyridoxine)	1.6–2 mg/day or 0.038 mg/g protein intake	Angular stomatitis, chelosis, glossitis, neuropathy, sideroblastic anaemia	Isoniazid, hydralazine and penicillamine are antagonists
Niacin	6.6 mg NE*	Pellagra (classically dermatitis 'Casal's necklace', diarrhoea, dementia)	Found in areas where maize is main dietary constituent (biologically unavailable niacin and low in precursor tryptophan)
Biotin	0.03–0.1 mg/day	Mental changes, myalgia, dermatitis	Deficiency rare
B$_{12}$ (cobalamin)	2 µg/day	Megaloblastic anaemia, glossitis, stomatitis peripheral neuropathy, subacute combined degeneration of the spinal cord	Found in meat, fish, dairy produce but not plants. May occur in vegans, pernicious anaemia, gastrectomy, coeliac disease, bacterial overgrowth, ileal disease/resection, Zollinger–Ellison syndrome. Average adult stores may last up to 5 years before deficiency develops. Treat with 3-monthly vitamin B$_{12}$ injections
Folic acid	3 µg/kg/day	Megaloblastic anaemia, glossitis, stomatitis	Found in green, leafy vegetables and offal. Main cause of deficiency is poor intake. May occur in small bowel disease (e.g. coeliac disease). Phenytoin and methotrexate are antifolate drugs

* NE = niacin + tryptophan (mg)/60.

Table 44 List of minerals and trace elements required in diet.

Mineral	Requirement	Effect of deficiency	Notes
Iron	1 mg/day	Microcytic anaemia, glossitis, cheilosis, koilonychias	Iron deficiency is very common. Prevalence is 0.2% men, 1.9% postmenopausal women, 2.6% menstruating women. May be due to poor intake or excess loss (GI tract most commonly)
Calcium	800–1000 mg/day is normal Western intake	Weakness, proximal myopathy, perioral paraesthesia, tetany	Correct for albumin level (add 0.02 × 40 minus serum albumin)
Copper	2–4 mg/day	Hypochromic anaemia, leucopenia, osteoporosis	
Magnesium		Myopathy	
Zinc	15 mg/day	Rash (nasolabial, hands), hair loss, infections, diarrhoea	
Selenium		Muscle pain and weakness, cardiomyopathy	
Chromium		Glucose intolerance, neuropathy	

GI, gastrointestinal.

Body mass index

A nutritional assessment also involves calculating the body mass index (BMI) from the height (m) and weight (kg):

$$BMI = weight/(height)^2$$

The World Health Organization classifies BMI as follows:

<18.5	underweight
18.5–24.9	normal
25.0–30	overweight
>30	obese

Investigations

Blood tests

Malnutrition is indicated by:
- albumin <30 g/L (but often reflects coexistent disease)
- lymphocytes <1.5 × 10^9/L
- transferrin <2 g/L.

Albumin, thyroxine-binding prealbumin, retinol-binding protein, transferrin, and lymphocyte counts have all been used as indicators of protein–energy malnutrition, but all may be affected by other conditions.

Although low albumin levels may indicate protein–energy malnutrition, albumin concentration often reflects disease activity and may be regarded as 'the reciprocal of the ESR'. Albumin has a plasma half-life of 21 days and although fasting affects albumin synthesis within 24 h, this has little impact on albumin levels because of the low turnover rate and large pool size. Infection, malignancy, inflammation, and gastrointestinal, renal and liver disease may all depress albumin levels, and yet most anorexic patients have a normal serum albumin.

Anthropometric measurements

These include the triceps and subscapular skinfold thickness, which provide an index of body fat, and the midarm circumference which provides a measure of muscle mass. There are, however, problems with both the reference database and considerable interobserver measurement variability.

Dynamometry

This refers to the use of hand grip strength, which has been shown to predict postoperative complications in surgical patients. Other more objective tests have used electrical stimulation of the adductor pollicis muscle in the hand to measure force–frequency curves, fatiguability and relaxation. These have been shown to predict postoperative surgical complications.

Others

Total lymphocyte count and delayed cutaneous hypersensitivity tests may also be used as indicators of nutritional status.

Total body water

Body composition may be divided into four compartments: water, protein, fat and mineral. Total body water may be measured by isotope dilution techniques using tritium, deuterium or ^{18}O-labelled water. Water has a relatively stable relationship to fat-free body mass (protein), with the proportion of water taken to be a constant at 0.732. Thus the following can be calculated:
- protein = fat-free body mass
- fat = [total body weight – (fat-free body mass + water)].

Combined non-invasive methods for measuring the following are in developmental stages:
- protein (total body nitrogen)
- fat (dual photon absorptiometry)
- mineral (dual photon absorptiometry and delayed gamma neutron activation)
- water (isotope water dilution).

Prognosis

There is a near linear relationship of increasing BMI with morbidity and mortality. A BMI <15 kg/m² is also associated with increased mortality.

2.14.2 PROTEIN–CALORIE MALNUTRITION

Kwashiorkor and marasmus are the two classical primary nutrition disorders seen in children. Although described as distinct entities, features of both are often present. Marasmus is defined as present when weight is <60% that expected for the age, and is termed marasmic kwashiorkor when oedema is additionally present. Less severe protein–calorie malnutrition is present when weight is 60–80% that expected for age, and is termed undernutrition in the absence of oedema, and kwashiorkor in its presence.

Other causes of undernutrition include:
- anorexia nervosa (see *Psychiatry*, Section 1.5)
- intestinal disorders (e.g. Crohn's, coeliac)
- infections (including parasites)
- neoplasms
- severe inflammatory disorders.

2.14.3 OBESITY

 'Sudden death is more common in those who are naturally fat than in the lean.' (Hippocrates)

Aetiology/pathophysiology

Obesity, defined as a BMI >30 kg/m², is a large and increasing problem. In addition to the total body-fat mass (estimated by the BMI), the distribution of fat is also important. Centralization of body fat is associated with dyslipidaemia, hypertension, insulin resistance, diabetes mellitus, cardiovascular disease and stroke. In clinical practice, distribution can be simply assessed by the waist : hip circumference ratio (WHR). The WHR should not exceed 1.0 in men and 0.85 in women. Genetic factors are involved. A signal protein, leptin, produced by adipose tissue, has recently been discovered which may modulate bodyweight and energy expenditure.

Epidemiology

In the UK, the prevalence of obesity increased from 8% in 1980 to 15% by 1995. In Europe and the USA the figures are 15–25%. As the BMI increases, so does morbidity and mortality. Obesity is a result of energy input exceeding output.

Treatment

Dietary

The principle of treatment is to induce negative energy balance, which should be by a combination of long-term low-intensity exercise and diet (500–600 kcal daily deficit), which should be low in fat.

Other

Other cardiovascular risk factors present should be addressed (e.g. smoking, hypertension, diabetes, hyperlipidaemia). Alcohol intake should be minimized (7 kcal/g), and hypothyroidism excluded.

Behaviour modification

Behaviour modification is important and includes a diary of food intake, meal frequency and separating eating from other activities.

Drug treatments

These are considered if diet, exercise, and behaviour modification has failed, and the risks of obesity outweigh the risks of the drug in that individual.

Serotoninergic agonists

These suppress appetite but may cause pulmonary hypertension and pulmonary valve disease.

Orlistat

This is a potent pancreatic lipase inhibitor, recently shown to be effective in weight reduction management.

Surgery

Vertical banded gastroplication, reducing the reservoir capacity of the stomach, is reserved for seriously obese patients (BMI >35 kg/m^2).

2.14.4 ENTERAL AND PARENTERAL NUTRITION

Principle

Nutritional support is indicated for malnourished patients since studies have shown poorer outcome in those suffering protein–calorie malnutrition. Support may be given enterally (gastrointestinal) or parenterally (intravenous).

Indications

Enteral nutrition

Enteral nutrition is the preferred option in all malnourished patients who have a normal or near normal, functioning, accessible gut. It is trophic for the upper intestinal mucosa, maintains epithelial barrier integrity, and is cheaper and safer than parenteral feeding [1].

Parenteral nutrition

Parenteral nutrition is indicated in those malnourished patients who have a non-functioning gut (e.g. short bowel syndrome, prolonged ileus). Traditionally, parenteral nutrition is administered via the large central veins (subclavian or internal jugular) which allow rapid dilution of the hyperosmolar solutions and reduces the incidence of thrombophlebitis and subsequent line failure.

Contraindications

Enteral nutrition

This is contraindicated in paralytic ileus, mechanical obstruction and major intra-abdominal sepsis, and in those with complex fluid balance problems.

Practical details

Enteral nutrition

Many patients can take oral supplements (e.g. Fortisip, Fortijuice) by mouth. In those with swallowing problems, or those who lack appetite, nasogastric feeding may be initiated via a fine bore feeding tube. In patients in whom aspiration is a potential problem (e.g. gastric dysmotility) nasojejunal feeding may be the preferred option. If long-term enteral feeding is required, then a percutaneous endoscopic gastrostomy tube, or jejunostomy tube may be sited, as these are more convenient and comfortable, and not prone to removal/displacement.

Parenteral nutrition

Central venous catheterization can lead to complications and hence many clinicians use peripheral lines (15–20-cm catheters inserted via the antecubital veins) if they anticipate a return to enteral feeding within 14 days or so.

Complications

Parenteral nutrition

The complications of parenteral nutrition include central venous access-related complications, metabolic complications, vitamin and trace element deficiencies and hepatobiliary dysfunction [2].

Complications of central venous cannulation are:
- arterial puncture
- pneumothorax
- haemothorax
- air embolism
- central venous thrombosis
- infection.

Metabolic complications include:
- hyper-/hypoglycaemia
- hyper-/hyponatraemia
- hyper-/hypocalcaemia
- hypophosphataemia
- mineral/vitamin/trace element deficiency.

Nutrition Support Teams have been shown to dramatically reduce infective complications related to parenteral nutrition, can provide informed advice on nutritional support, and carefully monitor patients receiving such treatment.

1 Nicholson FB, Korman MG, Richardson MA. Percutaneous endoscopic gastrostomy: review of indications, complications and outcome. *J Gastroenterol Hepatol* 2000; 15: 21–25.
2 Quigley EMM, Marsh MN, Shaffer JL, Markin RS. Hepatobiliary complications of total parenteral nutrition. *Gastroenterol* 1993; 104: 286–301.

2.14.5 DIETS

Elemental diet

This comprises low molecular weight nutrients, usually with 10% free amino acids, 85% oligosaccharides and <5% fat. Studies show that this diet is as effective as steroids in the treatment of active Crohn's disease, but many patients find it distasteful and need nasogastric feeding over a 6-week period [1]. Its mechanism of action is unknown but it may have an effect by reducing immunogenic load and altering bacterial flora.

Exclusion diet

The most common conditions requiring exclusion of specific foods from the diet are coeliac disease (where gluten provokes an immunological response), cow's milk protein intolerance, and hypolactasia. Some patients with irrit-

able bowel syndrome seem to benefit from avoiding certain foods.

1 King TS, Woolner JT, Hunter JO. Review article: the dietary management of Crohn's. *Aliment Pharmacol Ther* 1997; 11: 17–31.

2.15 Liver transplantation

Principle

About 600 adult orthotopic liver transplantations are carried out per year in the UK. Donor livers are matched to the recipient on the basis of size and ABO blood group.

The numbers performed are limited by donor shortage. Ways of trying to increase organ availability are as follows:

- *Living related transplantation.* Either a right or left lobe is used primarily in children who need small grafts and in adults in Japan where cadaveric organs are not available.
- *Split liver transplantation.* This provides two grafts from a single donor and is useful in children.
- *Xenotransplantation.* This approach using pig livers is the subject of laboratory research and ethical debate.

Indications

The main indications for liver transplantation
- End-stage chronic liver disease
- Acute hepatic failure
- Metabolic liver disease—oxalosis, glycogen storage disease.

Ethical issues

These are largely related to donor shortage and include [1–3]:
- Should patients with liver failure due to paracetamol overdose or alcohol be transplanted?
- Should patients who have a worse post transplant prognosis be transplanted (i.e. acute liver failure vs chronic liver disease)?
- Should patients with acute liver failure take priority over other patients already on a waiting list?
- What is the role of xenotransplantation?

Emergency transplantation

There are two liver transplant waiting lists in the UK:
- acute liver failure
- chronic liver disease.

Table 45 King's College Hospital criteria for listing for urgent liver transplantation in acute liver failure.

Paracetamol	pH <7.3 or prothrombin time >100 s + creatinine >300 µmol/L + grade 3/4 encephalopathy

Non-paracetamol	Prothrombin time >100 s or
	any three of the following:
	    aetiology: drug reactions or non-A non-B hepatitis
	    age <10 or >40
	    jaundice to encephalopathy in less than 7 days
	    prothrombin time >50 s
	    serum bilirubin >300 µmol/L

Certain strict criteria need to be met before an individual can be placed on the acute waiting list as these patients take priority over all other waiting list patients (Table 45).

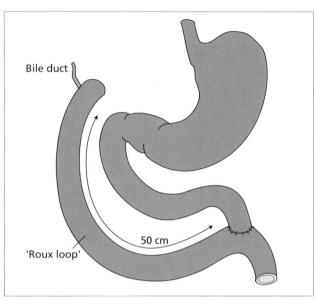

Fig. 72 Roux-en-Y biliary anastomosis.

Extent of liver dysfunction

The indication for liver transplantation in chronic liver disease is cirrhosis in the presence of hepatic decompensation, e.g. diuretic-resistant ascites, one episode of bacterial peritonitis, uncontrolled oesophageal variceal or gastric variceal bleeding, hepatic encephalopathy or a hepatocellular carcinoma <5 cm in diameter.

Quality of life is also an important consideration.

Timing of transplantation

Timing is a balance of risk of death without transplantation against risk with transplantation. Prognostic scores to assess mortality in chronic liver disease have been developed (e.g. Mayo score for primary biliary cirrhosis depending on albumin, PT and bilirubin) but are of limited value in individual patients.

Donor issues

A decision to list a patient for liver transplantation is also determined by the ease of organ procurement (worse if small size, blood group O or AB, needing more than one organ, e.g. cystic fibrosis). Individuals may wait up to a year for liver transplantation once listed.

Contraindications

• These include alcohol intake within the last 6 months as liver function can improve on abstinence, and this is also a risk factor for recidivism after transplantation. Consideration should be given to patients who deteriorate before 6 months has elapsed if they are likely to remain abstinent.

• Other absolute contraindications are cholangiocarcinoma, e.g. complicating primary sclerosing cholangitis, and active bacterial infection.

• Increasing age, advanced end-stage disease, poor nutrition and cardiorespiratory disease are all relative contraindications.

• The presence of psychiatric disease and absence of social support may adversely affect compliance with immunosuppressive medication.

Practical details

Biliary anastomosis is usually a duct to duct anastomosis but in the presence of recipient biliary disease (e.g. cystic fibrosis, PSC) a roux-en-Y biliary anastomosis is fashioned (Fig. 72).

 The waiting list is long (up to 12 months) and so early referral to a liver transplant centre is important. Patients with chronic liver disease do poorly if transplanted from the ICU.

Postoperative immunosuppression is usually a combination of prednisolone/azathiaprine and cyclosporin or tacrolimus. All patients require long-term immunosuppression but this can be achieved with monotherapy and often less is needed than with other organ transplants.

Outcome

The 1-year survival rate following transplantation for chronic liver disease is 80–95%, falling to 80% at 5 years primarily due to recurrent disease. The 1-year survival is only 61% following transplantation for acute liver failure, reflecting the presence of infection and multiorgan failure at the time of transplantation. Survival is lower following retransplantation.

Complications

Early complications

These include graft non-function and hepatic arterial or portal vein thrombosis, problems which usually require retransplantation. Up to 60% of individuals have at least one episode of acute cellular rejection, usually occurring in the first few weeks, but unlike in renal transplantation this is not a predictor of chronic rejection, which only affects 5–10% of recipients.

Biliary complications

These affect 10–20% of patients and include anastomatic biliary strictures and biliary leaks.

Disease recurrence

The most important late complication is disease recurrence; this may lead to graft loss before 5 years in hepatitis B and C.

1 The British Society of Gastroenterology. Indications for referral and assessment in adult liver transplantation. *Gut* 1999; Suppl. VI.
2 Neuberger J, James O. Guidelines for selection of patients for liver transplantation in the era of donor-organ shortage. *Lancet* 1999; 354: 1636–1639.
3 Masterton G. Psychological factors in selection for liver transplantation. *BMJ* 2000; 320: 263–264.

2.16 Screening, case finding and surveillance

Colorectal carcinoma

Attempting to identify asymptomatic individuals harbouring an important pathology is becoming an increasing challenge in gastroenterology. Overall the term screening tends to be applied to all such activities, although in some respects it is useful to distinguish:
• 'targeted' screening on the basis of a pre-existing disease (i.e. surveillance) or positive family history (i.e. case finding) (see *Oncology*, Sections 1.7 and 3.2)
• population screening of individuals of average risk.
Colorectal cancer is a significant cause of mortality in the UK and the adenoma to carcinoma sequence (Fig. 55, p. 94) provides the theoretical opportunity for early interven-

tion at the adenoma stage. Furthermore there are clearly identifiable 'at-risk' groups on the basis of either pre-existing disease or positive family history. Colorectal cancer therefore provides good examples of surveillance, case finding and potentially population screening.

2.16.1 SURVEILLANCE

Principle

Colonoscopy may identify adenomatous polyps in patients with a prior history of colorectal carcinoma or a previous high-risk polyp. Colonoscopy and colonic biopsy may identify high-grade dyplasia predicting the imminent development of carcinoma in patients with longstanding ulcerative colitis.

Indications

These include:
• previous diagnosis of colorectal carcinoma (CRC) (secondary prevention)
• previous high-risk colonic polyp (>1 cm, >20% villous architecture or severe dysplasia)
• longstanding (greater than 10 years) total (i.e. as opposed to distal or left-sided) ulcerative colitis (UC)
• familial colon cancer syndrome, familial adenomatous polyposis (FAP) or hereditary non-polyposis cancer syndromes (HNPCC).

Practical details

Total colonoscopy with biopsies looking for dysplasia is needed in the case of UC.
   Colonoscopy should be repeated at the following intervals:
• yearly for HNPCC
• 2-yearly for UC surveillance
• 5-yearly for polyps/previous CRC.

 Genetic testing for mutations in *h*MLH1 and *h*MSH2 may be of use in some kindreds with HNPCC.

Complications

Colonic perforation occurs in 1 : 1000. Bleeding occurs in 5 : 1000. Both complications are more likely after colonoscopic polypectomy.

Important information for patients

• Identification of a polyp warrants colonoscopic polypectomy which increases the risk of the procedure.

• Identification of high-grade dysplasia in longstanding UC is an indication for colectomy.

Clinic-based surveillance is also undertaken to detect:
• *Oesophageal carcinoma* by repeated endoscopy and biopsy, looking for dysplasia in Barrett's oesophagus.
• *Hepatocellular carcinoma* by repeated ultrasound and AFP measurement in cirrhotic patients.

2.16.2 CASE FINDING

Principle

Even in the absence of a familial cancer syndrome many individuals have an increased risk of CRC on the basis of a positive family history.

Indications

Colonoscopic surveillance is justified for lifetime risk of colorectal cancer of 1 : 10 or greater (e.g. one first-degree relative developing colorectal cancer <45 years or two first-degree relatives) (see Table 30).

Practical details

Regular colonoscopy and removal of any identified polyps. No hard evidence exists to support the recommended interval between examinations, but in most cases this is performed on a 3–5 yearly basis.

Case finding is also undertaken to detect:
• *haemochromatosis* by analysis for HFE mutation or measurement of iron indices in first-degree relatives of patients with haemochromatosis
• *Wilson's disease* by measurement of caeruloplasmin and 24 h urinary copper in first-degree relatives of patients with Wilson's disease.

2.16.3 POPULATION SCREENING

Principle

This is a very controversial topic. Many expect that screening the adult population in general might reduce the death rate from colorectal cancer and reduce morbidity (i.e. identification of disease at an earlier pathological stage) [1,2].

Indications

Most of the pilot studies have been directed at asymptomatic adults in midlife (usually around 50 years of age).

Practical details

Various approaches have been proposed:
• regular testing for faecal occult blood
• flexible sigmoidoscopy
• colonoscopy
• any combination of the above.

Comment

Given the time necessary to achieve the study end-points (i.e. development of a colon cancer or death) it may yet be many years before it is possible to say whether population screening is justified.

Atkin W. Implementing screening for colorectal cancer. *BMJ* 1999; 319: 1212–1213.
1 Rhodes JM. Colorectal cancer screening in the UK: Joint position statement by the British Society of Gastroenterology, the Royal College of Physicians, and the Association of Coloproctology of Great Britain and Ireland. *Gut* 2000; 46: 746–748.
2 Hardcastle J, Chamberlain JO, Robinson MK *et al.* Randomised control trial of faecal occult blood screening for colorectal cancer. *Lancet* 1996; 348: 1472–1477.

3 Investigations and practical procedures

3.1 General investigations

Biliary tract

Jaundice (hyperbilirubinaemia) and elevated 'biliary enzymes' (alkaline phosphatase, ALP and γ-glutamyl transferase, GGT) suggest biliary disease. Passage of gallstones may also cause pancreatitis, which should prompt further biliary investigation. Major pancreaticobiliary investigations are summarized in Table 46. Figure 73 shows an MRCP and Fig. 74 shows an ultrasound of the liver.

Luminal radiology

The lumen of the intestine can be imaged by introduction of radio-opaque contrast or air. Although still images are usually studied, much of the information comes from dynamic changes, so consultation with the radiologist

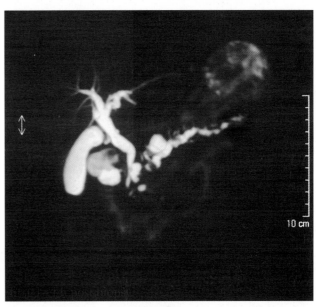

10 cm

Fig. 73 MRCP. The common bile duct and pancreatic duct are clearly seen with a filling defect in the pancreatic duct (a stone).

Table 46 Pancreaticobiliary investigations.

Investigation	Indications/abnormalities	Contraindications/notes
Ultrasound scan	Dilated intrahepatic ducts Dilated extrahepatic ducts Stones Gallbladder wall abnormalities Pancreatic abnormalities	Initial investigation of choice for suspected biliary and pancreatic disease Fasting avoids postprandial gallbladder emptying and increases sensitivity CT and MRI scanning may add further information, especially with intravenous contrast agents
Endoscopic retrograde cholangiopancreatography (ERCP)	Dilated or strictured ducts Typical features of PSC (beads on a string stricturing) Carcinoma of the head of the pancreas Stones	Contraindications as for any upper gastrointestinal endoscopy Side-viewing endoscope allows cannulation of the ampulla of Vater Radiocontrast injection delineates the biliary tract on fluoroscopy May be therapeutic (e.g. retrieval of stones, sphincterotomy, insertion of stent) Allows collection of cytological and microbiological samples
Percutaneous transhepatic cholangiography (PTC)	Dilated or strictured ducts	Caution if there is disordered coagulation or low platelet count Radiocontrast is introduced into the biliary system by percutaneous injection Indicated when ERCP is difficult or impossible May be therapeutic as well as diagnostic (e.g. allows cutaneous drainage of bile from an obstructed system and stent insertion)

Magnetic resonance cholangiopancreatography (MRCP)	Intra- and extrahepatic biliary and
	  pancreatic anatomy
	Can also detect solid parenchymal
	  lesions and thickening of the
	  bile ducts
		Cannot be performed in some patients with metallic implants
		  and electrical devices
		Claustrophobia is a relative contraindication
		Increasingly used as it is non-invasive and does not use X-rays
		Imaging is improving as software and machines evolve

Functional testing	HIDA (radionucleide) scanning Bromosulphthan excretion test	HIDA scanning demonstrates functional biliary excretion and is useful for delineating complicated surgical anastomoses, biliary leaks, etc. Bromosulphthalein excretion is a measure of biliary excretory function

CT, computed tomography; MRI, magnetic resonance imaging; PSC, primary sclerosing cholangitis.

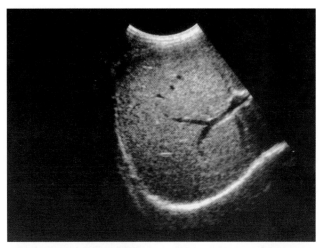

Fig. 74 Normal ultrasound of the liver. The liver has normal texture and the bile ducts are not dilated.

supervising the procedure is essential to obtain maximal diagnostic information (Fig. 47).

Major investigations are summarized in Table 47.

Endoscopy

Endoscopy of the intestinal tract is one of the most powerful diagnostic and therapeutic manoeuvres available to the physician, and can be safely performed under light sedation even in frail and ill patients. Originally flexible fibreoptic devices with a light source and a channel for suction, insufflation and instrumentation were used, but these are now increasingly replaced by devices that collect visual information through a charge-coupled device located at the end of the instrument. Channels for insufflation, suction and instrumentation are still present, but the visual information is transmitted electronically and viewed on a video-display unit. The main endoscopic procedures (apart from ERCP) are shown in Table 48.

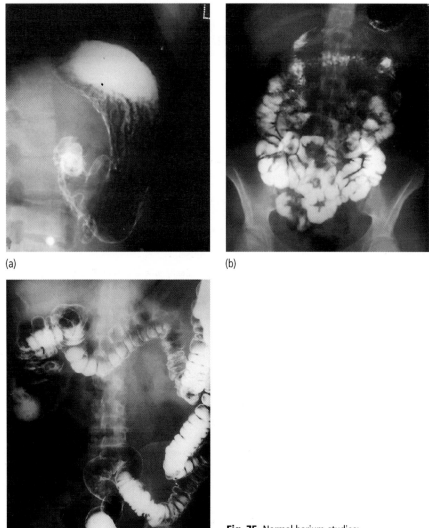

(a)

(b)

(c)

Fig. 75 Normal barium studies:
(a) barium meal; (b) barium follow-through;
and (c) barium enema.

Table 47 Radiological investigation of the gastrointestinal lumen.

Investigation	Indications/abnormalities	Contraindications/notes
Barium or gastrograffin swallow	Oesophageal dysmotility, stricture, neoplasia, and rupture or fistula are typically sought	Barium should be avoided if there is high suspicion of rupture, fistula or potential for aspiration, when gastrograffin (water-soluble contrast) is preferred Barium swallow should precede endoscopy in investigating dysphagia
Barium meal	Oral contrast is allowed to enter the stomach Can delineate stomach and duodenal ulcers Usually used to investigate gastric outlet obstruction, surgical anastomoses	Endoscopy is the preferred modality to investigate most gastric and duodenal pathology, but barium meal may be useful particularly in the postsurgical stomach
Barium meal and follow-through or small bowel enema	Diseases of the small intestine: lymphoma, tumours, Crohn's disease, Meckel's diverticulum	At present the only standard technique for imaging the small intestine Relatively insensitive and non-specific, and dependent on expert interpretation
Barium enema	Colorectal carcinoma, polyps, diverticulosis, complications of inflammatory bowel disease	Contraindicated in frail or immobile patients who are unable to position themselves on the radiology table, and who may be overcome by the strong purgative necessary beforehand Contraindicated for 24 h after rectal or colonic biopsy Alternative to colonoscopy that does not allow therapeutic manoeuvres such as polypectomy, or collection of tissue for histology
Contrast CT scanning and virtual colonoscopy	Colorectal carcinoma, polyps, diverticulosis, complications of inflammatory bowel disease	Used interchangeably with barium enema Air insufflation of the colon is well tolerated and allows delineation of the lumen Abnormalities of the wall can be detected Imaging is improving rapidly as image-processing software evolves

CT, computed tomography.

Table 48 Endoscopic techniques for examining the intestinal lumen.

Investigation	Indications/abnormalities	Contraindications/notes
Oesophagogastroduodenoscopy (OGD) (upper gastrointestinal endoscopy)	Causes of dyspepsia including peptic ulcer Causes of heartburn, including gastroesophageal reflux disease Causes of haematemesis, melaena, and iron-deficiency anaemia	Ensure that endoscopy is safe (e.g. that the patient's airway is protected, and the patient understands the procedure) A frail patient with cardiac failure or respiratory compromise should not be endoscoped without due attention to these problems Dysphagia may be caused by carcinoma of the oesophagus, which could be perforated on endoscopy: consider a barium or gastrograffin swallow first Endoscopy may be therapeutic as well as diagnostic (e.g. bonding of bleeding varices) Biopsy obtained for urease assay (CLO test) can diagnose *Helicobacter pylori* infection at the bedside. Patients should preferably abstain from acid-suppressing medications prior to the test Duodenal biopsy should always be performed when investigating iron-deficiency anaemia, to exclude coeliac disease
Enteroscopy	A special long endoscope may be introduced beyond the duodenum, but the technique is unreliable	There is no reproducible and reliable endoscopic means of examining the small intestine between the second part of the duodenum and the terminal ileum
Colonoscopy and terminal ileoscopy	Colitis, colorectal polyps, carcinoma, diverticulosis Terminal ileitis, ileal Crohn's disease and tuberculosis Mucosal lesions such as angiodysplasia that are not detected radiologically	Requires adequate colonic clearance (e.g. with polyethylene glycol containing purgative) Patients should be adequately informed about the procedure There is a risk of colonic perforation and bleeding, particularly if laser treatment, electrocautery or polypectomy is performed May be therapeutic and diagnostic
Flexible sigmoidoscopy	Colonic lesions distal to the splenic flexure	Does not require extensive colonic purging: may be performed after an enema. May be useful as a screening test, or to assess the extent of ulcerative colitis

Table 49 Investigation of occult gastrointestinal blood loss.

Investigation	Indications/abnormalities	Notes
Red cell scanning	The patient's red cells are radiolabelled and reinjected. A gamma camera is used to locate the site of radioactive accumulation, which corresponds to extravasation of blood	Requires relatively brisk bleeding, e.g. 100 mL/24 h May not provide sufficient anatomical detail to direct therapy
Meckel's scanning	Technetium label directed to parietal cells	Detects ectopic gastric mucosa, which may be associated with a Meckel's diverticulum
Selective visceral angiography	Brisk bleeding from the coeliac or mesenteric arterial territories	Requires fairly brisk bleeding to be detected, e.g. 750 mL/day May be therapeutic (embolization of vascular lesion)
Exploratory laparotomy	Reserved for young patients where an anatomical lesion such as Meckel's diverticulum is more likely	Often inadequate to locate subtle mucosal abnormalities such as angiodysplasia May be combined with 'on table' endoscopy, especially for the small intestine

Table 50 Functional and breath tests used in gastroenterology.

Investigation	Indications	Substrate	Metabolite/read-out	Notes
Urease breath test	*Helicobacter pylori* infection	^{13}C-labelled urea	^{13}C-labelled CO_2	Most sensitive and specific test for *H. pylori* infection
Lactose breath test	Hypolactasia	Lactose	Excess H_2 from bacterial fermentation of lactose	
Lactulose breath test	Intestinal bacterial overgrowth and intestinal hurry	Lactulose	Early release of excess H_2 by bacteria in the small intestine, or as a result of rapid intestinal transit	Lactulose is not absorbed or metabolized by the intestine, and normally reaches the large intestine intact
Glycocholate breath test	Intestinal bacterial overgrowth	Labelled glycine-glycocholate	Early release of labelled glycine by bacteria in the small intestine results in absorption of glycine and release of labelled CO_2 in the breath	
Xylose excretion test	Malabsorption due to small intestinal disease	Xylose	Urinary xylose excretion	The majority of ingested xylose is normally excreted unchanged by the kidneys, unless it is not absorbed
Schilling test	Cause of vitamin B_{12} deficiency	Labelled hydroxocobalamin (vitamin B_{12}) tracer administered after body stores are saturated by an intramuscular dose of unlabelled vitamin B_{12}	Urinary excretion of labelled vitamin B_{12}	Normal: complete absorption and excretion of vitamin B_{12} Pernicious anaemia: incomplete absorption and excretion of vitamin B_{12}, corrected by coadministration of intrinsic factor Terminal ileal disease: incomplete absorption and excretion of vitamin B_{12}, not corrected by coadministration of intrinsic factor

Oesophageal manometry and pH monitoring

Gastroesophageal reflux and associated pathology (especially Barrett's oesophagus and oesophageal adenocarcinoma) are assuming greater public health importance. Measuring gastroesophageal motility and acid reflux are important adjuncts to endoscopy and radiology and can be performed simply in an outpatient setting. A nasogastric tube is passed and pH or pressure measurements taken through an appropriate transducer and recording apparatus. The results are used to determine whether oesophageal symptoms (heartburn, pain, dysphagia or odynophagia) are related to acid reflux or abnormal oesophageal motility.

Gastrointestinal blood loss and iron-deficiency anaemia

Gastrointestinal bleeding resulting in overt melaena or rectal bleeding, or occult bleeding resulting in anaemia, may be difficult to localize in a minority of patients. Upper gastrointestinal endoscopy (OGD) and colonoscopy will provide a diagnosis in the majority of patients but may need to be repeated if the bleeding is intermittent or due to a small, easily missed lesion. Other techniques (Table 49) may also be used, particularly for blood loss from the small intestine, which is inaccessible to endoscopy.

Functional and breath tests

Bacterial metabolism or intestinal absorption of orally administered substrates forms the basis of a number of functional tests. In some cases the products of metabolism result in the release of H_2 or CO_2 gas which is detected on the breath. Alternatively, renal excretion of substrate is measured. Some commonly performed tests are described in Table 50.

Complications of gastrointestinal investigations

Some of the main complications of gastrointestinal investigations are:
- All tests requiring sedation carry the risk of hypoxia and aspiration pneumonia due to impaired consciousness.
- Inadvertent intubation of the respiratory tract can cause serious laryngeal spasm.
- Endoscopy and barium enema can increase cardiovascular stress and could induce angina in susceptible patients.
- Perforation of the intestine is a risk with all endoscopic examinations, particularly where the intestine is abnormal (e.g. if there is neoplastic tissue), or where a procedure such as polypectomy or sclerotherapy is performed.
- ERCP can cause acute pancreatitis, particularly if the pancreatic duct is cannulated.
- Extensive radiological investigation, particularly CT scanning and barium studies, result in high cumulative doses of radiation.

Bateson M, Bouchier I. *Clinical Investigations in Gastroenterology*, 2nd edn. Dordrecht: Kluwer Academic Publishers, 1997.

3.2 Rigid sigmoidoscopy and rectal biopsy

Principle

The rectum and proximal sigmoid colon can be viewed directly with a rigid instrument and a light source. Many symptomatic colorectal carcinomas occur distally, and patients with ulcerative colitis almost universally have rectal involvement.

Indications

These include:
- altered bowel habit
- rectal bleeding of unknown cause
- diarrhoea and rectal bleeding in patients with ulcerative colitis
- tenesmus, proctalgia
- to obtain rectal mucosal biopsy, e.g. for diagnosis of schistosomiasis, amyloidosis.

Contraindications

It cannot be performed if:
- the patient is unwilling, apprehensive or uncooperative
- there are inadequate facilities: lack of privacy, nurse escort or chaperone, biopsy forceps
- severe anorectal pain: consider examination under anaesthetic
- biopsy contraindicated in prescence of bleeding diathesis.

Practical details

Before the procedure

Patient

The procedure can usually be performed without an enema beforehand. Ensure that the patient's clotting and platelet count are satisfactory. Sedation or intravenous cannula are unnecessary.

Equipment

Essential equipment (Fig. 76) includes a sigmoidoscope with obturator, light source, insufflating bulb with functioning ball valve, and biopsy forceps. Lubricating jelly, swabs, towels, gloves and a specimen pot with histological fixative should be at hand.

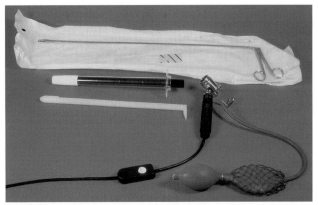

Fig. 76 Disposable plastic sigmoidoscope with obturator removed, light source and insufflator with rubber bulb, and sterilized packaged 'crocodile' biopsy forceps.

Personnel

Ensure that the patient understands the procedure, and that a nurse or assistant is present to reassure the patient, hand you additional equipment, and act as a chaperone.

The procedure

1 Explain the procedure and place the patient comfortably in the left lateral position, with the buttocks close to the edge of the couch and the knees slightly extended.
2 Perform a gentle rectal digital examination.
3 Lubricate the sigmoidoscope and obturator.
4 With the obturator fully inserted in the sigmoidoscope, insert the first 5 cm of the instrument into the anus, pointing anteriorly and cranially (towards the umbilicus).
5 Withdraw the obturator and attach the light-source head and insufflator.
6 Gently insufflate air and direct the instrument posteriorly (towards the sacro-iliac joint) until a luminal view is obtained.
7 Insert the instrument gently, insufflating and manoeuvring to maintain a luminal view.
8 Examine the mucosa in all directions by angling the instrument gently. The instrument may safely be inserted to 20 cm provided a mucosal view is maintained and the patient does not complain of discomfort.
9 If indicated obtain a mucosal biopsy by inserting a forceps through the viewing port, and gently shearing a sample of mucosa under direct vision.
10 Withdraw the instrument to 5 cm, carefully examining the mucosa. Replace the obturator and remove the instrument.

 It is safest to take a biopsy posteriorly and from the distal 10 cm where the rectum lies outside the peritoneum. Provided the anal mucosa is avoided, the procedure should be painless.

After the procedure

Medical

Warn the patient that there may be minor rectal bleeding for about 24 h if a biopsy has been taken.

Complications

Complications are rare, and may include:
• pain
• bleeding
• perforation.

 Bateson M, Bouchier I. *Clinical Investigations in Gastroenterology,* 2nd edn. Dordrecht: Kluwer Academic Publishers, 1997.

3.3 Paracentesis

Principle

Paracentesis can be diagnostic or therapeutic. A diagnostic paracentesis involves the removal of 50 mL ascitic fluid using a sterile green needle and syringe. The fluid should be analysed for albumin, amylase, cytology and a quantitative white count. If the fluid is cloudy chylous ascites is confirmed by an ascitic triglyceride level greater than the serum level.

Indications

 All patients with ascites must have a diagnostic ascitic tap.

Therapeutic paracentesis is used as treatment of tense diuretic-resistant ascites in patients with portal hypertension.

Contraindications

Small or large bowel obstruction with dilated loops of bowel.

Practical details

Before the procedure

Lie the patient flat on their back. Prepare the following equipment:
• suprapubic bladder drainage catheter or paracentesis catheter (Fig. 77)
• lignocaine 1 or 2%
• blade
• suture
• urine catheter bag
• 10 mL syringe and 18G needle.

The procedure

Insert the catheter into either the right or left iliac fossa. Clean the skin and infiltrate with lignocaine through to the peritoneum. Do not continue with the procedure if you are not able to draw back ascitic fluid while anaesthetizing. Make an incision in the skin.

 Insert the catheter through the skin and under the skin for 1-cm so, entering the peritoneum at 90 degrees to the skin and a little way from the skin entry site. This reduces the risk of an ascitic leak on removal of the catheter.

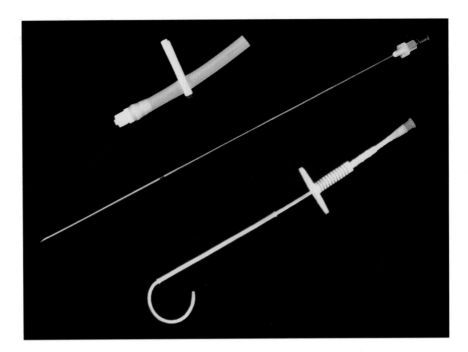

Fig. 77 Paracentesis catheter. Normally used for suprapubic catheterization, the catheter is easily introduced and when inserted the end of the catheter curls up in the abdominal cavity. Fluid drains through side holes in the distal catheter.

Suture a purse string around the catheter. Attach the end of the catheter to the urine bag. Tap the catheter securely to the abdominal wall.

After the procedure

Nursing

Allow 5–10 L of ascites to drain over 1–6 h. In patients with portal hypertension give 6 g albumin intravenously per litre of fluid drained (100 mL 4.5% albumin = 4.5 g; 100 mL 20% albumin = 20 g). If the fluid does not drain change the patient's position.

Medical

 Remove catheter after 6 h irrespective of the amount of fluid drained to reduce the risk of bacterial peritonitis.

Tighten the purse string around the exit site.

Complications

Major

• Peritoneal varices are rare but can be ruptured by the insertion of an ascitic drain.

Minor

• Failure to drain ascites. If the patient has had previous paracenteses the abdominal fluid often becomes loculated and the drain may need to be inserted under ultrasound guidance. The end of a suprapubic catheter is coiled and exudative malignant ascites may be more difficult to drain.
• Infection at exit site.

Fernandez-Esparrach G, Guevara M, Sort P *et al.* Diuretic requirements after therapeutic paracentesis in nonazotaemic patients with cirrhosis. A randomised double-blind trial of spironolactone vs placebo. *J Hepatol* 1997; 26: 616–620. [Diuretics should be continued in patients after paracentesis.]
Gines A, Fernandez-Esparrach G, Monescillo A *et al.* Randomised trial comparing albumin, dextran 70, and polygeline in cirrhotic patients with ascites treated by paracentesis. *Gastroenterol* 1996; 111: 1002–1110. [Albumin prevents postparacentesis circulatory dysfunction in cirrhosis.]

3.4 Liver biopsy

Principle

The aim is to obtain a core of liver tissue of sufficient length (about 2 cm, containing >4 portal tracts) to allow the histopathologist to establish a diagnosis. The procedure can be done 'blind' without imaging at the bedside, ultrasound guided or via the transjugular route.

 Liver biopsy can be performed as a day case in individuals who are non-cirrhotic with normal coagulation.

There is a move away from performing 'blind' biopsies to all biopsies being ultrasound guided; the latter are associated with less morbidity, e.g. pain.

Indications

Indications for liver biopsy:
- acute hepatitis
- drug-related hepatitis
- chronic liver disease
- cirrhosis
- post liver transplantation
- space-occupying lesions
- unexplained hepatomegaly or liver enzyme elevations.

Ultrasound guided

Specifically indicated in
- Focal liver lesion
- Small liver
- Emphysema.

Transjugular liver biopsy

Specifically indicated in
- Ascites
- Prolonged prothrombin time >4 s
- Platelet count <60 × 10⁹/L.

See Fig. 78.

Contraindications

A percutaneous liver biopsy is contraindicated in the case of:
- ascites
- coagulopathy
- an uncooperative patient.

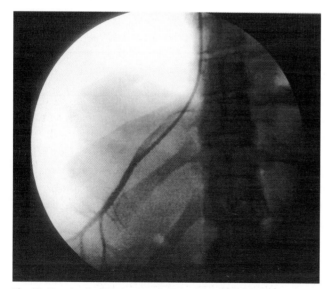

Fig. 78 Transjugular biopsy. Contrast is seen in a hepatic vein with the biopsy needle in the vein.

Practical details

Details are for percutaneous non-radiologically guided liver biopsies.

Before the procedure

Patient

Platelet count should be >60 × 10⁹/L; PT <3 s prolonged. If 3–4 s prolonged give fresh frozen plasma just prior to procedure. Sedation is usually avoided as the patient has to cooperate with breathing, but if sedation is required then use midazolam with monitoring of oxygen saturations. If the patient has renal failure then desmopressin acetate (DDAVP) should be given.

Personnel

An assistant is needed.

Equipment

- Menghini 1.9 mm diameter × 80–100 mm length needle or a Tru-cut needle (Fig. 79).
- saline 10 mL
- blade
- lignocaine 1or 2%, 10 mL
- formalin in a sterile container.

The procedure

1 Lie the patient flat on their back.
2 Mark the first dull intercostal space on expiration in the midaxillary line. The needle should be inserted over the top of a rib, avoiding the intercostal vessels below the rib.
3 Clean the skin with antiseptic.
4 Anaesthetize down to the liver capsule with lignocaine. Do this by advancing the needle slowly perpendicular to the skin with the patient holding their breath in expiration. You will feel the needle pass through skin and muscle and over the rib. You will hear the needle moving against the liver capsule when the patient breathes. It is important that you fully anaesthetize the liver capsule.

 If you cannot identify the capsule do not continue.

5 If using the Menghini needle a cut is made in the skin.
6 A track is then made down to the liver capsule using the metal needle in the Menghini pack.
7 The biopsy is now peformed by inserting the Menghini

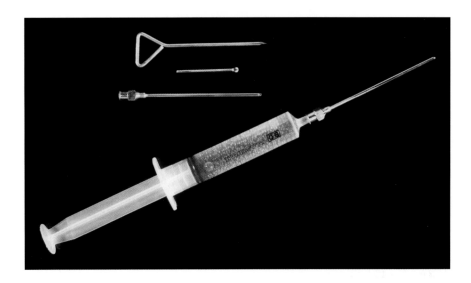

Fig. 79 Menghini biopsy needle.

needle (attached to a syringe of saline) down the preformed track as far as the liver capsule.

8 Then, while the patient is holding their breath in expiration, the needle is advanced quickly 2–3 cm in and out of the liver while continuously aspirating back on the syringe.

> ⚡ No more than two passes into the liver should be made.

After the procedure

Medical

Ensure analgesia (paracetamol or codeine; narcotics occasionally needed).

Nursing

The patient lies flat for 2 h with 6 h bed rest. Blood pressure and pulse recorded every 15 min for first 2 h and then half hourly for 2 h and then hourly.

Handling of specimens

The tissue should go into formaldehyde for routine histology. If Wilson's disease is suspected part of the biopsy is sent fresh for biochemical analysis. If tuberculosis is suspected part of the biopsy should be placed in a sterile vial for microbiology.

Complications

Mortality

Mortality rate is 0.01%.

Major

Haemorrhage

Occurs in 0.5%, usually occurs in first 3–4 h post biopsy. There is a higher rate in malignancy and it is rare in the non-jaundiced patient. If there is major bleeding, angiography followed by transcatheter hepatic embolization may be needed.

Intrahepatic haematomas

Rare. Consider if severe pain, fever, right upper quadrant tenderness. May be seen 24 h after biopsy.

Pneumothorax

Uncommon. May be complicated by haemothorax.

Minor

Pain

A small amount of bleeding is universal and minor discomfort is common. Pain is more likely during and after the procedure if the capsule is inadequately anaesthetized.

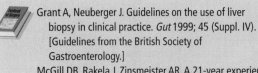 Grant A, Neuberger J. Guidelines on the use of liver biopsy in clinical practice. *Gut* 1999; 45 (Suppl. IV). [Guidelines from the British Society of Gastroenterology.]
McGill DB, Rakela J, Zinsmeister AR. A 21-year experience with major haemorrhage after percutaneous liver biopsy. *Gastroenterol* 1990; 99: 1396–1400. [Incidence of bleeding after a liver biopsy.]

Answers on pp. 145–155.

Question 1
Gastrinoma (T/F):
A Causes constipation
B May be associated with hypercalcaemia
C If sporadic is usually single
D Is always easy to identify
E Is diagnosed by a fasting gastrin level when taking a proton pump inhibitor.

Question 2
H. pylori infection (T/F):
A Is more prevalent in the UK than in central Africa
B Is associated with T-cell gastric lymphoma
C Produces a urease
D Eradication can be confirmed by serology
E Resistance to clarithromycin and metronidazole occurs.

Question 3
A Primary sclerosing cholangitis
B Primary biliary cirrhosis
C Choledocholithiasis
D Cholangiocarcinoma.
Which is the single most useful test in making the above diagnoses? The tests can be used once, more than once or not at all.
1 Liver biopsy
2 CA19-9
3 Antimitochondrial antibody
4 Endoscopic retrograde cholangiopancreatography (ERCP)
5 Abdominal CT scan.

Question 4
Common bile duct stones may present with (T/F):
A Non-dilated common bile duct on ultrasound
B Macrocytic anaemia
C Chronic pancreatitis
D Hypotension
E Cholestatic liver biochemistry in the absence of jaundice.

Question 5
Acute liver failure is commonly complicated by (T/F):
A Gastrointestinal haemorrhage
B Acute tubular necrosis
C Bacterial infections
D Hypotension
E Haemolysis.

Question 6
A Acute hepatitis B
B Liver failure from acute hepatitis B
C Hepatitis B vaccination
D Chronic hepatitis B.
Which of the following serological patterns are seen in the above states of hepatitis B infection? Each option may be used once, more than once or not at all.
1 HBsAg and e Ag
2 Hepatitis B core IgM alone
3 HBsAb and HBcAb
4 HBsAb alone
5 HBcAb (IgG) alone.

Question 7
A Paracetamol
B Flucloxacillin
C Rifampicin
D Amioderone
E Non-steroidal anti-inflammatory drugs
F Co-proxamol.
For each of the drugs select the commonest type of liver damage caused by the drug. Each option may be used once, more than once or not at all.
1 Acute hepatitis
2 Acute cholestasis
3 No liver damage
4 Steatohepatitis
5 Granuloma.

Question 8
A Phenytoin
B Augmentin
C Ibuprofen
D Methotrexate
E Isoniazid.
In a hepatic drug toxicity which of the above drugs causes the pattern of liver biochemistry shown below? Each option may be used once, more than once or not at all.
1 Elevated transaminases (ALT and AST)
2 Elevated alkaline phosphatase and GGT
3 Normal liver biochemistry
4 Elevated GGT alone.

Question 9
The indications for liver transplantation are (T/F):
A Primary biliary cirrhosis in a 75-year-old

B A 3-cm hepatocellular carcinoma complicating hepatitis
C cirrhosis
C Spontaneous bacterial peritonitis
D Acute alcoholic hepatitis
E Haemophilia with end-stage hepatitis C.

Question 10
The following conditions may recur following liver transplantation (T/F):
A Hepatitis C
B Non-A non-B non-C hepatitis (cryptogenic)
C Autoimmune chronic active hepatitis
D Primary sclerosing cholangitis
E Wilson's disease.

Question 11
A *Campylobacter*
B *Clostridium difficile*
C *Salmonella*
D *Shigella*
E HIV
F *Yersinia enterocolitica*
G *Escherichia coli.*
For each statement, select the most appropriate organism from the list of options above. Each option may be used once, more than once or not at all.
1 Metronidazole is an effective treatment
2 May result in asymptomatic gall bladder carriage
3 Guillain–Barré is a rare complication
4 Causes a terminal ileitis which may mimic Crohn's disease.

Question 12
A Vitamin A
B Thiamine (vitamin B_1)
C Pyridoxine (vitamin B_6)
D Cobalamin (Vitamin B_{12})
E Vitamin C
F Iron
G Folic acid
H Niacin (nicotinamide)
I Magnesium.
Deficiencies of the above vitamins/trace elements may cause various defects. From the above list, select the most likely vitamin/trace element causing the conditions listed below.
1 Nystagmus
2 Perifollicular haemorrhages
3 Bitot's spots
4 Sideroblastic anaemia.

Question 13
The following are associated with an increased risk of oesophageal carcinoma (T/F):
A Barrett's oesophagus

B NSAIDs
C Hypercalcaemia
D Achalasia
E Familial tylosis.

Question 14
Achalasia (T/F):
A Has characteristic features on manometry
B Is associated with the presence of hiatus hernias
C Responds to botulinum toxin injections
D Is a risk factor for the development of oesophageal carcinoma
E Is associated with gastroesophageal reflux disease.

Question 15
The following are characteristics of the MMC (migrating motor complex) (T/F):
A It is most prominent immediately after eating
B It is abolished by sleep
C The major propulsive wave is during phase III
D It is abolished by eating
E It is confined to the small intestine.

Question 16
Which of the following are true of bile salts?
A Preferentially absorbed from the colon
B Malabsorption causes constipation
C Malabsorption may be caused by right hemicolectomy
D Malabsorption is treated with ursodeoxycholic acid
E SeHCAT test showing <20% retention at 7 days is abnormal.

Question 17
Which of the following are true of idiopathic inflammatory bowel disease?
A Rectal sparing is a recognized feature of Crohn's disease
B 5-aminosalicylic acid compounds induce remission in the majority of patients
C The ESR and CRP are early markers of flares of ulcerative colitis
D The incidence of Crohn's disease is increasing worldwide
E Rigid sigmoidoscopy is contraindicated in an acute flare of ulcerative colitis.

Question 18
Consider whether the following statements concerning a patient with chronic diarrhoea are true.
A Infectious diarrhoea is excluded if symptoms have continued for longer than 4 weeks.
B The stool leucocyte count is a reliable test for inflammatory bowel disease.
C HIV infection is commonly associated with recurrent bacterial dysentery.
D Amoebiasis is reliably diagnosed on routine stool culture.

E Metronidazole is a recognized part of the treatment of exacerbations of Crohn's disease.

Question 19

Match the following diseases with the most appropriate test result.

A Alpha 1-antitrypsin deficiency
B Wilson's disease
C Genetic haemochromatosis
D Primary biliary cirrhosis
E Primary sclerosing cholangitis.
1 Highly typical genetic abnormality
2 'Beads on a string' sign
3 Positive antiliver and kidney microsomal antibody
4 Reduced serum copper
5 Raised serum copper
6 Raised serum immunoglobulin level
7 Abnormal serum electrophoresis
8 Positive antimitochondrial antibody.

Question 20

Regarding the complications of chronic liver disease (T/F):
A Ascites may be precipitated by portal vein thrombosis
B Variceal haemorrhage and ascites should prompt consideration of liver transplantation
C Maintaining a low protein diet is critical
D The diagnosis of spontaneous bacterial peritonitis should be based on a positive ascites culture
E Coagulation abnormalities are caused exclusively by decreased hepatic function.

Question 21

For each scenario, select the most likely cause of a single focal lesion noted on ultrasound of the liver.

A A 24-year-old married female with tender right upper quadrant pain
B A 24-year-old male with jaundice and a history of chronic bloody diarrhoea
C A 60-year-old male with a recent history of altered bowel habit
D A 60-year-old healthy male with no medical history and normal blood tests
E A 60-year-old male with a history of hepatitis B infection.
1 Focal nodular hyperplasia
2 Hepatocellular carcinoma (HCC)
3 Colorectal carcinoma
4 Haemangioma
5 Cholangiocarcinoma
6 Pyogenic liver abscess
7 Amoebic liver abscess
8 Hepatic adenoma.

Question 22

Choose the most appropriate answer.

A Cirrhosis is the most important risk for primary liver cancer.
B HCC is the most common malignant lesion in the liver.
C Gallstones may cause cholangiocarcinoma.
D Hepatic adenomas should be treated with wide segmental resection as there is a high risk of malignant transformation.
E Hepatic adenomas never require resection.

Question 23

Choose the most appropriate diagnostic test for each condition.

A Progressive dysphagia for solids
B Iron, B_{12} and folate deficiency
C Persistent epigastric pain in an otherwise healthy 30-year-old male
D Jaundice in a patient with ulcerative colitis
E Exacerbation of ulcerative colitis.
1 Oesophagogastroduodenoscopy
2 Barium meal and follow-through or small bowel enema
3 Colonoscopy
4 Barium enema
5 ERCP
6 Barium swallow
7 Schilling test
8 Urease breath test.

Question 24

Which of the following statements regarding gastro-intestinal investigations are true?

A Urease breath test is the most sensitive and specific test of HP infection.
B The CLO test is based on a solid phase ELISA test for the most common HP-associated antigens.
C The Schilling test can distinguish pernicious anaemia from small intestinal malabsorption as a cause of vitamin B_{12} deficiency.
D Enteroscopy is a promising alternative to small bowel radiology that allows direct visualization and biopsy of the mucosa.
E Virtual colonoscopy is based on computer-generated three-dimensional reconstruction of the colon from high-resolution air-contrast CT scan images.

Question 25

In acute pancreatitis (T/F):

A The prognosis is poor if the serum amylase is greater than 2000
B A CT scan should be performed in all cases
C Early feeding is contraindicated
D Cholecystectomy should be deferred for at least 6 weeks in cases of severe gallstone pancreatitis;
E If caused by ERCP it has a good prognosis.

Question 26
The following are recognized presentations of chronic pancreatitis (T/F):
A Jaundice
B Weight loss
C Abdominal pain
D Ascites
E Iron deficiency.

Question 27
The following clinical features favour a diagnosis of colorectal cancer over that of diverticular change (T/F):
A An acute lower gastrointestinal haemorrhage
B Change in bowel habit
C Iron deficiency
D A tender left iliac fossa mass
E A sigmoid stricture demonstrated on barium enema.

Question 28
Match the inherited gastrointestinal condition to the most appropriate statement relating to the potential for genetic testing of first-degree relatives.
A Familial adenomatous polyposis (FAP)
B Hereditary non-polyposis colon cancer (HNPCC)
C Peutz–Jeghers syndrome
D Hereditary pancreatitis
E Haemochromatosis.
1 Clinical phenotype only
2 Genetic mutation analysis
3 Haplotype analysis
4 Family history only.

Question 29
The following are all characteristic features of a functional bowel disorder (T/F):
A Abdominal pain that disturbs sleep
B Intolerance of dairy products
C The passage of blood per rectum
D The passage of mucus per rectum
E Diurnal mood variation.

Question 30
Regarding sphincter of Oddi dysfunction (T/F):
A It can cause biliary colic
B It can cause liver blood test abnormalities
C It is associated with significant mortality
D ERCP and endoscopic sphincterotomy provides the best treatment
E ERCP and sphincterotomy is safe.

Question 31
The following scenarios suggest an increased lifetime risk of colorectal cancer (T/F):
A A 1.5-cm villous adenoma of the rectum
B Multiple hyperplastic rectal polyps
C Distal ulcerative colitis
D Two first-degree relatives with colorectal cancer presenting after the age of 70
E A single first-degree relative with colorectal cancer presenting before the age of 45.

Question 32
Which of the following statements relating to surveillance and screening for colorectal cancer are true?
A Yearly flexible sigmoidoscopy is necessary in patients with a history suggesting hereditary non-polyposis colon cancer (HNPCC).
B Barium enema is a suitable alternative method for screening patients at low to moderate risk.
C The sensitivity of colonoscopy may be increased by the use of dye spraying.
D Faecal occult blood (FOB) testing is cheap and very sensitive.
E Genetic mutation analysis is at present only likely to be beneficial in less than 5% of cases.

Question 33
A 42-year-old man presents with a 2-week history of painless jaundice.
Investigations show:
bilirubin 200 μmol/L
alkaline phosphatase 800 IU/L
aspartate transaminase 120 IU/L
gamma glutamyl transferase 100 IU/L
prothrombin time 18 s.
Which of the following diagnoses are consistent with this clinical picture?
A Acute hepatitis A
B Acute alcoholic hepatitis
C Primary sclerosing cholangitis
D Acute hepatitis B
E Paracetamol hepatoxicity.

Question 34
Consider the CT scan in Fig. 80.
1 What is the diagnosis?
2 What three abnormalities are shown on the CT scan?
3 How is the condition inherited?

Question 35
A 23-year-old girl presents with non-specific symptoms of lethargy and impaired concentration. She thinks her sister has liver disease. On examination she has a small liver and a palpable spleen and is in grade 1 hepatic encephalopathy. Investigations show:
Hb 8 g/dL
MCV 102fL
Platelets 80 × 109/L

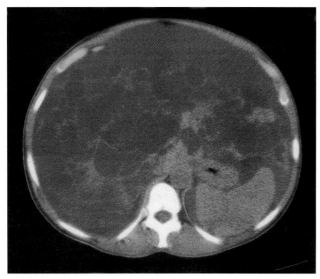

Fig. 80 Question 34.

Reticulocyte count 6%
Bilirubin 200 μmol/L
Alkaline phosphatase 100 IU/L
Aspartate transaminase 200 IU/L
Prothrombin time 25 s.
1 Why is it important to look in her eyes?
2 Why is she anaemic?
3 What is the diagnosis?
4 How can this condition present?

Question 36
Chronic hepatitis C infection (T/F):
A Is a risk factor for hepatocellular carcinoma in the absence of cirrhosis
B Can be transmitted vertically from an infected mother
C Is a contraindication to breast feeding
D Is more likely to result in progressive liver damage if acquired after the age of 40
E Should be treated with interferon monotherapy.

Question 37
Concerning bacterial overgrowth (T/F):
A A low folate is a common finding
B It is a recognized complication of systemic sclerosis
C It is associated with the use of proton pump inhibitors
D Diagnosis is usually made by a lactose hydrogen breath test
E Cholestyramine is a useful treatment.

Question 38
With regard to gut motility (T/F):
A Erythromycin accelerates gastric emptying
B The MMC (migrating motor complex) propels colonic contents aborally
C Small bowel transit is around 10 h in health

D The colon exhibits cyclical motor activity
E Simultaneous high-amplitude contractions occur in the normal oesophagus.

Question 39
A Elemental diet
B Percutaneous endoscopic gastrostomy (PEG) feeding tube
C Total parenteral nutrition (TPN)
D Oral supplements (e.g. Fortijuice)
E Percutaneous endoscopic jejunostomy (PEJ) feeding tube.
Choose the most appropriate nutritional support from the above for the indications listed below.
1 Persistent dysphagia following a stroke
2 Massive small bowel resection following mesenteric infarction
3 Preoperative work up of oropharyngeal carcinoma patients
4 Active small bowel Crohn's disease
5 Postoperative nutrition in patients with gastroparesis.

Question 40
With regard to gut hormones (T/F):
A CCK is secreted from the duodenal mucosa and causes gall bladder contraction
B Proton pump inhibitors cause hypogastrinaemia
C Somatostatin inhibits release of gastrin
D VIPomas classically present with watery diarrhoea and a hypokalaemic alkalosis
E Secretin is released from the pancreas in response to exposure of the duodenum to acid.

Question 41
Crohn's disease (T/F):
A Is associated with smoking
B May cause bile salt malabsorption
C Predisposes to DVTs
D Never affects the lips
E Should be considered in resistant duodenal ulcers.

Question 42
A Duodenal biopsies
B Small bowel meal
C Rectal biopsy
D Lactose hydrogen breath test
E CLO test
F Glucose hydrogen breath test
G SeHCAT test.
Choose the most helpful investigation from the above for each of the four scenarios described below. Each investigation may be chosen once, more than once or not at all.
1 A young woman with abdominal pain, diarrhoea and weight loss
2 A middle-aged man with diarrhoea who suffers from CREST syndrome

3 A middle-aged women who is found to have a dimorphic blood film

4 A young male who is found to have a 'beaded' intrahepatic biliary tree at ERCP following the work up of abnormal LFTs.

Question 43

Gilbert's syndrome (T/F):

A Is present in about 4% of the population

B Characteristically results in an isolated conjugated hyperbilirubinaemia

C Results in a decreased haptoglobin concentration

D Is associated with an increased incidence of bile pigment gallstones

E Causes elevation of the serum bilirubin during fasting.

Question 44

In ulcerative colitis (T/F):

A Bloody diarrhoea is a late sign

B Skin rashes are common, and pyoderma gangrenosum is the commonest

C Joint symptoms are rare, and should prompt the clinician to exclude other diseases such as infectious diarrhoea

D Primary sclerosing cholangitis is an infrequent complication of poorly controlled disease

E About 15% of patients have an affected first-degree relative.

Question 45

Match the following.

A Clinical response to oral metronidazole

B Increased incidence of colorectal carcinoma

C Vesicular skin rash

D Chronic abdominal pain radiating through to the back

E Middle-aged Caucasian males most affected.

1 Coeliac disease

2 Crohn's disease

3 Whipple's disease

4 Ulcerative pancolitis

5 Chronic pancreatitis.

Question 46

Hepatitis C virus infection (T/F):

A Is most commonly transmitted sexually or from mother to child

B Persists only in those patients who do not develop acute hepatitis

C Often causes hepatocellular carcinoma even in the absence of cirrhosis

D Is caused by an RNA virus

E May be associated with autoimmune phenomena.

Question 47

In chronic liver disease (T/F):

A Spontaneous bacterial peritonitis is less common than in acute liver failure

B Gallstones are common but usually asymptomatic

C Coronary artery disease is more common

D Liver transplantation should be offered as soon as practical providing the patient is not a chronic alcohol abuser or otherwise unfit

E Hepatic encephalopathy can progress rapidly to coning and death.

Question 48

Which of the following are true?

A Magnetic resonance imaging of the abdomen has limited resolution because of the presence of air in the bowel.

B Contrast-enhanced ultrasound scanning increases the sensitivity of detection of hepatic mass lesions.

C Plain abdominal radiograph can detect 90% of gallstones.

D ERCP is generally safe, but should not be performed in patients with known obstruction of the biliary tract.

E Pancreatic calcification is diagnostic of acute pancreatitis.

Question 49

Match the following:

A Extremely sensitive and specific serological test

B Non-specific finding in many upper GI disorders

C Invalidated if the patient is on a gastric acid-suppressing medication

D Indicative of a systemic vasculitic disorder, and may be associated with inflammatory bowel disease

E Strongly differentiates Crohn's disease from ulcerative colitis.

1 Positive ANCA

2 Positive antiendomysial antibody

3 Urease breath test

4 Submucosal granulomas

5 Serum amylase raised to twice the upper limit of normal.

Question 50

The following statements relate to the clinical assessment of pancreatic disease (T/F):

A A normal serum amylase excludes a diagnosis of chronic pancreatitis

B Abdominal CT is useful in diagnosis of pancreas divisum

C ERCP is useful in the assessment of hereditary pancreatitis

D A 3-day faecal fat estimation remains the only reliable method for diagnosing pancreatic malabsorption

E A successful pancreolauryl test requires a reliable 24-hour urine collection.

Question 51

The following clinical features would suggest that a right iliac fossa mass is more likely to be malignant than due to an inflammatory process such as Crohn's disease (T/F):

143

A Raised ESR

B Anaemia

C Thrombocytosis

D Weight loss

E Symptoms of subacute intestinal obstruction (i.e. postprandial bloating with nausea and colicky abdominal pain).

Question 52

Intestinal obstruction complicating colorectal cancer (T/F):

A Carries a poor prognosis

B May be safely demonstrated by double contrast barium enema

C Is an indication for urgent colonoscopy

D Can commonly be alleviated by stenting

E Requires a CT or ultrasound scan for staging of disease before consideration of surgery.

Question 53

Suspecting alcohol as a significant contribution to a patient's presenting complaint, it is useful to do the following (T/F):

A Check MCV

B Check GGT

C Check random ethanol level

D Confront the patient

E Seek corroborative evidence from other sources such as the GP or other family members.

Question 54

Diarrhoea of more than 6 weeks' duration (T/F):

A May warrant an empirical course of antibiotics

B May be due to NSAIDs

C Is never due to dietary factors alone

D May require upper gastrointestinal endoscopy as part of the assessment

E May require colonoscopy and colonic biopsies.

Question 55

The following statements relate to the clinical evaluation of suspected iron deficiency (T/F):

A Transferrin saturation should always be performed on a fasting sample

B A low serum ferritin is very specific

C Coeliac disease is unlikely in the absence of weight loss or malabsorption

D May require bone marrow examination

E Investigation is not required if the patient is taking a diet poor in iron.

Answers to Self-assessment

Answers to Question 1
F, T, T, F, F
- Classically associated with profuse watery diarrhoea.
- Gastrinoma may occur in individuals with MEN type 1. Hyperparathyroidism which is associated with hypercalcaemia is part of this syndrome.
- Gastrinomas are either sporadic or associated with MEN type 1. Sporadic gastrinomas are more likely to be benign and solitary.
- Occur in the pancreas and duodenum. They can be difficult to localize even with CT or MRI scanning.
- Proton pump inhibitors cause elevations in serum gastrin. The diagnosis is made by the finding of an elevated fasting serum gastrin while off a proton pump inhibitor.

Answers to Question 2
F, F, T, F, T
- Prevalence is associated with socioeconomic class. The prevalence is falling in the UK.
- The organism's ability to produce a urease is used in diagnostic tests such as the urea breath test and CLO test.
- Infection is associated with low-grade B-cell lymphoma of the stomach (MALT lymphoma).
- Serology is only useful in diagnosis. Antibodies persist after the eradication of infection.
- Eradication occurs in 90% of individuals who take two antibiotics and a proton pump inhibitor for a week. These regimes are either clarithromycin or metronidazole based. Retreatment may be needed if there is selective antibiotic resistance.

Answers to Question 3
A4 B3 C4 D4
In early primary sclerosing cholangitis a liver biopsy may be normal. High-titre antimitochondrial antibodies are specific for primary biliary cirrhosis (PBC) and present in 95% of patients with PBC. In cholangiocarcinoma the tumour is confined to the bile duct and so a CT scan may show no tumour mass and the tumour marker CA19-9 is not sensitive or specific enough to use diagnostically.

Answers to Question 4
T, T, F, T, T
- The common bile duct may not dilate in acute biliary obstruction. In the presence of cholestatic liver biochemistry, stones in the gall bladder and a history of pain ERCP is indicated.
- Haemolysis causes macrocytosis and pigmented gallstones.
- CBD stones often present with acute pancreatitis. In chronic pancreatitis stones form in the pancreatic duct. CBD stones occur above a lower common bile duct stricture due to chronic pancreatitis causing jaundice.
- Acute cholangitis is a cause of septic shock.
- If bile duct obstruction is incomplete or intermittent jaundice is absent.

Answers to Question 5
F, F, T, T, F
- Although prothrombin time is usually greater than 50 s spontaneous bleeding is rare. Hepatorenal failure is the most common cause of renal failure. Acute tubular necrosis may complicate paracetamol overdose.
- Up to 70% of patients with acute liver failure develop bacterial infections and 30–40% fungal sepsis.
- Haemolysis complicates Wilson's disease but this is a rare cause of acute liver failure.

Answers to Question 6
A1 B2 C4 D1

Answers to Question 7
A1 B2 C3 D4 E1 F2

Answers to Question 8
A4 B2 C1 D3 E1

Answers to Question 9
F, T, T, F, T
- Liver transplantation is rarely performed in patients over 65 years of age.
- Primary hepatocellular carcinoma less than 3 cm can be cured by transplantation.
- The 1-year survival following first episode of spontaneous bacterial peritonitis is less than 50% and so such patients should be considered for transplantation.
- The outcome of liver transplantation for acute alcoholic hepatitis is poor with 1-year survival of less than 50%.
- Liver transplantation can safely be performed in haemophilia, which is cured.

Answers to Question 10
T, F, T, T, F
- All patients with hepatitis C become HCV RNA positive again following liver transplantation and 15–20% are cirrhotic within 5 years.
- Acute liver failure due to non-A non-B non-C (or cryptogenic) hepatitis does not recur following liver transplantation although a mild hepatitis is often observed histologically.
- Although primary sclerosing cholangitis recurs following transplantation it does not adversely affect graft or patient survival in the short term (5–10 years).
- Liver transplantation cures Wilson's disease as the metabolic defect is in the liver. The effect of liver transplantation on the neurological complications of Wilson's disease is variable.

Answers to Question 11
1B 2C 3A 4F
- The use of broad-spectrum antibiotics diminishes the normal colonic flora and allows proliferation of *Clostridium*

difficile. It liberates toxins causing diarrhoea, inflammation and classically pseudomembranes, hence 'pseudomembranous colitis'. Clindamycin and cephalosporin usage are particularly implicated, although the infection can result from any antibiotic. Metronidazole is effective treatment and should be given for 1 week. Oral vancomycin is an alternative (more expensive), and may be used to treat relapses.

• *Salmonella* may be carried in the gall bladder in asymptomatic individuals. Any person involved with the food industry must have three negative stool cultures following *Salmonella* infection before returning to work.

• *Campylobacter* is probably the most common cause of bacterial gastroenteritis in the UK. It may cause Reiter's syndrome, and rarely Guillain–Barré.

• *Yersinia enterocolitica* invades and proliferates in the Peyer's patches in the distal small bowel, causing mesenteric adenitis and a terminal ileitis, which may mimic terminal ileal Crohn's disease on barium studies. Stool cultures and antibody titres will differentiate.

Answers to Question 12

1B 2E 3A 4C

• Thiamine deficiency leads to Wernicke's encephalopathy, characterized by confusion, ataxia, nystagmus and ophthalmoplegia. Wernicke's encephalopathy develops acutely and arises from poor nutrition, e.g. associated with alcoholism and hyperemesis gravidarum. Haemorrhages occur in the mammillary bodies, walls of the third ventricle, thalamus and periaqueductal grey matter. Red cell transketolase is elevated. Urgent treatment with i.v. thiamine is indicated to prevent the development of Korsakoff's psychosis (inability to lay down new memory, confabulation). Beware giving i.v. dextrose if Wernicke's is a possibility, as it consumes the remaining thiamine.

• Scurvy, due to vitamin C deficiency, is characterized by bleeding gums, loose teeth, perifollicular haemorrhages and 'corkscrew' hair and easy bruising.

• Vitamin A deficiency leads to night blindness. Bitot's spots are whitish plaques of keratinized epithelial cells on the conjunctiva, and are associated with vitamin A deficiency.

• Erythroblasts (sideroblasts) normally contain two or three granules of iron around the nucleus. Ringed sideroblasts are pathological and show a 'collar' of iron granules around the nucleus. Sideroblastic anaemia is characterized by hypochromic peripheral erythrocytes, with increased bone marrow iron and ringed sideroblasts. Causes are hereditary or acquired. Aquired may be primary due to somatic mutations, associated with myelodysplastic syndromes, or secondary to drugs, e.g. isoniazid (B_6 antagonist), alcohol, lead poisoning or pyridoxine (vitamin B_6) deficiency.

Answers to Question 13

T, F, F, T, T

• Barrett's oesophagus is associated with a relative risk of

approximately ×40 for oesophageal carcinoma. Male gender, smoking, length of Barrett's epithelium, and ulceration are associated with increased risk. Achalasia is likewise a risk factor for oesophageal carcinoma.

• NSAIDs may cause oesophageal damage and ulceration, especially if they lodge in the gullet.

• Hypercalcaemia is a risk factor for ulcer disease and pancreatitis ('abdominal moans, groans, bones and stones'). It does not increase the risk of oesophageal carcinoma.

• Familial hyperkeratosis of the palms of the hands and soles of the feet is strongly associated with the development of oesophageal carcinoma.

Answers to Question 14

T, F, T, T, F

• Achalasia is diagnosed by a typical history, usually of slowly progressive dysphagia for both solids and liquids, a dilated oesophagus with distal smooth tapered appearance ('bird's beak'), and manometry which shows a hypertensive lower oesophageal sphincter which fails to relax upon swallowing.

• Aetiology is unknown. Chagas' disease may mimic it. There is no association with hiatus hernias.

• Injection of botulinum toxin into the lower oesophageal sphincter is effective but often further injections are required. The traditional methods are balloon dilatation or surgical myotomy.

• It is not associated with reflux disease, but patients often suffer from this following balloon dilatation or surgical intervention. It confers a relative risk of approximately 15-fold for the development of oesophageal carcinoma.

Answers to Question 15

F, F, T, T, F

The migrating motor complex describes an electrical (and motor) pattern of activity which traverses the gastrointestinal tract in an aboral direction in the fasted state. It usually begins in the oesophagus, but may start in the stomach or small intestine, and has generally petered out before reaching the terminal ileum. It is thought to act as the 'housekeeper', keeping the small intestinal lumen clear of debris and bacteria. It is abolished by eating and returns some 3–4 h postprandially. The most intense electrical activity is classified as phase III and corresponds to a contraction which sweeps down the small intestine. Sleep slows the velocity of propagation of the MMC, shortens the periodicity and reduces phase II activity, but does not abolish it.

Answers to Question 16

F, F, T, F, F

Bile salts are passively and actively absorbed from the distal ileum and recirculated, forming the enterohepatic circulation. Bile salt malabsorption may be idiopathic, or secondary to damage to the terminal ileum (e.g. Crohn's disease) or resection. It is also occasionally provoked by cholecystectomy, probably due to increased production and cycling of bile salts which overwhelm the absorptive capacity of the ileum. Failed uptake by the distal ileum results in passage into the colon where they are irritant and cause diarrhoea. Ursodeoxycholic acid is a synthetic bile acid which may be used for dissolution of gallstones and is also often used in primary biliary cirrhosis. Cholestyramine binds bile salts and prevents their irritative effect on the colonic mucosa and ameliorates bile salt diarrhoea. Retention of >10% of the synthetic bile salt SeHCAT is normal; <5% is abnormal; 5–10% is borderline.

Answers to Question 17
T, F, F, T, F

- Rectal involvement is almost universal in ulcerative colitis, where inflammation extends continuously from the rectum to variable distances proximally, up to the caecum. In Crohn's disease, however, inflammation may be patchy, affecting variable parts of the intestine. In a third of cases the anorectum is involved, but in other patients the rectum may be spared.

- Remission is usually induced by steroid treatment. 5 aminosalicylic acid compounds (sulphasalazine, mesalazine, olsalazine and balsalazide) have a recognized role in maintaining remission.

- The CRP and ESR are usually only raised in very severe ulcerative colitis, and patients may have significant inflammation without a systemic response. The response is more pronounced and early in Crohn's disease.

- The reasons are not known, but Crohn's disease appears to be increasing in incidence worldwide, and is recognized to occur in populations previously thought to be rarely affected (e.g. patients from Asia and Africa).

- Rigid sigmoidoscopy is indicated in patients who may have a flare of ulcerative colitis in order to rapidly confirm the diagnosis, and obtain histological confirmation.

Answers to Question 18
F, F, F, F, T

- Infectious diarrhoea may cause prolonged symptoms, particularly in immunocompromised individuals, while even immunocompetent patients may suffer prolonged symptoms in cases of giardiasis and amoebiasis.

- The stool leucocyte count is raised in all causes of inflammatory diarrhoea, including bacterial and amoebic dysentery.

- Chronic diarrhoea in HIV infection is usually caused by opportunistic pathogens such as atypical mycobacteria, protozoa such as microsporidia and cryptosporidium, and viruses such as CMV.

- Amoebiasis may be missed in routine stool culture and microsporidia as the trophozoites die rapidly. A hot stool specimen should be examined in all suspected cases.

- Metronidazole may be beneficial in acute exacerbations of Crohn's disease, but not in ulcerative colitis.

Answers to Question 19
A7 B5 C1 D8 E2

- Abnormal α_1-antitrypsin protein, which is synthesized by and accumulates in hepatocytes, can be detected on serum electrophoresis.

- Wilson's disease is caused by an inherited abnormality in the hepatic copper transporter, resulting in hepatic, neurological and serum accumulation of copper. Urinary copper excretion is also increased.

- Genetic haemochromatosis is an autosomal recessive condition caused by a mutation in the HFE gene, which has been cloned. About 95% of cases are caused by a mutation resulting in substitution of cysteine by tyrosine at position 282 of the polypeptide chain.

- Primary biliary cirrhosis is reliably diagnosed by a positive antimitochondrial antibody test.

- ERCP in PSC gives rise to a typical pattern of intra- and extrahepatic biliary strictures and dilatation, giving rise to a 'beads on a string' appearance.

Answers to Question 20
T, T, F, F, F

- Ascites results from a combination of portal hypertension and hypoalbuminaemia associated with cirrhosis. In a previously stable patient, the development of ascites should prompt a search for a precipitating cause, which may include worsening liver function, growth of hepatocellular carcinoma and portal vein thrombosis.

- Ascites and variceal haemorrhage are signs of decompensated liver disease, and should prompt adequate secondary prevention, and consideration of whether liver transplantation would be appropriate for the patient.

- Patients with cirrhosis are chronically malnourished, and maintaining adequate calorie and protein intake is critical to long-term survival. The risks of precipitating hepatic encephalopathy on a diet containing moderate quantities of protein are overestimated.

- SBP is a medical emergency that requires rapid diagnosis and treatment. The diagnosis should be based on a white cell count of the ascites fluid. Positive cultures are not always obtained.

- Coagulation abnormalities may be aggravated in jaundiced patients who may malabsorb vitamin K and other fat-soluble vitamins.

Answers to Question 21
A8 B5 C3 D4 E2

- Hepatic adenoma is the most common focal liver lesion in young women on the oral contraceptive pill.

- Chronic bloody diarrhoea may be a sign of IBD, which is a risk factor for the development of PSC, which is a risk factor for cholangiocarcinoma. The history is also compatible with pyogenic or amoebic abscess, but cholangiocarcinoma typically causes obstructive jaundice.

• Altered bowel habit raises the suspicion of colorectal carcinoma, particularly in patients over the age of 50.

• Hepatic haemangioma is a relatively common incidental finding, and should be considered before a biopsy is performed, in case severe haemorrhage is precipitated. Focal nodular hyperplasia and simple cysts are also diagnostic possibilities.

• Cirrhosis caused by chronic viral hepatitis carries the greatest risk of HCC. HCC can also develop in patients with haemochromatosis and alcoholic liver disease, but is rare in women and in patients with PBC.

Answers to Question 22

A

• Patients with cirrhosis may benefit from screening to detect early HCC.

• Secondary deposits are the most common malignant lesion in the liver.

• Cholangiocarcinoma is associated with PSC. Gallstones are associated with an increased risk of carcinoma of the gall bladder.

Hepatic adenomas are associated with oral contraceptive use, and may require resection if they are very large. There is also a small risk of malignant transformation. The tumours regress after cessation of oral contraceptive use.

Answers to Question 23

A6 B1 C8 D5 E3

• Contrast swallow should be the first investigation in all patients with significant dysphagia.

• Multiple nutrient deficiency suggests severe nutritional deficiency or malabsorption. Upper GI endoscopy allows examination of the duodenum for biopsy and diagnosis of coeliac disease, small intestinal Crohn's disease and bacterial overgrowth.

• Dyspepsia in young patients is rarely associated with organic pathology unless the patient is *Helicobacter pylori* (HP) positive. It is reasonable to test such patients for HP status non-invasively, and treat HP infection if it is present. If symptoms regress, no further investigations are required.

• PSC should be considered and excluded, and ERCP is the diagnostic test of choice.

• Exacerbation of ulcerative colitis may be treated empirically, but if confirmation is required, colonoscopy and biopsy are preferred to radiological investigation.

Answers to Question 24

T, F, T, F, T

• The urease breath test does not suffer from sampling error associated with endoscopic biopsies, and is rapidly and easily performed in an outpatient setting.

• The CLO test is based on the urease activity of gastric helicobacters in a biopsy specimen.

• The Schilling test is used to distinguish whether abnormal vitamin B_{12} absorption is corrected by adding exogenous intrinsic factor.

• Enteroscopy is not reliable at present, as it is not possible to guarantee that the instrument has been passed beyond the second part of the duodenum.

• Virtual colonoscopy images have the advantage over conventional barium enema and colonoscopy that the colonic wall can also be reconstructed.

Answers to Question 25

F, F, F, F, T

• Although a raised serum amylase is important in making the diagnosis of acute pancreatitis it carries no prognostic value.

• An ultrasound should be performed in all cases of acute pancreatitis to identify gallstones. CT should be performed between days 3 and 10 in cases of severe acute pancreatitis as determined by the Glasgow criteria.

• Although historically patients with acute pancreatitis were fasted early enteral feeding is now encouraged.

• There is no advantage to deferring cholecystectomy after gallstone pancreatitis.

• ERCP carries a risk of pancreatitis. This risk is increased with procedures such as endoscopic sphincterotomy. Although many patients may have an elevated amylase the day after the procedure the prognosis is generally good.

Answers to Question 26

T, T, T, F, F

• Mild jaundice and cholestatic abnormalities of liver blood tests may occur with chronic pancreatitis, although deep jaundice should always raise the suspicion of choledocolithiasis or the presence of a pancreatic carcinoma.

• Weight loss may be due to either malabsorption associated with pancreatic exocrine insufficiency or a new presentation of diabetes.

• Severe epigastric pain often radiating through to the back is one of the more common presentations of chronic pancreatitis.

• Acute pancreatitis is a rare cause of ascites but this is not a recognized presentation of chronic pancreatitis.

• Iron absorption occurs independent of pancreatic enzymes and the presence of iron deficiency should always prompt consideration of an additional diagnosis (e.g. coeliac disease, colorectal cancer, etc.).

Answers to Question 27

F, F, T, F, F

• Acute lower GI bleeding is a frequent presentation of diverticula. This should be distinguished from chronic persistant rectal bleeding.

- Patients with diverticular change will often report a change in bowel habit.
- Iron deficiency associated with positive faecal occult blood should always prompt a thorough exclusion of a gastrointestinal malignancy.
- Diverticular change complicated by abscess may often present with a palpable mass.
- Chronic inflamed diverticular change may result in stricture formation.

Answers to Question 28

A1 B4 C1 D2 E2

Answers to Question 29

F, T, F, T, F

- Pain disturbing sleep is not typical of the functional gastrointestinal disorders and an alternative cause for the symptoms should be sought.
- Intolerance of dairy products is not specific to hypolactasia and many patients with more non-specific gastrointestinal symptoms may feel better on an empirical low lactose diet regardless of the result of a lactose breath test.
- Rectal bleeding requires further investigation. Although in many cases this may ultimately be due to haemorrhoidal bleeding associated with poor defecatory habits this should not be assumed without sigmoidoscopy.
- The passage of mucus per rectum is frequently reported by patients with functional symptoms.
- Diurnal mood variation and early morning wakening should alert the physician to a coexistent depressive illness which may warrant independent evaluation and treatment.

Answers to Question 30

T, T, F, T, F

- Sphincter of Oddi dysfunction typically causes biliary colic but, by definition, in the absence of gallstones.
- The presence of abnormal liver blood tests is one of the more specific features of sphincter of Oddi dysfunction and provides the basis of the morphine provocation test.
- Sphincter of Oddi dysfunction causes significant morbidity but is not in itself associated with a shortened life expectancy.
- Endoscopic sphincterotomy may provide good relief of symptoms in well selected patients but carries an increased risk of pancreatitis.

Answers to Question 31

T, F, F T, T

- Colonic adenomas carry an increased lifetime risk of the future development of colorectal cancer. This is particularly the case for adenomas greater than 1 cm and for villous histology (as opposed to tubular).
- Hyperplastic polyps do not carry a significantly increased risk of colorectal cancer.

- The increased risk associated with ulcerative colitis is associated with longstanding total colitis.
- The risk of colorectal cancer if two first-degree relatives have the condition is 1 : 6.
- A single first-degree relative presenting before the age of 45 incurs a risk of 1 : 10.

Answers to Question 32

F, F, T, T, T

- Patients with a history suggestive of HNPCC are at particular risk of right-sided (i.e. proximal) cancers and total colonoscopy is the only appropriate investigation.
- The low sensitivity and associated radiation dose of contrast radiology precludes its use as a form of screening.
- In selected circumstances dye spraying may be used to identify 'flat' carcinomas that may be present particularly in the proximal colon.
- FOB testing is cheap and sensitive. Its performance is limited by its lack of specificity.
- Hereditary colon cancer only constitutes a very small proportion of patients with colorectal cancer.

Answers to Question 33

A, B, C

A Acute hepatitis A is associated with high serum transaminases but may be followed by a cholestatic phase with rising alkaline phosphatase and bilirubin.

B Acute alcoholic hepatitis is often associated with a raised alkaline phosphatase due to bile duct damage or because of associated pancreatic disease with a lower common bile duct stricture. High levels of serum transaminases are uncommon. There is often an underlying cirrhosis and so alcoholic hepatitis may just present as an elevated bilirubin with only minor elevation of transaminases and alkaline phosphatase.

C Cholangitis, common bile duct stones, biliary strictures and cholangiocarcinoma can all lead to jaundice in patients with primary sclerosing cholangitis.

D Acute hepatitis B is associated with high serum transaminases but unlike hepatitis A it is not followed by a cholestatic phase.

E Paracetamol causes high serum transaminases. Jaundice only occurs in severe injury and would not persist at 2 weeks in the presence of a relatively normal prothrombin time.

Answers to Question 34

1 Adult polycystic liver disease.

2 Multiple liver cysts, ascites, absent kidneys. The patient was in renal failure and because of the abdominal discomfort had had both kidneys removed prior to renal transplantation.

3 Autosomal dominant.

Answers to Question 35

1 To look for Kayser–Fleischer rings. A slit lamp examination is necessary to exclude KF rings.

2 Haemolysis. She also has splenomegaly which may also partly account for her low haemoglobin.

3 Wilson's disease. It is always important to exclude Wilson's in a young person (less than 40 years) presenting with liver failure. The clue to the diagnosis is the presence of haemolysis which occurs due to copper release.

4 Acute liver failure. Cirrhosis is usually present at the time of presentation and so prothrombin time is not as high as seen in paracetamol and non-A non-B acute liver failure. Haemolysis is often present and contributes to the elevated bilirubin levels.

• Abnormal liver blood tests. A liver biopsy shows chronic hepatitis. The serum caeruloplasmin is usually low and a dry weight liver copper is high.

• An established cirrhosis. Wilson's must always be considered in a young person. The results of treatment with penicillamine are excellent even in the presence of cirrhosis with patients surviving beyond 20 years. Stopping therapy can rapidly lead to liver failure.

• Screening. The condition is autosomal recessive and it is important to screen sibs with serum caeuruloplasmin, copper and liver biochemistry.

• Neurological symptoms of Wilson's.

Answers to Question 36
F, T, F, T, F

A In contrast to hepatitis B hepatocellular carcinoma only complicates hepatitis C in the presence of cirrhosis.

B The risk of a women transmitting hepatitis C to her baby during pregnancy is about 6%.

C Hepatitis C infection is not a contraindication to breast feeding.

D The risk factors for disease progression in hepatitis C infection are: (i) acquisition of the infection over 40 years of age; (ii) excess alcohol use; (iii) immunosuppression; and (iv) male sex. Thus a women acquiring infection through intravenous drug use in her late teens who does not drink is much less likely to develop progressive fibrosis than a man acquiring the infection in the same way who is an alcoholic.

E The current first-line treatment for chronic hepatitis C is a combination of alpha interferon and ribavirin given for 6–12 months depending on viral genotype. This leads to an overall sustained loss of virus of 40% 6 months after completing therapy.

Answers to Question 37
F, T, F, F, F

Red cell folate levels are usually normal, but B_{12} levels may be low due to utilization by the bacteria.

Hypomotility, which is a feature of systemic sclerosis, predisposes to bacterial overgrowth. Blind loops following gastric surgery, jejunal diverticula and autonomic neuropathy are other predisposing factors. There appears to be an increased incidence of gastroenteritis with the use of proton pump inhibitors (presumably due to loss of the sterilizing effect of gastric acid), but they are not associated with chronic small bowel bacterial overgrowth.

Diagnosis is usually made by clinical suspicion plus a glucose or lactulose hydrogen breath test. The lactose hydrogen breath test identifies lactase deficiency. Treatment is with cyclical antibiotics.

Answers to Question 38
T, F, F, F, T

Erythromycin acts as a motilin agonist, promoting gastric emptying and may be helpful in the gastroparesis seen in diabetes.

The MMC is a well defined cyclical pattern of motor activity which starts in the upper GI tract (oesophagus or duodenum) and propagates along the small intestine. It is not seen in the colon, where the motor activity is by and large erratic and follows no particular pattern.

Contractions usually progress aborally along the oesophagus. Simultaneous high-amplitude contractions are seen in diffuse oesophageal spasm.

Answers to Question 39
1B 2C 3B 4A 5E

• Dysphagia with risk of aspiration following a stroke is probably the most common indication for the placement of a PEG feeding tube. Patients about to undergo major surgery for oropharyngeal carcinomas may have a PEG feeding tube inserted prior to surgery to allow adequate nutrition during the postoperative healing phase.

• A PEJ feeding tube is suitable for patients who are suffering from gastroparesis or who are at high risk of aspiration and therefore need 'bypassing' of the stomach.

• An elemental diet is a useful treatment option in patients with active Crohn's disease, and may be as effective as steroids.

• Total gut failure, as in mesenteric infarction, usually requires TPN support if the patient survives the initial insult.

Answers to Question 40
T, F, T, F, F

• CCK causes contraction of the gall bladder and inhibits gastric emptying.

• Proton pump inhibitors, by reducing acid output, inhibit the negative feedback of acid on gastrin production, and result in hypergastrinaemia. This is important to bear in mind in the investigation of possible Zollinger–Ellison syndrome if the patient is on a proton pump inhibitor.

• Somatostatin, released from D cells in the gastric antrum, inhibits many GI hormones including gastrin.

• VIPomas are extremely rare neuroendocrine tumours often located in the pancreas. They result in copious watery diarrhoea. Large amounts of potassium and bicarbonate are secreted from the gastrointestinal tract, resulting in a hypokalaemic acidosis.

- Secretin is released from the duodenal mucosa and causes pancreatic exocrine secretion.

Answers to Question 41

T, T, T, F, T

- Crohn's disease is associated with smokers; ulcerative colitis with non-smokers. Cessation of smoking improves disease activity and risk of relapse.
- Crohn's disease often affects the terminal ileum, which is involved in both bile salt and vitamin B_{12} absorption, hence bile salt diarrhoea and B_{12} deficiency may occur with active ileal disease or following a right hemicolectomy for ileocaecal disease.
- Crohn's disease may affect any part of the GI tract from the lips to the anus. Crohn's disease should be considered in duodenal ulceration resistant to conventional treatment.
- The risk of deep vein thrombosis is high in patients with active ulcerative colitis and Crohn's disease, and patients admitted to hospital should be on prophylactic heparin.

Answers to Question 42

1B 2G 3A 4C

- Abdominal pain, diarrhoea and weight loss are typical presenting features of Crohn's disease. The lack of blood and weight loss point towards small bowel rather than colonic involvement. A small bowel meal may show characteristic stricturing in the terminal ileum, rosethorn ulceration, or enteroenteric fistulae compatible with a diagnosis of Crohn's disease.
- Scleroderma, as part of the CREST syndrome, may result in hypomotility of the small bowel predisposing to bacterial overgrowth. Glucose is normally rapidly absorbed in the upper small intestine. Bacteria generate hydrogen in their utilization of glucose, and this results in an early rapid rise in breath hydrogen.
- A dimorphic blood film indicates the presence of two distinct sizes of red cell. Combined iron and B_{12} or folate deficiency will give rise to this picture. Coeliac disease, by impairing absorption of iron and folate (and occasionally B_{12}), may result in a dimorphic blood film with the presence of Howell–Jolly bodies (due to associated hyposplenism). It is diagnosed by finding partial villous atrophy and intraepithelial lymphocytes on duodenal biopsies.
- A beaded intrahepatic tree, with stricturing and dilatation, is suggestive of primary sclerosing cholangitis. Between 70 and 80% of patients with PSC have associated (often mild or covert) ulcerative colitis which may be diagnosed by sigmoidoscopy and rectal biopsy.

Answers to Question 43

T, F, F, F, T

Gilbert's syndrome is extremely common, affecting approximately 4% of the population. It is caused by a deficiency in glucuronyl transferase resulting in elevation of unconjugated bilirubin. The other liver enzymes are normal. It has no effect on morbidity or mortality. Fasting or intercurrent illness causes an elevation of the bilirubin level and may result in frank jaundice.

The other usual cause of an isolated hyperbilirubinaemia is haemolytic anaemia, in which the reticulocyte count is usually raised (increased production of red cells) and the serum haptoglobin levels reduced (bind to released haemoglobin). Haemolytic anaemias are associated with development of pigmented gallstones.

Answers to Question 44

F, F, F, F, T

A Bloody diarrhoea is the commonest presentation, and it occurs early.

B Skin manifestations are uncommon.

C Joint symptoms, particularly painful but not obviously inflamed joints are common.

D PSC is rare, and is unrelated to ulcerative colitis disease activity, sometimes occurring after colectomy.

E There is a strong heritable component in ulcerative colitis and Crohn's disease.

Answers to Question 45

A2 Acute flares of Crohn's disease may respond to treatment with metronidazole.

B4 There is an increased risk of colorectal cancer in ulcerative colitis, and it is most pronounced in patients with long-standing pancolitis. The relative risk of cancer in Crohn's disease is less well defined.

C1 Coeliac disease may be associated with a pruritic, vesicular skin rash (dermatitis herpetiformis) that resolves on a gluten-free diet.

D5 This is the classical symptomatology of chronic pancreatitis.

E3 Whipple's disease, caused by *Tropheryma whippelii* infection of the small intestine, is most common in this group, and causes a multisystem inflammatory disorder and small bowel malabsorption.

Answers to Question 46

FFFTT

A HCV infection is only rarely transmitted sexually, although it is transmitted in blood and bodily fluids. The most common defined mode of transmission is by needle-stick inoculation, although in the majority of cases worldwide, the definite mode of transmission is not known.

B Acute hepatitis is rare or non-existent in HCV infection, and spontaneous clearance of the virus is rare, but not related to the clinical manifestation of the disease.

C HCV infection definitely increases the risk of hepatocellular carcinoma, but hepatocellular carcinoma without cirrhosis is almost non-existent.

D And viral persistence is not related to integration into the host genome.

E The main autoimmune phenomena are cryoglobulinaemia leading to skin rashes, arthralgia and arthritis.

Answers to Question 47

F, T, F, F, F

A Spontaneous bacterial peritonitis is a common complication with cirrhosis and ascites, and is less often seen in acute liver failure.

B The reason is unknown.

C Possibly as a result of altered plasma lipid profiles, coronary artery disease is less common.

D Liver transplantation is only appropriate when the patient's life expectancy is reduced to less than 2 years due to progressive liver failure, as many patients with cirrhosis can survive with a good quality of life given the appropriate conservative management.

E Chronic hepatic encephalopathy, as seen in chronic liver disease, is rarely associated with the gross disruption of the blood–brain barrier and cortical swelling that accompanies fulminant liver failure and causes coma and death from coning.

Answers to Question 48

F, T, F, F, F

A MRI of the abdomen is increasingly useful, as it is not limited by the presence of air or fat. However, in the presence of gross ascites, some MRI algorithms cannot be reliably performed.

B Intravenous contrast, usually in the form of microscopic air bubbles, increases the sensitivity and resolution of ultrasound scanning.

C About 10% of gallstones are radio-opaque, while 90% of renal stones are radio-opaque.

D ERCP carries a significant risk to the patient, with the main complications being acute pancreatitis, ascending cholangitis and gastrointestinal haemorrhage following sphincterotomy. However, biliary obstruction by stones or tumour is an indication for ERCP in some patients, where endoscopic therapy to relieve the obstruction (e.g. retrieval of stones, stenting of tumour, or sphincterotomy to the sphincter of Oddi), may be feasible.

E Pancreatic calcification is diagnostic of chronic pancreatitis, which may present with bouts of acute on chronic pancreatitis.

Answers to Question 49

A2 Greater than 90% sensitivity and specificity for coeliac disease.

B5 Is raised to 1000 IU/L or more in acute pancreatitis, but may also be mildly or moderately raised in peptic ulcer disease and other upper GI disorders.

C3 *Helicobacter pylori* growth and survival is inhibited by acid suppression.

D1 A positive ANCA titre should raise the strong suspicion of systemic vasculitis in the appropriate clinical context, but may also be associated with inflammatory bowel disease, particularly ulcerative colitis.

E4 Submucosal granulomas are strongly indicative of Crohn's disease as opposed to ulcerative colitis, where granuloma-like lesions may develop around a ruptured crypt abscess.

Answers to Question 50

F, F, F, F, T

• Amylase may be modestly elevated in chronic pancreatitis but a normal value does not exclude significant pancreatic disease.

• Pancreas divisum may cause recurrent pancreatitis and pancreatic pain but can only confidently be demonstrated with ERCP.

• A calcified pancreas demonstrated on plain abdominal radiograph or CT is usually sufficient indication of parenchymal pancreatic damage that further imaging of the duct is unnecessary.

• Increasingly less labour-intensive tests such as the pancreolauryl test and measurement of faecal elastase are replacing the quantification of faecal fats.

Answers to Question 51

F, F, F, F, F

None of the above clinical features would clearly distinguish a malignant from an inflammatory mass.

Answers to Question 52

T, F, F, F, F

• Peritoneal leakage of barium can be problematic and if imaging is necessary in this setting a water-soluble contrast is preferable.

• Colonoscopy is extremely hazardous in obstruction and stenting remains suitable for only a limited number of cancers at present.

• In the situation of an obstructed colon the staging of the tumour is less relevant than relieving the obstruction, whether that be by primary resection or a defunctioning procedure.

Answers to Question 53

F, F, T, T, T

• Neither MCV nor GGT are sensitive or specific for alcohol ingestion whereas a raised ethanol level is.

• Confronting the patient is reasonable, although the timing of this has to be sensitive.

- Seeking corroborative evidence is very useful but caution must be exercised not to breach patient confidentiality.

Answers to Question 54

T, T, F, T, T

- Although diarrhoea of this duration is unlikely to be due to food poisoning, small bowel bacterial overgrowth and giardiasis remain important if infrequent causes that will respond to antibiotic treatment.
- The effect of NSAIDs on the stomach and duodenum are well recognized but the association with microscopic colitis and worsening of inflammatory bowel disease is all too often forgotten.
- Hypolactasia or lactose intolerance may cause persisting diarrhoea.
- Endoscopy and duodenal biopsy remain the diagnostic test for the exclusion of villous atrophy or coeliac disease and may identify giardia.
- A full colonic series of biopsies remains the only way to formally exclude microscopic colitis (i.e. lymphocytic or collagenous colitis).

Answers to Question 55

T, T, F, T, F

- Transferrin saturation is rather labile and a fasting sample is ideal.
- Although there are many non-specific causes of a raised ferritin, a low level is specific for iron deficiency.
- Coeliac disease may cause iron deficiency in the absence of overt malabsorption.
- A bone marrow examination remains one of the most sensitive tests for iron deficiency and remains very useful in circumstances where blood tests such as ferritin and transferrin saturation may be difficult to interpret such as chronic disease.
- Intestinal mechanisms of iron absorption are very efficient and to ascribe iron deficiency to dietary factors without further investigation is not reasonable.

The Medical Masterclass series

Scientific Background to Medicine 1

Genetics and Molecular Medicine

1 Nucleic acids and chromosomes
2 Techniques in molecular biology
3 Molecular basis of simple genetic traits
4 More complex issues

Biochemistry and Metabolism

1 Requirement for energy
2 Carbohydrates
3 Fatty acids and lipids
4 Cholesterol and steroid hormones
5 Amino acids and proteins
6 Haem
7 Nucleotides

Cell Biology

1 Ion transport
2 Receptors and intracellular signalling
3 Cell cycle and apoptosis
4 Haematopoiesis

Immunology and Immunosuppression

1 Overview of the immune system
2 The major histocompatibility complex, antigen presentation and transplantation
3 T cells
4 B cells
5 Tolerance and autoimmunity
6 Complement
7 Inflammation
8 Immunosuppressive therapy

Anatomy

1 Heart and major vessels
2 Lungs
3 Liver and biliary tract
4 Spleen
5 Kidney
6 Endocrine glands
7 Gastrointestinal tract
8 Eye
9 Nervous system

Physiology

1 Cardiovascular system
  1.1 The heart as a pump
  1.2 The systemic and pulmonary circulations
  1.3 Blood vessels
  1.4 Endocrine function of the heart
2 Respiratory system
  2.1 The lungs
3 Gastrointestinal system
  3.1 The gut
  3.2 The liver
  3.3 The exocrine pancreas
4 Brain and nerves
  4.1 The action potential
  4.2 Synaptic transmission
  4.3 Neuromuscular transmission
5 Endocrine physiology
6 Renal physiology
  6.1 Blood flow and glomerular filtration
  6.2 Function of the renal tubules
  6.3 Endocrine function of the kidney

Scientific Background to Medicine 2

Statistics, Epidemiology, Clinical Trials, Meta-analyses and Evidence-based Medicine

1 Statistics
2 Epidemiology
  2.1 Observational studies
3 Clinical trials and meta-analyses
4 Evidence-based medicine

Clinical Pharmacology

1 Introducing clinical pharmacology
  1.1 Preconceived notions versus evidence
  1.2 Drug interactions and safe prescribing
2 Pharmacokinetics
  2.1 Introduction
  2.2 Drug absorption
  2.3 Drug distribution
  2.4 Drug metabolism
  2.5 Drug elimination
  2.6 Plasma half-life and steady-state plasma concentrations
  2.7 Drug monitoring
3 Pharmacodynamics
  3.1 How drugs exert their effects
  3.2 Selectivity is the key to the therapeutic utility of an agent
  3.3 Basic aspects of a drug's interaction with its target
  3.4 Heterogeneity of drug responses, pharmacogenetics and pharmacogenomics
4 Adverse drug reactions
  4.1 Introduction
  4.2 Definition and classification of adverse drug reactions
  4.3 Dose-related adverse drug reactions

4.4 Non-dose-related adverse drug reactions
4.5 Adverse reactions caused by long-term effects of drugs
4.6 Adverse reactions caused by delayed effects of drugs
4.7 Teratogenic effects
5 Prescribing in special circumstances
  5.1 Introduction
  5.2 Prescribing and liver disease
  5.3 Prescribing in pregnancy
  5.4 Prescribing for women of child-bearing potential
  5.5 Prescribing to lactating mothers
  5.6 Prescribing in renal disease
6 Drug development and rational prescribing
  6.1 Drug development
    6.1.1 Identifying molecules for development as drugs
    6.1.2 Clinical trials: from drug to medicine
  6.2 Rational prescribing
    6.2.1 Clinical governance and rational prescribing
    6.2.2 Rational prescribing, irrational patients?

Clinical Skills

General Clinical Issues

1 The importance of general clinical issues
2 History and examination
3 Communication skills
4 Being a doctor
  4.1 Team work and errors
  4.2 The 'modern' health service
  4.3 Rationing beds
  4.4 Stress

Pain Relief and Palliative Care

1 Clinical presentations
  1.1 Back pain
  1.2 Nausea and vomiting
  1.3 Breathlessness
  1.4 Confusion
2 Diseases and treatments
  2.1 Pain
  2.2 Breathlessness
  2.3 Nausea and vomiting
  2.4 Bowel obstruction
  2.5 Constipation
  2.6 Depression
  2.7 Anxiety
  2.8 Confusion
  2.9 The dying patient: terminal phase
  2.10 Palliative care services in the community

Medicine for the Elderly

1 Clinical presentations
  1.1 Frequent falls
  1.2 Sudden onset of confusion
  1.3 Urinary incontinence and immobility
  1.4 Collapse
  1.5 Vague aches and pains
  1.6 Swollen legs and back pain
  1.7 Gradual decline
2 Diseases and treatments
  2.1 Why elderly patients are different
  2.2 General approach to managment
  2.3 Falls
  2.4 Urinary and faecal incontinence
    2.4.1 Urinary incontinence
    2.4.2 Faecal incontinence
  2.5 Hypothermia
  2.6 Drugs in elderly people
  2.7 Dementia
  2.8 Rehabilitation
  2.9 Aids and appliances
  2.10 Hearing impairment
  2.11 Nutrition
  2.12 Benefits
  2.13 Legal aspects of elderly care
3 Investigations and practical procedures
  3.1 Diagnosis vs common sense
  3.2 Assessment of cognition, mood and function

Emergency Medicine

1 Clinical presentations
  1.1 Cardiac arrest
  1.2 Collapse with hypotension
  1.3 Central chest pain
  1.4 Tachyarrythmia
  1.5 Nocturnal dyspnoea
  1.6 Bradydysrhythmia
  1.7 Acute severe asthma
  1.8 Pleurisy
  1.9 Community-acquired pneumonia
  1.10 Chronic airways obstruction
  1.11 Upper gastrointestinal haemorrhage
  1.12 Bloody diarrhoea
  1.13 'The medical abdomen'
  1.14 Hepatic encephalopathy/alcohol withdrawal
  1.15 Renal failure, fluid overload and hyperkalaemia
  1.16 Diabetic ketoacidosis
  1.17 Hypoglycaemia
  1.18 Hypercalcaemia and hyponatraemia
  1.19 Metabolic acidosis
  1.20 An endocrine crisis
  1.21 Another endocrine crisis
  1.22 Severe headache with meningism
  1.23 Acute spastic paraparesis
  1.24 Status epilepticus
  1.25 Stroke
  1.26 Coma
  1.27 Fever in a returning traveller
  1.28 Septicaemia
  1.29 Anaphylaxis
2 Diseases and treatments
  2.1 Overdoses

3 Investigations and practical procedures
  3.1 Femoral vein cannulation
  3.2 Central vein cannulation
  3.3 Intercostal chest drain insertion
  3.4 Arterial blood gases
  3.5 Lumbar puncture
  3.6 Pacing
  3.7 Haemodynamic monitoring
  3.8 Ventilatory support
  3.9 Airway management

Infectious Diseases and Dermatology

Infectious Diseases

1 Clinical presentations
  1.1 Fever
  1.2 Fever, hypotension and confusion
  1.3 A swollen red foot
  1.4 Fever and cough
  1.5 A cavitating lung lesion
  1.6 Fever, back pain and weak legs
  1.7 Fever and lymphadenopathy
  1.8 Drug user with fever and a murmur
  1.9 Fever and heart failure
  1.10 Still feverish after six weeks
  1.11 Persistent fever in ICU
  1.12 Pyelonephritis
  1.13 A sore throat
  1.14 Fever and headache
  1.15 Fever with reduced conscious level
  1.16 Fever in the neutropenic patient
  1.17 Fever after renal transplant
  1.18 Chronic fatigue
  1.19 Varicella in pregnancy
  1.20 Imported fever
  1.21 Eosinophilia
  1.22 Jaundice and fever after travelling
  1.23 A traveller with diarrhoea
  1.24 Malaise, mouth ulcers and fever
  1.25 Needlestick exposure
  1.26 Breathlessness in an HIV+ patient
  1.27 HIV+ and blurred vision
  1.28 Starting anti-HIV therapy
  1.29 Failure of anti-HIV therapy
  1.30 Don't tell my wife
  1.31 A spot on the penis
  1.32 Penile discharge
  1.33 Woman with a genital sore
  1.34 Abdominal pain and vaginal discharge
  1.35 Syphilis in pregnancy
  1.36 Positive blood cultures
  1.37 Therapeutic drug monitoring—antibiotics
  1.38 Contact with meningitis
  1.39 Pulmonary tuberculosis—follow-up failure
  1.40 Penicillin allergy
2 Pathogens and management

2.1 Antimicrobial prophylaxis
2.2 Immunization
2.3 Infection control
2.4 Travel advice
2.5 Bacteria
  2.5.1 Gram-positive bacteria
  2.5.2 Gram-negative bacteria
2.6 Mycobacteria
  2.6.1 *Mycobacterium tuberculosis*
  2.6.2 *Mycobacterium leprae*
  2.6.3 Opportunistic mycobacteria
2.7 Spirochaetes
  2.7.1 Syphilis
  2.7.2 Lyme disease
  2.7.3 Relapsing fever
  2.7.4 Leptospirosis
2.8 Miscellaneous bacteria
  2.8.1 *Mycoplasma* and *Ureaplasma*
  2.8.2 Rickettsiae
  2.8.3 *Coxiella burnetii* (Q fever)
  2.8.4 Chlamydiae
2.9 Fungi
  2.9.1 *Candida* SPP.
  2.9.2 *Aspergillus*
  2.9.3 *Cryptococcus neoformans*
  2.9.4 Dimorphic fungi
  2.9.5 Miscellaneous fungi
2.10 Viruses
  2.10.1 Herpes simplex virus types 1 and 2
  2.10.2 Varicella-zoster virus
  2.10.3 Cytomegalovirus
  2.10.4 Epstein–Barr virus
  2.10.5 Human herpes viruses 6 and 7
  2.10.6 Human herpes virus 8
  2.10.7 Parvovirus
  2.10.8 Hepatitis viruses
  2.10.9 Influenza virus
  2.10.10 Paramyxoviruses
  2.10.11 Enteroviruses
2.11 Human immunodeficiency virus
2.12 Travel–related viruses
  2.12.1 Rabies
  2.12.2 Dengue
  2.12.3 Arbovirus infections
2.13 Protozoan parasites
  2.13.1 Malaria
  2.13.2 Leishmaniasis
  2.13.3 Amoebiasis
  2.13.4 Toxoplasmosis
2.14 Metazoan parasites
  2.14.1 Schistosomiasis
  2.14.2 Strongyloidiasis
  2.14.3 Cysticercosis
  2.14.4 Filariasis
  2.14.5 Trichinosis
  2.14.6 Toxocariasis
  2.14.7 Hydatid disease
3 Investigations and practical procedures
  3.1 Getting the best from the laboratory
  3.2 Specific investigations

Dermatology

1 Clinical presentations
 1.1 Blistering disorders
 1.2 Acute generalized rashes
 1.3 Erythroderma
 1.4 A chronic, red facial rash
 1.5 Pruritus
 1.6 Alopecia
 1.7 Abnormal skin pigmentation
 1.8 Patches and plaques on the lower legs
2 Diseases and treatments
 2.1 Alopecia areata
 2.2 Bullous pemphigoid and pemphigoid gestationis
 2.3 Dermatomyositis
 2.4 Mycosis fungoides and Sézary syndrome
 2.5 Dermatitis herpetiformis
 2.6 Drug eruptions
 2.7 Atopic eczema
 2.8 Contact dermatitis
 2.9 Erythema multiforme, Stevens–Johnson syndrome, toxic epidermal necrolysis
 2.10 Erythema nodosum
 2.11 Lichen planus
 2.12 Pemphigus vulgaris
 2.13 Superficial fungal infections
 2.14 Psoriasis
 2.15 Scabies
 2.16 Urticaria and angio-oedema
 2.17 Vitiligo
 2.18 Pyoderma gangrenosum
 2.19 Cutaneous vasculitis
 2.20 Acanthosis nigricans
3 Investigations and practical procedures
 3.1 Skin biopsy
 3.2 Direct and indirect immunofluorescence
 3.3 Patch testing
 3.4 Topical therapy: corticosteroids
 3.5 Phototherapy
 3.6 Systemic retinoids

Haematology and Oncology

Haematology

1 Clinical presentations
 1.1 Microcytic hypochromic anaemia
 1.2 Chest syndrome in sickle cell disease
 1.3 Normocytic anaemia
 1.4 Macrocytic anaemia
 1.5 Hereditary spherocytosis and failure to thrive
 1.6 Neutropenia
 1.7 Pancytopenia
 1.8 Thrombocytopenia and purpura
 1.9 Leucocytosis
 1.10 Lymphocytosis and anaemia
 1.11 Spontaneous bleeding and weight loss
 1.12 Menorrhagia and anaemia
 1.13 Thromboembolism and fetal loss
 1.14 Polycythaemia
 1.15 Bone pain and hypercalcaemia
 1.16 Cervical lymphadenopathy and weight loss
 1.17 Isolated splenomegaly
 1.18 Inflammatory bowel disease with thrombocytosis
 1.19 Transfusion reaction
 1.20 Recurrent deep venous thrombosis
2 Diseases and treatments
 2.1 Causes of anaemia
  2.1.1 Thalassaemia syndromes
  2.1.2 Sickle cell syndromes
  2.1.3 Enzyme defects
  2.1.4 Membrane defects
  2.1.5 Iron metabolism and iron-deficiency anaemia
  2.1.6 Vitamin B_{12} and folate metabolism and deficiency
  2.1.7 Acquired haemolytic anaemia
  2.1.8 Bone-marrow failure and infiltration
 2.2 Haemic malignancy
  2.2.1 Multiple myeloma
  2.2.2 Acute leukaemia—acute lymphoblastic leukaemia and acute myeloid leukaemia
  2.2.3 Chronic lymphocytic leukaemia
  2.2.4 Chronic myeloid leukaemia
  2.2.5 Malignant lymphomas—non-Hodgkin's lymphoma and Hodgkin's disease
  2.2.6 Myelodysplastic syndromes
  2.2.7 Non-leukaemic myeloproliferative disorders
  2.2.8 Amyloidosis
 2.3 Bleeding disorders
  2.3.1 Inherited bleeding disorders
  2.3.2 Acquired bleeding disorders
  2.3.3 Idiopathic thrombocytopenic purpura
 2.4 Thrombotic disorders
  2.4.1 Inherited thrombotic disease
  2.4.2 Acquired thrombotic disease
 2.5 Clinical use of blood products
 2.6 Haematological features of systemic disease
 2.7 Haematology of pregnancy
 2.8 Iron overload
 2.9 Chemotherapy and related therapies
 2.10 Principles of bone-marrow and peripheral blood stem-cell transplantation
3 Investigations and practical procedures
 3.1 The full blood count and film
 3.2 Bone-marrow examination
 3.3 Clotting screen
 3.4 Coombs' test (direct antiglobulin test)
 3.5 Erythrocyte sedimentation rate vs plasma viscosity
 3.6 Therapeutic anticoagulation

Oncology

1 Clinical presentations
 1.1 A lump in the neck
 1.2 Breathlessness and a pelvic mass
 1.3 Breast cancer and headache
  1.3.1 Metastatic disease
 1.4 Cough and weakness
  1.4.1 Paraneoplastic conditions

1.5 Breathlessness after chemotherapy
1.6 Hip pain after stem cell transplantation
1.7 A problem in the family
  1.7.1 The causes of cancer
1.8 Bleeding, breathlessness and swollen arms
  1.8.1 Oncological emergencies
1.9 The daughter of a man with advanced prostate cancer
2 Diseases and treatments
  2.1 Breast cancer
  2.2 Central nervous system cancers
  2.3 Digestive tract cancers
  2.4 Genitourinary cancer
  2.5 Gynaecological cancer
  2.6 Head and neck cancer
  2.7 Skin tumours
  2.8 Paediatric solid tumours
  2.9 Lung cancer
  2.10 Liver and biliary tree cancer
  2.11 Bone cancer and sarcoma
  2.12 Endocrine tumours
3 Investigations and practical procedures
  3.1 Tumour markers
  3.2 Screening
  3.3 Radiotherapy
  3.4 Chemotherapy
  3.5 Immunotherapy
  3.6 Stem-cell transplantation

Cardiology and Respiratory Medicine

Cardiology

1 Clinical presentations
  1.1 Paroxysmal palpitations
  1.2 Palpitations with dizziness
  1.3 Syncope
  1.4 Stroke and a murmur
  1.5 Acute central chest pain
  1.6 Breathlessness and ankle swelling
  1.7 Hypotension following myocardial infarction
  1.8 Breathlessness and haemodynamic collapse
  1.9 Pleuritic pain
  1.10 Breathlessness and exertional presyncope
  1.11 Dyspnoea, ankle oedema and cyanosis
  1.12 Chest pain and recurrent syncope
  1.13 Fever, weight loss and new murmur
  1.14 Chest pain following a 'flu-like illness
  1.15 Elevated blood pressure at routine screening
  1.16 Murmur in pregnancy
2 Diseases and treatments
  2.1 Coronary artery disease
    2.1.1 Stable angina
    2.1.2 Unstable angina
    2.1.3 Myocardial infarction
  2.2 Cardiac arrhythmia
    2.2.1 Bradycardia
    2.2.2 Tachycardia
  2.3 Cardiac failure
  2.4 Diseases of heart muscle
    2.4.1 Hypertrophic cardiomyopathy
    2.4.2 Dilated cardiomyopathy
    2.4.3 Restrictive cardiomyopathy
    2.4.4 Acute myocarditis
  2.5 Valvular heart disease
    2.5.1 Aortic stenosis
    2.5.2 Aortic regurgitation
    2.5.3 Mitral stenosis
    2.5.4 Mitral regurgitation
    2.5.5 Tricuspid valve disease
    2.5.6 Pulmonary valve disease
  2.6 Pericardial disease
    2.6.1 Acute pericarditis
    2.6.2 Pericardial effusion
    2.6.3 Constrictive pericarditis
  2.7 Congenital heart disease
    2.7.1 Tetralogy of Fallot
    2.7.2 Eisenmenger's syndrome
    2.7.3 Transposition of the great arteries
    2.7.4 Ebstein's anomaly
    2.7.5 Atrial septal defect
    2.7.6 Ventricular septal defect
    2.7.7 Patent ductus arteriosus
    2.7.8 Coarctation of the aorta
  2.8 Infective diseases of the heart
    2.8.1 Infective endocarditis
    2.8.2 Rheumatic fever
  2.9 Cardiac tumours
  2.10 Traumatic heart disease
  2.11 Diseases of systemic arteries
    2.11.1 Aortic dissection
  2.12 Diseases of pulmonary arteries
    2.12.1 Primary pulmonary hypertension
    2.12.2 Secondary pulmonary hypertension
  2.13 Cardiac complications of systemic disease
    2.13.1 Thyroid disease
    2.13.2 Diabetes
    2.13.3 Autoimmune rheumatic diseases
    2.13.4 Renal disease
  2.14 Systemic complications of cardiac disease
    2.14.1 Stroke
  2.15 Pregnancy and the heart
  2.16 General anaesthesia in heart disease
  2.17 Hypertension
    2.17.1 Accelerated phase hypertension
  2.18 Venous thromboembolism
    2.18.1 Pulmonary embolism
  2.19 Driving restrictions in cardiology
3 Investigations and practical procedures
  3.1 ECG
    3.1.1 Exercise ECGs
  3.2 Basic electrophysiology studies
  3.3 Ambulatory monitoring
  3.4 Radiofrequency ablation and implantable cardioverter defibrillators
    3.4.1 Radiofrequency ablation
    3.4.2 Implantable cardioverter defibrillator
  3.5 Pacemakers
  3.6 The chest radiograph in cardiac disease

3.7 Cardiac biochemical markers
3.8 Cardiac catheterization, percutaneous transluminal coronary angioplasty and stenting
   3.8.1 Cardiac catheterization
   3.8.2 Percutaneous transluminal coronary angioplasty and stenting
3.9 Computed tomography and magnetic resonance imaging
   3.9.1 Computed tomography
   3.9.2 Magnetic resonance imaging
3.10 Ventilation–perfusion isotope scanning ($\dot{V}/\dot{Q}$)
3.11 Echocardiography
3.12 Nuclear cardiology
   3.12.1 Myocardial perfusion imaging
   3.12.2 Positron emission tomography

Respiratory Medicine

1 Clinical presentations
  1.1 New breathlessness
  1.2 Solitary pulmonary nodule
  1.3 Exertional dyspnoea with daily sputum
  1.4 Dyspnoea and fine inspiratory crackles
  1.5 Pleuritic chest pain
  1.6 Unexplained hypoxia
  1.7 Nocturnal cough
  1.8 Daytime sleepiness and morning headache
  1.9 Haemoptysis and weight loss
  1.10 Pleural effusion and fever
  1.11 Lung cancer with asbestos exposure
  1.12 Lobar collapse in non-smoker
  1.13 Breathlessness with a normal radiograph
  1.14 Upper airway obstruction
  1.15 Difficult decisions
2 Diseases and treatments
  2.1 Upper airway
    2.1.1 Obstructive sleep apnoea
  2.2 Atopy and asthma
    2.2.1 Allergic rhinitis
    2.2.2 Asthma
  2.3 Chronic obstructive pulmonary disease
  2.4 Bronchiectasis
  2.5 Cystic fibrosis
  2.6 Occupational lung disease
    2.6.1 Asbestosis and the pneumoconioses
  2.7 Diffuse parenchymal (interstitial) lung disease
    2.7.1 Cryptogenic fibrosing alveolitis
    2.7.2 Bronchiolitis obliterans and organizing pneumonia
  2.8 Miscellaneous conditions
    2.8.1 Extrinsic allergic alveolitis
    2.8.2 Sarcoidosis
    2.8.3 Pulmonary vasculitis
    2.8.4 Pulmonary eosinophilia
    2.8.5 Iatrogenic lung disease
    2.8.6 Smoke inhalation
    2.8.7 Sickle cell disease and the lung
    2.8.8 HIV and the lung
  2.9 Malignancy
    2.9.1 Lung cancer

    2.9.2 Mesothelioma
    2.9.3 Mediastinal tumours
  2.10 Disorders of the chest wall and diaphragm
  2.11 Complications of respiratory disease
    2.11.1 Chronic respiratory failure
    2.11.2 Cor pulmonale
  2.12 Treatments in respiratory disease
    2.12.1 Domiciliary oxygen therapy
    2.12.2 Continuous positive airways pressure
    2.12.3 Non-invasive ventilation
  2.13 Lung transplantation
3 Investigations and practical procedures
  3.1 Arterial blood gas sampling
  3.2 Aspiration of pleural effusion or pneumothorax
  3.3 Pleural biopsy
  3.4 Intercostal tube insertion
  3.5 Fibreoptic bronchoscopy and transbronchial biopsy
    3.5.1 Fibreoptic bronchoscopy
    3.5.2 Transbronchial biopsy
  3.6 Interpretation of clinical data
    3.6.1 Arterial blood gases
    3.6.2 Lung function tests
    3.6.3 Overnight oximetry
    3.6.4 Chest radiograph
    3.6.5 Computed tomography scan of the thorax

Gastroenterology and Hepatology

1 Clinical presentations
  1.1 Chronic diarrhoea
  1.2 Heartburn and dysphagia
  1.3 Melaena and collapse
  1.4 Haematemesis and jaundice
  1.5 Abdominal mass
  1.6 Jaundice and abdominal pain
  1.7 Jaundice in a heavy drinker
  1.8 Abdominal swelling
  1.9 Abdominal pain and vomiting
  1.10 Weight loss and tiredness
  1.11 Diarrhoea and weight loss
  1.12 Rectal bleeding
  1.13 Severe abdominal pain and vomiting
  1.14 Chronic abdominal pain
  1.15 Change in bowel habit
  1.16 Acute liver failure
  1.17 Iron-deficiency anaemia
  1.18 Abnormal liver function tests
  1.19 Progressive decline
  1.20 Factitious abdominal pain
2 Diseases and treatments
  2.1 Inflammatory bowel disease
    2.1.1 Crohn's disease
    2.1.2 Ulcerative colitis
    2.1.3 Microscopic colitis
  2.2 Oesophagus
    2.2.1 Barrett's oesophagus
    2.2.2 Oesophageal reflux and benign stricture

2.2.3 Oesophageal tumours
2.2.4 Achalasia
2.2.5 Diffuse oesophageal spasm
2.3 Gastric and duodenal disease
  2.3.1 Peptic ulceration and *Helicobacter pylori*
  2.3.2 Gastric carcinoma
  2.3.3 Rare gastric tumours
  2.3.4 Rare causes of gastrointestinal haemorrhage
2.4 Pancreas
  2.4.1 Acute pancreatitis
  2.4.2 Chronic pancreatitis
  2.4.3 Pancreatic cancer
  2.4.4 Neuroendocrine tumours
2.5 Biliary tree
  2.5.1 Choledocholithiasis
  2.5.2 Cholangiocarcinoma
  2.5.3 Primary sclerosing cholangitis
  2.5.4 Primary biliary cirrhosis
  2.5.5 Intrahepatic cholestasis
2.6 Small bowel
  2.6.1 Coeliac
  2.6.2 Bacterial overgrowth
  2.6.4 Other causes of malabsorption
2.7 Large bowel
  2.7.1 Adenomatous polyps of the colon
  2.7.2 Colorectal carcinoma
  2.7.3 Diverticular disease
  2.7.4 Intestinal ischaemia
  2.7.5 Anorectal disease
2.8 Irritable bowel
2.9 Acute liver disease
  2.9.1 Hepatitis A
  2.9.2 Hepatitis B
  2.9.3 Other viral hepatitis
  2.9.4 Alcohol and alcoholic hepatitis
  2.9.5 Acute liver failure
2.10 Chronic liver disease
2.11 Focal liver lesions
2.12 Drugs and the liver
  2.12.1 Hepatic drug toxicity
  2.12.2 Drugs and chronic liver disease
2.13 Gastrointestinal infections
  2.13.1 Campylobacter
  2.13.2 Salmonella
  2.13.3 Shigella
  2.13.4 Clostridium difficile
  2.13.5 Giardia lamblia
  2.13.6 Yersinia enterocolitica
  2.13.7 Escherichia coli
  2.13.8 Entamoeba histolytica
  2.13.9 Traveller's diarrhoea
  2.13.10 Human immunodeficiency virus (HIV)
2.14 Nutrition
  2.14.1 Defining nutrition
  2.14.2 Protein-calorie malnutrition
  2.14.3 Obesity
  2.14.4 Enteral and parenteral nutrition
  2.14.5 Diets
2.15 Liver transplantation

2.16 Screening, case finding and surveillance
  2.16.1 Surveillance
  2.16.2 Case finding
  2.16.3 Population screening
3 Investigations and practical procedures
  3.1 General investigations
  3.2 Rigid sigmoidoscopy and rectal biopsy
  3.3 Paracentesis
  3.4 Liver biopsy

Neurology, Ophthalmology and Psychiatry

Neurology

1 Clinical presentations
  1.1 Numb toes
  1.2 Back and leg pain
  1.3 Tremor
  1.4 Gait disturbance
  1.5 Dementia and involuntary movements
  1.6 Muscle pain on exercise
  1.7 Increasing seizure frequency
  1.8 Sleep disorders
  1.9 Memory difficulties
  1.10 Dysphagia
  1.11 Weak legs
  1.12 Neck/shoulder pain
  1.13 Impotence and urinary difficulties
  1.14 Diplopia
  1.15 Ptosis
  1.16 Unequal pupils
  1.17 Smell and taste disorders
  1.18 Facial pain
  1.19 Recurrent severe headache
  1.20 Funny turns
  1.21 Hemiplegia
  1.22 Speech disturbance
  1.23 Visual hallucinations
  1.24 Conversion disorders
  1.25 Multiple sclerosis
2 Diseases and treatments
  2.1 Peripheral neuropathies and diseases of the lower motor neurone
    2.1.1 Peripheral neuropathies
    2.1.2 Guillain–Barré Syndrome
    2.1.3 Motor neuron disease
  2.2 Diseases of muscle
    2.2.1 Metabolic muscle disease
    2.2.2 Inflammatory muscle disease
    2.2.3 Inherited dystrophies (myopathies)
    2.2.4 Channelopathies
    2.2.5 Myasthenia gravis
  2.3 Extrapyramidal disorders
    2.3.1 Parkinson's disease
  2.4 Dementias
    2.4.1 Alzheimer's disease
  2.5 Multiple sclerosis

2.6   Causes of headache
    2.6.1   Migraine
    2.6.2   Trigeminal neuralgia
    2.6.3   Cluster headache
    2.6.4   Tension-type headache
2.7   Epilepsy
2.8   Cerebrovascular disease
    2.8.1   Stroke
    2.8.2   Transient ischaemic attacks
    2.8.3   Intracerebral haemorrhage
    2.8.4   Subarachnoid haemorrhage
2.9   Brain tumours
2.10 Neurological complications of infection
    2.10.1 New variant Creutzfeldt–Jakob disease
2.11 Neurological complications of systemic disease
    2.11.1 Paraneoplastic conditions
2.12 Neuropharmacology
3 Investigations and practical procedures
3.1   Neuropsychometry
3.2   Lumbar puncture
3.3   Neurophysiology
    3.3.1   Electroencephalography
    3.3.2   Evoked potentials
    3.3.3   Electromyography
    3.3.4   Nerve conduction studies
3.4   Neuroimaging
    3.4.1   Computed tomography and computed
        tomographic angiography
    3.4.2   MRI and MRA
    3.4.3   Angiography
3.5   SPECT and PET
    3.5.1   SPECT
    3.5.2   PET
3.6   Carotid Dopplers

Ophthalmology

1 Clinical presentations
1.1   An acutely painful red eye
1.2   Two painful red eyes and a systemic disorder
1.3   Acute painless loss of vision in one eye
1.4   Acute painful loss of vision in a young woman
1.5   Acute loss of vision in an elderly man
1.6   Difficulty reading
1.7   Double vision
2 Diseases and treatments
2.1   Iritis
2.2   Scleritis
2.3   Retinal artery occlusion
2.4   Retinal vein occlusion
2.5   Optic neuritis
2.6   Ischaemic optic neuropathy in giant cell arteritis
2.7   Diabetic retinopathy
3 Investigations and practical procedures
3.1   Examination of the eye
    3.1.1   Visual acuity
    3.1.2   Visual fields
    3.1.3   Pupil responses
    3.1.4   Ophthalmoscopy
    3.1.5   Eye movements

3.2   Biopsy
    3.2.1   Temporal artery biopsy
    3.2.2   Conjunctival biopsy for diagnosis of sarcoidosis
3.3   Fluorescein angiography

Psychiatry

1 Clinical presentations
1.1   Acute confusional state
1.2   Panic attack and hyperventilation
1.3   Neuropsychiatric aspects of HIV and AIDS
1.4   Deliberate self-harm
1.5   Eating disorders
1.6   Medically unexplained symptoms
1.7   The alcoholic in hospital
1.8   Drug abuser in hospital
1.9   The frightening patient
2 Diseases and treatments
2.1   Dissociative disorders
2.2   Dementia
2.3   Schizophrenia and antipsychotic drugs
    2.3.1   Schizophrenia
    2.3.2   Antipsychotics
2.4   Personality disorder
2.5   Psychiatric presentation of physical disease
2.6   Psychological reactions to physical illness
    (adjustment disorders)
2.7   Anxiety disorders
    2.7.1   Generalised anxiety disorder
    2.7.2   Panic disorder
    2.7.3   Phobic anxiety disorders
2.8   Obsessive–compulsive disorder
2.9   Acute stress reactions and post-traumatic stress disorder
    2.9.1   Acute stress reaction
    2.9.2   Post-traumatic stress disorder
2.10 Puerperal disorders
    2.10.1 Maternity blues
    2.10.2 Post-natal depressive disorder
    2.10.3 Puerperal psychosis
2.11 Depression
2.12 Bipolar affective disorder
2.13 Delusional disorder
2.14 The Mental Health Act (1983)

Endocrinology

1 Clinical presentations
1.1   Hyponatraemia
1.2   Hypercalcaemia
1.3   Polyuria
1.4   Faints, sweats and palpitations
1.5   Crystals in the knee
1.6   Hirsutism
1.7   Post-pill amenorrhoea
1.8   Short girl with no periods
1.9   Young man who has 'not developed'
1.10 Depression and diabetes

1.11 Acromegaly
1.12 Postpartum amenorrhoea
1.13 Weight loss
1.14 Tiredness and lethargy
1.15 Flushing and diarrhoea
1.16 'Off legs'
1.17 Avoiding another coronary
1.18 High blood pressure and low serum potassium
1.19 Hypertension and a neck swelling
1.20 Tiredness, weight loss and amenorrhoea
2 Diseases and treatments
  2.1 Hypothalamic and pituitary diseases
    2.1.1 Cushing's syndrome
    2.1.2 Acromegaly
    2.1.3 Hyperprolactinaemia
    2.1.4 Non-functioning pituitary tumours
    2.1.5 Pituitary apoplexy
    2.1.6 Craniopharyngioma
    2.1.7 Hypopituitarism and hormone replacement
  2.2 Adrenal disease
    2.2.1 Cushing's syndrome
    2.2.2 Primary adrenal insufficiency
    2.2.3 Primary hyperaldosteronism
    2.2.4 Congenital adrenal hyperplasia
    2.2.5 Phaeochromocytoma
  2.3 Thyroid disease
    2.3.1 Hypothyroidism
    2.3.2 Thyrotoxicosis
    2.3.3 Thyroid nodules and goitre
    2.3.4 Thyroid malignancy
  2.4 Reproductive diseases
    2.4.1 Oligomenorrhoea/amenorrhoea and the premature menopause
    2.4.2 Polycystic ovarian syndrome
    2.4.3 Erectile dysfunction
    2.4.4 Gynaecomastia
    2.4.5 Delayed growth and puberty
  2.5 Metabolic and bone diseases
    2.5.1 Hyperlipidaemia
    2.5.2 Porphyria
    2.5.3 Haemochromatosis
    2.5.4 Osteoporosis
    2.5.5 Osteomalacia
    2.5.6 Paget's disease
    2.5.7 Primary hyperparathyroidism
    2.5.8 Hypercalcaemia
    2.5.9 Hypocalcaemia
  2.6 Diabetes mellitus
  2.7 Other endocrine disorders
    2.7.1 Multiple endocrine neoplasia
    2.7.2 Autoimmune polyglandular endocrinopathies
    2.7.3 Ectopic hormone syndromes
3 Investigations and practical procedures
  3.1 Stimulation tests
    3.1.1 Short synacthen test
    3.1.2 Corticotrophin-releasing hormone (CRH) test
    3.1.3 Thyrotrophin-releasing hormone test
    3.1.4 Gonadotrophin-releasing hormone test
    3.1.5 Insulin tolerance test
    3.1.6 Pentagastrin stimulation test
    3.1.7 Oral glucose tolerance test
  3.2 Suppression tests
    3.2.1 Low-dose dexamethasone suppression test
    3.2.2 High-dose dexamethasone suppression test
    3.2.3 Oral glucose tolerance test in acromegaly
  3.3 Other investigations
    3.3.1 Thyroid function tests
    3.3.2 Water deprivation test

Nephrology

1 Clinical presentations
  1.1 Routine medical shows dipstick haematuria
  1.2 Pregnancy with renal disease
  1.3 A swollen young woman
  1.4 Rheumatoid arthritis with swollen legs
  1.5 A blood test shows renal failure
  1.6 A worrying ECG
  1.7 Postoperative acute renal failure
  1.8 Diabetes with impaired renal function
  1.9 Renal impairment and a multi-system disease
  1.10 Renal impairment and fever
  1.11 Atherosclerosis and renal failure
  1.12 Renal failure and haemoptysis
  1.13 Renal colic
  1.14 Backache and renal failure
  1.15 Is dialysis appropriate?
  1.16 Patient who refuses to be dialysed
  1.17 Renal failure and coma
2 Diseases and treatments
  2.1 Major renal syndromes
    2.1.1 Acute renal failure
    2.1.2 Chronic renal failure
    2.1.3 End-stage renal failure
    2.1.4 Nephrotic syndrome
  2.2 Renal replacement therapy
    2.2.1 Haemodialysis
    2.2.2 Peritoneal dialysis
    2.2.3 Renal transplantation
  2.3 Glomerular diseases
    2.3.1 Primary glomerular disease
    2.3.2 Secondary glomerular disease
  2.4 Tubulointerstitial diseases
    2.4.1 Acute tubular necrosis
    2.4.2 Acute interstitial nephritis
    2.4.3 Chronic interstitial nephritis
    2.4.4 Specific tubulointerstitial disorders
  2.5 Diseases of renal vessels
    2.5.1 Renovascular disease
    2.5.2 Cholesterol atheroembolization
  2.6 Postrenal problems
    2.6.1 Obstructive uropathy
    2.6.2 Stones
    2.6.3 Retroperitoneal fibrosis or periaortitis
    2.6.4 Urinary tract infection
  2.7 The kidney in systemic disease
    2.7.1 Myeloma

2.7.2 Amyloidosis
2.7.3 Haemolyticuraemic syndrome
2.7.4 Sickle cell disease
2.7.5 Autoimmune rheumatic disorders
2.7.6 Systemic vasculitis
2.7.7 Diabetic nephropathy
2.7.8 Hypertension
2.7.9 Sarcoidosis
2.7.10 Hepatorenal syndrome
2.7.11 Pregnancy and the kidney
2.8 Genetic renal conditions
2.8.1 Autosomal dominant polycystic kidney disease
2.8.2 Alport's syndrome
2.8.3 X-linked hypophosphataemic vitamin D-resistant rickets
3 Investigations and practical procedures
3.1 Examination of the urine
3.1.1 Urinalysis
3.1.2 Urine microscopy
3.2 Estimation of renal function, 106
3.3 Imaging the renal tract
3.4 Renal biopsy

Rheumatology and Clinical Immunology

1 Clinical presentations
1.1 Recurrent chest infections
1.2 Recurrent meningitis
1.3 Recurrent facial swelling and abdominal pain
1.4 Fulminant septicaemia
1.5 Recurrent skin abscesses
1.6 Chronic atypical mycobacterial infection
1.7 Collapse during a restaurant meal
1.8 Flushing and skin rash
1.9 Drug induced anaphylaxis
1.10 Arthralgia, purpuric rash and renal impairment
1.11 Arthralgia and photosensitive rash
1.12 Systemic lupus erythematosus and confusion
1.13 Cold fingers and difficulty in swallowing
1.14 Dry eyes and fatigue
1.15 Breathlessness and weakness
1.16 Prolonged fever and joint pains
1.17 Back pain
1.18 Acute hot joints
1.19 Recurrent joint pain and morning stiffness
1.20 Foot drop and weight loss
1.21 Fever, myalgia, arthralgia and elevated acute phase indices
1.22 Non-rheumatoid pain and stiffness
1.23 A crush fracture
1.24 Widespread pain
1.25 Fever and absent upper limb pulses

2 Diseases and treatments
2.1 Immunodeficiency
2.1.1 Primary antibody deficiency
2.1.2 Combined T- and B-cell defects
2.1.3 Chronic granulomatous disease
2.1.4 Cytokine and cytokine receptor deficiencies
2.1.5 Terminal pathway complement deficiency
2.1.6 Hyposplenism
2.2 Allergy
2.2.1 Anaphylaxis
2.2.2 Mastocytosis
2.2.3 Nut allergy
2.2.4 Drug allergy
2.3 Rheumatology
2.3.1 Carpal tunnel syndrome
2.3.2 Osteoarthritis
2.3.3 Rheumatoid arthritis
2.3.4 Seronegative spondyloarthritides
2.3.5 Idiopathic inflammatory myopathies
2.3.6 Crystal arthritis: gout
2.3.7 Calcium pyrophosphate deposition disease
2.4 Autoimmune rheumatic diseases
2.4.1 Systemic lupus erythematosus
2.4.2 Sjögren's syndrome
2.4.3 Systemic sclerosis (scleroderma)
2.5 Vasculitides
2.5.1 Giant cell arteritis and polymyalgia rheumatica
2.5.2 Wegener's granulomatosis
2.5.3 Polyarteritis nodosa
2.5.4 Cryoglobulinaemic vasculitis
2.5.5 Behçet's disease
2.5.6 Takayasu's arteritis
3 Investigations and practical procedures
3.1 Assessing acute phase response
3.1.1 Erythrocyte sedimentation rate
3.1.2 C-reactive protein
3.2 Serological investigation of autoimmune rheumatic disease
3.2.1 Antibodies to nuclear antigens
3.2.2 Antibodies to double-stranded DNA
3.2.3 Antibodies to extractable nuclear antigens
3.2.4 Rheumatoid factor
3.2.5 Antineutrophil cytoplasmic antibody
3.2.6 Serum complement concentrations
3.3 Suspected immune deficiency in adults
3.4 Imaging in rheumatological disease
3.4.1 Plain radiography
3.4.2 Bone densitometry
3.4.3 Magnetic resonance imaging
3.4.4 Nuclear medicine
3.5 Arthrocentesis
3.6 Corticosteroid injection techniques
3.7 Intravenous immunoglobulin

Index

Note: page numbers in *italics* refer to figures, those in **bold** refer to tables.

α-fetoprotein (AFP) 25, 28
  hepatocellular carcinoma 128
abdominal mass 17–20
  diagnostic tests 18–19
  examination 18
  investigations 18–19
abdominal scars 56
abdominal swelling 27–29
  communication with patient 29
  examination 27–8
  fluid aspiration 28–9
  imaging 28
  investigation 28–9
abdominal wall bruising 40
ablative therapy, endoscopic for Barrett's
  oesophagus 64
acamprosate 108
N-acetylcysteine 47, 109–10
achalasia 69–70
  dysphagia 7
  investigations 9
  treatment 70
acid reflux measurement 132
acidosis, acute liver failure 110
acute abdomen 42, 43
  peptic ulceration 71
acute fatty liver of pregnancy 51
Addison's disease
  chronic abdominal pain 43
    differential diagnosis 42
  weight loss 33
adenovirus 106
adult respiratory distress syndrome
  (ARDS) 77
albumin, nutritional status 122, 123
alcohol
  abstinence 41, 53, 77, 78, 79, 80, 108
    cirrhosis 116
    liver transplantation 126
  metabolism 106, *107*
  units *24*, 106
  withdrawal 17, 25, 41
    acute liver failure 45, 46
  see also hepatitis, alcoholic
alcohol use/abuse
  abnormal liver function tests 50, **51**
  cirrhosis 27
  detoxification 26
  history 23
  jaundice 21, 23–7
  liver disease 16, 26, 27, 106–8, 125
  management 25
  medical history 24
  melaena 10
  oesophageal variceal haemorrhage 14
  pancreatitis 4, 32
    acute 75, 78
    chronic 78
  portal hypertension 108
  safe limits 106
  severe abdominal pain with vomiting 39
  thiamine replacement 17
alcoholism 26
alendronate 66
alkaline phosphatase 50
  alcoholic hepatitis 108

Alosetron 102
alverine 45
  irritable bowel syndrome 102
amino acids, essential 121
5-aminosalicylic acid
  Crohn's disease treatment 59
  inflammatory bowel disease management
    6
  microscopic colitis 63
amitriptyline 102
amoxycillin
  H. pylori eradication 72
  salmonella infection 119
  Shigella infection 119
anaemia
  coeliac disease 91
  haemolytic 84
  iron-deficiency 8, 33, 48–9
    coeliac disease differential diagnosis
    91
    examination 48–9
    gastric carcinoma 73
    investigations 49, 132–3
    management 49
    oesophageal carcinoma 67
    peptic ulceration 71
    pernicious 74
anal fissure 100, 101
analgesia
  chronic pancreatitis 79
  liver biopsy 137
  severe abdominal pain 41
angina 7
  diarrhoea and weight loss 34
  mesenteric 99
angiodysplasia 37, 75
  colonic 48
  rectal bleeding differential diagnosis
    36
angiography, visceral **132**
angular stomatitis 121
anorectal disease 100–1
anorexia, nutritional state 121
anorexia nervosa 55
Antabuse 108
anthropometric measurements 123
anti-reflux surgery
  Barrett's oesophagus 64, 65
  gastro-oesophageal reflux 66
antibiotics
  acute pancreatitis 41
  alcoholic hepatitis 26
  prophylaxis for oesophageal variceal
    haemorrhage 15
anticoagulation, melaena 10
antigliadin antibodies 91
antimitochondrial antibody 88
antispasmodics 45
  irritable bowel syndrome 102
anxiety, bowel habit change 43
anxiolytics 118
aortic dissection 76
aphthous ulcers in Crohn's disease 4, 18,
  58
appendicitis 116
arthralgia
  chronic diarrhoea 3, 4
  Crohn's disease 18, 60
  drug hepatotoxicity 117

arthritis
  Crohn's disease 60
  Yersinia enterocolitica 120
ascites
  abdominal swelling 27
  acute liver failure 47, 109
  acute pancreatitis 77
  chronic liver disease complications 112,
    113
  differential diagnosis **27**
  diuretics 29
  examination 28
  fluid aspiration 28–9
  gastric carcinoma 73
  liver biopsy contraindication 136
  management 29
  oesophageal variceal haemorrhage 14
  pancreatic carcinoma 80
  paracentesis 134, 135
  transjugular intrahepatic portosystemic
    shunt (TIPSS) 29
ataxia 121
atheromatous vascular disease 43
atherosclerosis 42
Augmentin 35
azathioprine
  acute pancreatitis 75
  bone marrow suppression 48
  Crohn's disease 20, 59
  inflammatory bowel disease management 6
  liver transplantation 126

β-blockers 112
bacteria, enteric 118–19, 120
  ulcerative colitis 61
bacterial infection 110
bacterial overgrowth 35, 92–3
  causes **93**
  chronic pancreatitis differential
    diagnosis 79
  diagnosis 35
  diarrhoea and weight loss 34
  investigations 35
  management 35–6
  treatment 93
bacterial peritonitis 29, 112
balloon tamponade 15
Balthazar score 40
band ligation 15–16, 17
barium enema **131**
  Crohn's disease 19
barium studies *130*, **131**
Barrett's oesophagus 63–5
  complications 64
  endoscopic surveillance 69
  gastro-oesophageal motility 132
  long-term acid reflux 66
  prevention 66
  surveillance 128
benzodiazepines
  alcohol withdrawal 17
  biliary cirrhosis 89
bile acids 84
bile duct
  drug hepatotoxicity 117
  obstruction 20, 89
  stasis 84
  stents 22, 81, 85
biliary anastomosis 126

biliary cirrhosis
  coeliac disease 27
    associations 92
  liver transplantation 89
  primary **51**, 88–90
    abnormal liver function tests 51
  primary sclerosing cholangitis 88
biliary colic 39
  chronic abdominal pain 41
    differential diagnosis 42
  vomiting 42
biliary strictures 22
  primary sclerosing cholangitis 87
biliary tract investigations 129, *130*
biliary tree diseases 82–90
bisphosphonates 7
blindness, night 121
blood group matching for liver
  transplantation 125
body mass index 122, 123
bone marrow suppression 118
botulinum toxin 70
bowel
  functional disorders 101
  sounds 56
  see also inflammatory bowel disease; large
    bowel; small bowel
bowel habit change 43–5
  diet 45
  examination 44
  history 44
  investigations 44–5
  malignancy 45
  management 45
breath tests **132**, 133
Budd–Chiari syndrome 14, 109
  obstructive jaundice differential diagnosis 21
  pain 46
  presentation 27, 47

C-reactive protein 76
CA19–9 85
cachexia 113
caecal carcinoma **17**
caecal perforation risk 97
calcium supplementation 91
Campylobacter 118
candidiasis
  gastro-oesophageal reflux differential
    diagnosis 66
  oesophageal 7, 8
  oral in HIV infection 121
carcinoembryonic antigen (CEA) 96
carcinoid syndrome 4, 5
cardiac pain 39
  gastro-oesophageal reflux differential
    diagnosis 66
cardiomyopathy, alcoholic 108
case finding 128
central venous catheterization 124
cephalosporins
  acute liver failure 48
  bacterial peritonitis 29
cerebellar atrophy 108
cerebral atrophy 108
cerebral oedema 47, 110
Chagas' disease 69
Charcot's triad 20
cheilosis 121
chloramphenicol 119
chlordiazepoxide **26**, 41
chlormethiazole 17
chlorpromazine hepatotoxicity 117
cholangiocarcinoma 81, 83, 84–6, 114
  biliary strictures 22
  liver transplantation 85
    contraindication 126

obstructive jaundice differential
    diagnosis 21
  primary sclerosing cholangitis 86, 88
  surgical resection 85
cholangitis
  acute pancreatitis 75, 77
  ascending 20, 21, 22
  bacterial 85
  choledocholithiasis 83, 84
  pyogenic liver abscess 116
  recurrent bacterial 84
  see also sclerosing cholangitis
cholecystectomy 41
choledochal cysts 84
choledocholithiasis 82–4
  chronic abdominal pain 43
cholelithiasis
  jaundice 21
  pain 4
  see also gallstones
cholestasis
  acute 117
  chronic 117
  intrahepatic 89, 90
  of pregnancy 51
cholestyramine 89
cigarette smoking
  Crohn's disease 58, 60
  peptic ulceration 72
  ulcerative colitis 61, 62
ciprofloxacin
  Campylobacter infection 118
  Escherichia coli infection 120
  salmonella infection 119
  traveller's diarrhoea 120
  Yersinia enterocolitica 120
cirrhosis
  alcohol use/abuse 27, 116
  causes **111**
  hepatitis C progression **113**
  hepatocellular carcinoma 114, 116
  liver enzymes 50
  liver transplantation 126
  macronodular *28*
cisapride 65, 66
clarithromycin 72
clavulanic acid–amoxycillin
  hepatotoxicity 117
CLO test 71
Clonorchis infection 84
Clostridium difficile 119
  chronic diarrhoea **6**
clubbing in Crohn's disease 58
co-trimoxazole 120
coagulopathy
  acute liver failure 110
  chronic liver disease complications 112
  correction in oesophageal variceal
    haemorrhage 15
  liver biopsy contraindication 136
codeine 118
coeliac axis block 79
coeliac disease 3, 4, 90–2
  abnormal liver function tests 51
  aetiology 90
  anaemia 91
  biliary cirrhosis 27, 90
  chronic pancreatitis differential
    diagnosis 79
  clinical presentation 90–1
  complications 91–2
  diagnosis 5
  diet 125
  differential diagnosis 91
  disease associations 92
  epidemiology 90
  family history 32, 51

  immunosuppression 91
  investigations 33, 91
  iron-deficiency anaemia 32
  irritable bowel syndrome differential
    diagnosis 102
  management 33–4
  occult 49
  pathophysiology/pathology 90
  prognosis 92
  treatment 91
  villous atrophy 33, *34*
colectomy
  emergency 6
  ulcerative colitis 128
colic
  pain 41
  see also biliary colic
colitis 3, 4
  amoebic 116
  colonoscopy 45
  Crohn's 58, 61
  fulminant 4, 5
  haemorrhagic 120
  infectious 4, 61
    microscopic colitis differential
      diagnosis 63
  inflammatory pseudopolyps 95
  ischaemic 43, 99
  lymphocytic 61
  microscopic 4, 61, 63
  NSAID-induced 61
  see also ulcerative colitis
collapse, melaena 9–13
colonic adenoma *49*
colonic angiodysplasia 48, 49
colonic carcinoma
  Crohn's disease 60
  diverticular disease differential diagnosis 98
colonic ischaemia 98
colonic malignancy 34
  barium enema 45
  investigations 38
colonic obstruction 30
  investigations 31
  management 31–2
colonic perforation 127
colonic polyps
  adenomatous 94–5
  colonoscopy 45, 127, 128
  family history 37
  hamartomatous 95
colonic spasm 44
colonic strictures 43
colonoscopy 5, **131**
  colonic polyps 45, 127, 128
  colorectal carcinoma 127
  Crohn's disease 19
  familial adenomatous polyposis (FAP) 127
  familial colon cancer syndrome 127
  hereditary non-polyposis cancer syndromes
    (HNPCC) 127
  rectal bleeding 38
  ulcerative colitis 127
  virtual **131**
colorectal carcinoma 18, 95–7
  adenomatous polyp progression 94, 95
  barium enema 96
  case finding 128
  chemotherapy 97
  clinical presentation 95
  colonoscopy 96, 127
  complications 97
  differential diagnosis 96–7
  epidemiology 95
  family history 37, 95, 128
  intestinal ischaemia differential
    diagnosis 99

liver metastases 114
metastatic disease 96
population screening 128
prognosis 97
radiotherapy 97
rectal bleeding differential diagnosis 36
screening 127
signs 95–6
staging 96
surgery 97
surveillance 127–8
treatment 97
ulcerative colitis 95
colorectal neoplasia 116
colpermin 45
irritable bowel syndrome 102
common bile duct
obstruction 20, 79
stones 22, 23, 83
primary sclerosing cholangitis 87
removal 84
stricture 81
communication with patient
abdominal swelling 29
enteral feeding 54
computed tomography (CT)
abdominal 19
air-contrast 38
contrast scanning **131**
confusion and acute liver failure 45
constipation 100, 101
abdominal swelling 27
chronic 3
corticosteroids
alcoholic hepatitis 26, 108
Crohn's disease 20, 59
inflammatory bowel disease management 6
oesophageal candidiasis 8
Courvoisier's law 21
Courvoisier's sign 80
cow's milk protein intolerance 125
COX-2 inhibitors for peptic ulceration 72
Coxsackie B virus 75
CREST, biliary cirrhosis 90
Crohn's disease 58–60
abdominal pain 32
abnormal liver function tests 51
aetiology 58
bacterial overgrowth 92
chronic abdominal pain differential
diagnosis 42
clinical presentation 58
coeliac disease differential diagnosis 91
complications 60
diagnostic tests 18–19
differential diagnosis 59
disease associations 60
drug therapy 20
epidemiology 58
fistula-in-ano 101
history 18
ileocaecal 17
inflammatory pseudopolyps 95
investigations 33, 58–9
management 6, 19–20
mouth ulcers 4, 18
MRI scan 59
nutrition 19–20
platelet count 33
prevention 60
primary sclerosing cholangitis association 88
prognosis 60
rectal biopsy 59
short bowel syndrome 94
skin tags 37, 58
strictures 34, 41, 58, 59
surgery 20

symptoms 4
terminal ileitis 19
treatment 59–60
weight loss 32
cryptosporidium in HIV infection 121
Cullen's sign 40, 76
cyclosporin
inflammatory bowel disease management 6
liver transplantation 126
cystic fibrosis mutation 4
cytochrome P450 deficiency 116
cytokine antagonists 77
cytomegalovirus (CMV) 106
acute pancreatitis 75
HIV infection 121

decline, progressive 53–5
delayed hypersensitivity, cutaneous 123
depression
acute liver failure 45
irritable bowel syndrome 102
dextropropoxyphene hepatotoxicity 117
diabetes mellitus
abnormal liver function tests 49–53
artherosclerosis 42
bacterial overgrowth 35
chronic pancreatitis 79
coeliac disease associations 92
family history 32, 51
oesophageal candidiasis 8
pancreatic carcinoma 79
weight loss 32, 33
diarrhoea
bacterial overgrowth 92
bowel habit change 43
Campylobacter infection 118
chronic 3–7
causes **6**
differential diagnosis **3**
examination 4
investigations 4–5
management 5–6
nutrition 5
Clostridium difficile infection 119
Entamoeba histolytica infection 120
gastrointestinal infections 118
giardiasis 120
HIV infection 120, 121
infectious 4
ischaemic colitis 99
overflow 3
proton pump inhibitors 35
salmonella infection 118
secretory **6**
Shigella infection 119
traveller's 120
weight loss 34–6
examination 35
history 35
investigations 35
management 35–6
diet 125
bowel habit change 45
Crohn's disease treatment 59
diverticular disease 98
elemental 125
exclusion 125
irritable bowel syndrome 102
oesophageal carcinoma 69
dietary assessment 55
Dieulafoy lesion 74
diuretics
ascites 29
chronic liver disease 112
diverticula
sigmoid 38
small bowel 35, 36

diverticular disease 97–9
aetiology 97
chronic abdominal pain differential
diagnosis 42
clinical presentation 97–8
differential diagnosis 98
epidemiology 97
fistulae 98
intestinal ischaemia differential
diagnosis 99
investigations 38, 98
pain 37
pathophysiology/pathology 97
pyogenic liver abscess 116
rectal bleeding differential diagnosis 36
treatment 98–9
Down's syndrome 92
doxycycline 120
drugs
abnormal liver function tests 51
alcohol hepatitis differential diagnosis
108
chronic liver disease 118
gastro-oesophageal reflux differential
diagnosis 66
hepatotoxicity 46, 116–18
duodenal biopsy 91
duodenal disease 70–5
duodenal ulceration 108
alcoholic hepatitis association 108
H. pylori 70–2
dynamometry 123
dysphagia 7–9
achalasia 69
differential diagnosis **7**, 8
diffuse oesophageal spasm 70
examination 8
gastric carcinoma 73
investigations 8–9
management 9
nutritional state 121
oesophageal carcinoma 67
treatment 66

eating disorders
artificial feeding 55
weight loss 32, 33
encephalopathy
acute liver failure 109
chronic liver disease complications 112,
113
endomysial antibodies 33, 34, 44, 91
endoscopic retrograde
pancreaticocholangiography (ERCP)
20, 22, 41, **129**
acute pancreatitis 77
cholangiocarcinoma 85
choledocholithiasis 83
primary sclerosing cholangitis 87
endoscopy 130, **131**
Entamoeba histolytica infection 120
enteral feeding 53–5, 124
communication with patient 54
ethics 54
malnutrition 124
management approach 54–5
enteric fever, salmonella 119
enteritis, ulcerative 92
enterochromaffin cells 101
enteroclysis 19
enteroscopy **131**
epilepsy, coeliac disease associations 92
Epstein–Barr virus (EBV) 106
acute pancreatitis 75
ergotamine 37
erythema ab igne 56
chronic pancreatitis 78

erythema nodosum
  Campylobacter infection 118
  Yersinia enterocolitica 120
erythroderma 118
erythromycin 118
Escherichia coli infection 120
ethics
  alcoholism 26
  enteral feeding 54
  liver transplantation 125

factitious abdominal pain 55–7
factor VII, recombinant activated 15
familial adenomatous polyposis (FAP) 95
  colonoscopy 127
familial colon cancer syndrome 127
fatty acids, essential 121
fatty liver 52, *53*
  acute of pregnancy 51
febrile convulsions in *Shigella* infection 119
ferritin 49
ferrous sulphate 66
fever
  alcoholic hepatitis 25
  chronic abdominal pain 42
  drug hepatotoxicity 117
fistula-in-ano 100, 101
  Crohn's disease 101
flexible sigmoidoscopy **131**
flucloxacillin
  cholestasis 90
  hepatotoxicity 117
fluconazole 48
5-fluorouracil 97
folate/folic acid 93
  deficiency 35
  supplementation 91
food poisoning 118
fresh frozen plasma 15
frusemide
  acute pancreatitis 75
  ascites 29
functional bowel disorders 101
functional tests **132**, 133
furosemide *see* frusemide

gall bladder, palpable 80
gallstones
  acute pancreatitis 75, 77
  biliary obstruction 42
  choledocholithiasis 82–3
  cholestasis 90
  jaundice 21
  pain 4
  passage 129
gastrectomy, partial 10, *11*
  gastric carcinoma incidence 73
gastric carcinoma 7, 72, 73–4
gastric disease 70–5
gastric lymphoma 74
gastric outflow obstruction 10
gastric surgery
  bacterial overgrowth 35
  malabsorption 94
gastric tumours, rare 74
gastric varices 16
gastrin 5
gastrinoma 72, 74, 82
gastro-oesophageal junction *73*
gastro-oesophageal motility 132
gastro-oesophageal reflux 65–7
  acid reflux 132
  Barrett's oesophagus 63
  complications 66
  disease 8
  disease associations 67
  gastro-oesophageal motility 132

H. pylori eradication 72
  investigations 66
  presentation 65
  prevention 66
  prognosis 66
  proton pump inhibitors 65
  symptoms 65
  treatment 66
  see also reflux oesophagitis
gastrocolic reflex 102
gastroenteritis 42
gastrointestinal blood loss 132–3
  occult **132**
gastrointestinal haemorrhage 9–13
  angiodysplasia 75
  comorbidity 10
  Dieulafoy lesion 74
  endoscopy 12
  hereditary haemorrhagic telangiectasia 75
  iron-deficiency anaemia 49
  management 13
  Meckel's diverticulum 75
  oesophageal varices 14
  peptic ulceration **71**
    differential diagnosis 72
  severity assessment **12**
  vascular ectasia 75
gastrointestinal infections **6**, 118–21
gastrointestinal investigations 129–30, **131**, 132–3
  biliary tract 129, *130*
  complications 133
gastroplication, vertical banded 124
gentamicin 120
Giardia lamblia 93, 119–20
giardiasis
  coeliac disease differential diagnosis 91
  irritable bowel syndrome differential diagnosis 102
  malabsorption 93
Glasgow/Ranson criteria for pancreatitis 76
globus syndrome 8
glossitis 121
glucagoma 82
glucagon 5
glucose hydrogen breath test 93
gluten-free diet 34, 91, 92, 125
glyceryl trinitrate (GTN) paste 101
glycholate breath test **132**
glycogen storage disease 116
Graves' disease 33
Grey–Turner's sign 40, 76
Guillain–Barré syndrome 118

H₂ antagonists 66
haematemesis 10
  Barrett's oesophagus 64
  coffee grounds 39
  jaundice 13–17
  peptic ulceration 71
haematological disorders 21
haemochromatosis
  abnormal liver function tests **51**
  case finding 128
  chronic liver disease complications 113
  cirrhosis *28*
  liver biopsy 52
haemolytic uraemic syndrome
  Escherichia coli infection 120
  Shigella infection 119
haemorrhoids 100
  pain 37
  prolapsed 37
  rectal bleeding differential diagnosis **36**
halothane
  autoantibodies 116
  hepatotoxicity 117

heartburn 7–9
  examination 8
  investigations 8–9
  management 9
Helicobacter pylori 70–2
  detection 71–2
  eradication 72
  MALT lymphoma 74
hepatic adenoma 114
  benign 114
  glycogen storage disease 116
  see also liver
hepatic encephalopathy 25
  anxiolytics 118
  cerebral oedema 47
  consciousness level change 45
  grading **47**
  history 46
  oesophageal variceal haemorrhage 16
  ventilation 48
hepatic steatosis **51**, 52, *53*
hepatic vein occlusion 46, 47, 109
hepatitis
  acute 27
    drug hepatotoxicity 117
  alcoholic 23–6, 27, 106–8
    complications 108
    differential diagnosis 108
    disease associations 108
    drug hepatotoxicity 117
    histology *107*
    investigations 108
    physical signs *107*
    prevention 108
    treatment 108
  autoimmune chronic active 24, 29,46,51
    drug hepatotoxicity 117
  drug-induced 24
  viral 21, 22, 24, 25, 27, 103–6
    abnormal liver function tests 51
    alcohol hepatitis differential diagnosis 108
    drug hepatotoxicity 117
    hepatocellular carcinoma risk 116
    liver failure differential diagnosis 46
hepatitis A 21, 103–4
hepatitis B 29, **51**, 104–6
  clinical presentation 105
  complications 105
  epidemiology 104–5
  investigations 105
  prevention 105–6
  recurrence with liver transplantation 127
  vaccination 106
hepatitis C **51**
  natural history **113**
  recurrence with liver transplantation 127
hepatitis E 106
hepatocellular carcinoma 25, 28, 29, 114
  α-fetoprotein (AFP) 128
  chronic liver disease complications 113
  cirrhosis 116
  epidemiology 114
  hepatic bruit 115
  prevention 116
  surveillance 128
hepatomegaly
  acute liver failure 47, 109
  cholangiocarcinoma 84
  hepatitis A 103
  jaundice 25
hepatorenal failure 112
hepatotoxicity of drugs *see* drugs, hepatotoxicity
herbal remedies, hepatotoxicity 117
hereditary haemorrhagic telangiectasia 37, 75

hereditary non-polyposis cancer syndromes (HNPCC)
  colon 95
  colonoscopy 127
hernia, femoral 42
herpes simplex 106
  gastro-oesophageal reflux differential diagnosis 66
  oesophagitis in HIV infection 121
hiatus hernia 9
Hirschsprung's disease 27
HIV infection 120–1
  chronic diarrhoea **6**
  oesophageal candidiasis 8
HLA B27 60
HLA DQW2 90
HLA DR3 90
Hodgkin's lymphoma 18
Howell–Jolly bodies 91
hydatid cysts 113, 114, 115
5-hydroxyindoleacetic acid (5-HIAA) 5
5-hydroxytryptamine (5-HT) 101
5-hydroxytryptamine 3 receptor antagonists 102
hypercalcaemia in acute pancreatitis 75, 77
hyperlipidaemia 50
  family history 51
hyperparathyroidism
  acute pancreatitis 75
  pancreatic endocrine tumours 82
hypertriglyceridaemia 75
hypolactasia 94
  diet 125
  irritable bowel syndrome differential diagnosis 102
hyposplenism 92
hypothyroidism 90
hypovolaemic shock 77
hypoxia 77

ileal disease 84
  see also terminal ileitis
ileus, localized 40
ileus, paralytic 40
  abdominal swelling 27
  acute pancreatitis 77
immunization
  hepatitis A 104
  hepatitis B 106
immunoglobulin A (IgA)
  antibodies 5
  deficiency 92
  mesangial nephropathy 92
immunoglobulin M (IgM) 89
immunosuppression
  inflammatory bowel disease management 6
  liver transplantation 126
  oesophageal candidiasis 8
inflammatory bowel disease 58–63
  coeliac disease
    associations 92
    differential diagnosis 91
  diverticular disease differential diagnosis 98
  examination 5
  family history 18, 51
  idiopathic 3
  intestinal ischaemia differential diagnosis 99
  irritable bowel syndrome differential diagnosis 102
  management 6
  platelet count 33
  primary sclerosing cholangitis 27
  pyogenic liver abscess 116
  see also colitis, microscopic; Crohn's disease; ulcerative colitis
insulinoma 82

intestinal adhesions 42
intestinal infarction 76
  acute 43
intestinal infection **6**
intestinal ischaemia 99–100
  acute pancreatitis differential diagnosis 76
intestinal lumen radiology 129–30, **131**
intestinal neoplasia 3, 4
intestinal obstruction
  abdominal pain/vomiting 30–2
  abdominal swelling 27
  Crohn's disease 60
intestinal perforations in Crohn's disease 60
intestine *see* gastrointestinal *entries*; large bowel; small bowel
intracerebral haemorrhage 47
iron deficiency
  gastric surgery 94
  see also anaemia, iron-deficiency
iron replacement therapy 48, 49, 91
irritable bowel syndrome 101–2
  clinical presentation 102
  diet 125
  differential diagnosis 102
  epidemiology 101
  management 45
  treatment 102
isosorbide 70

jaundice
  abdominal pain 20–3
  abdominal swelling 27
  abnormal liver function tests 50
  acute liver failure 45, 46, 109
  alcohol use 21
  alcoholic hepatitis 23–6
  cholangiocarcinoma 84
  choledocholithiasis 83
  cholelithiasis 21
  differential diagnosis 21, 24
  drug hepatotoxicity 117
  examination 21, 25
  haematemesis 13–17
  heavy drinker 23–7
  hepatitis A 103
  hepatomegaly 25
  intrahepatic cholestasis 90
  investigations 21–2, 129, *130*
  management 22–3
  pain 20
  pancreatic carcinoma 80, 81
  pancreatitis 75

Kayser–Fleischer rings 47
Korsakoff's dementia 108
kwashiorkor 123

lactase deficiency 94
lactose breath test **132**
lactulose breath test 93, **132**
laparotomy/laparoscopy **132**
  Crohn's disease 19
large bowel disease 94–101
  anorectal disease 100–1
  familial cancer syndromes 95
  intestinal ischaemia 76, 99–100
  see also colonic *entries*; colorectal carcinoma; diverticular disease
leiomyoma 74
leptospirosis 46
leucocyte scan, radiolabelled 19
Levine shunt 29
Lexipafant 77
liver
  biopsy 52
  fatty 52, *53*, 117
  malignant infiltration 47

ultrasound *130*
  see also hepatic *entries*; hepatitis
liver abscess 113, 115
  amoebic 116
  Entamoeba histolytica infection 120
  pyogenic 116
liver biopsy 135–7
  transjugular 136
  ultrasound-guided 136
liver damage, acute/chronic 46
liver disease
  abnormal liver function tests 50
  acute 103–10
    differential diagnosis **104**
  alcoholic 16, 26, 27, 106
    liver transplantation ethics 125
  alcoholism 26
  autoimmune 108
  cause determination 28
  chronic 24, 25, 46, 110–13, *112*
    aetiology 110
    alcohol 27
    causes **111**
    clinical presentation 110–11
    complications 26, 112–13
    cutaneous stigmata 46
    diagnostic tests **52**
    drugs 118
    epidemiology 110
    investigations 111–12
    pathophysiology/pathology 110
    physical signs 111
    prognosis 113
    signs 21
    treatment 112
  detection 50
  family history 51
  management 16
  melaena 10
  metastatic 24, 25, 96, 114
  nutrition 17
  oesophageal variceal haemorrhage 14
  screen 109
  see also hepatitis
liver failure
  acute 45–8, 109–10
    complications 110
    drug hepatotoxicity 117
    examination 46–7
    hepatitis B 105
    investigations 47
    referral to specialist centre 47, **48**
    treatment 109–10
  chronic liver disease 113
  differential diagnosis 46
  signs 28
liver fluke 84
liver function tests, abnormal 49–53
  investigations 52
  management 52–3
  patient examination 51–2
  significance **50**
liver lesions, focal 113–16
  aetiology 113–14
  benign neoplastic 113–14, 115
  clinical presentation 114
  complications 115
  differential diagnosis 115
  disease associations 116
  epidemiology 114
  haemangioma 113, 114, 115
  investigations 115
  nodular hyperplasia 114
  pathophysiology/pathology 113–14
  physical signs 115
  prevention 116
  prognosis 116

liver lesions, focal (*continued*)
  regenerative hyperplasia 114
  surgery 115
  treatment 115
  tumour markers **114**
liver transplantation 125–7
  alcoholism 26
  ascites 29
  biliary cirrhosis 90
  cholangiocarcinoma 85
  chronic liver disease 112, 113
  complications 127
  contraindications 126
  disease recurrence 127
  emergency 125–6
  ethics 125
  hepatocellular carcinoma 115
  immunosuppression 126
  indications 125
  outcome 126–7
  sclerosing cholangitis 88
  timing 126
lower oesophageal sphincter, hypertensive 69
lymph node enlargement 18
lymphadenopathy
  bowel habit change 44
  chronic abdominal pain 42
lymphocyte count 123
lymphoma
  abnormal liver function tests 51
  coeliac disease 92
  Crohn's disease differential diagnosis 59
  gastric 74
  MALT 74
  strictures 41

magnetic resonance
  cholangiopancreatography (MRCP) 22,
    23, 83, **129**
major histocompatibility complex (MHC)
  class II markers 90
malabsorption 93–4
  chronic diarrhoea **6**
  chronic pancreatitis 79, 93
  Crohn's disease 60
  diarrhoea and weight loss 34
  examination 35
  giardiasis 93
  HIV infection 120
  hypolactasia 94
  investigations 35
  markers 33
  nutritional state 121
  post-gastric surgery 94
  short bowel syndrome 94
  tropical sprue 93
  weight loss 32
  Whipple's disease 93
malignancy
  abdominal mass **17**
  bowel habit change 45
  Budd–Chiari syndrome 21
  coeliac disease 92
  colonic 34
  Crohn's disease differential diagnosis 59
  dysphagia 9
  gastro-oesophageal junction 69
  irritable bowel syndrome differential
    diagnosis 102
  strictures 41
  weight loss 7, 32, 33
Mallory–Weiss tear 10
malnutrition 121
  blood counts 122–3
  nutritional support 124
MALT lymphoma 74
marasmus 123

mebeverine 45, 119
  irritable bowel syndrome 102
Meckel's diverticulum 75
Meckel's scanning **132**
melaena 9–13
  Barrett's oesophagus 64
  differential diagnosis **9**, 11, 12
  endoscopy 12
  examination 11–12
  gastrointestinal haemorrhage 14
  history 10
  investigations 12–13, 132–3
  management 13
  peptic ulceration 71
  rectal examination 40
  resuscitation 13
membranous colitis *see* colitis, microscopic
Menghini biopsy needle 136, *137*
meningitis 119
mesenteric adenitis 120
mesenteric angina 99
mesenteric ischaemia
  chronic abdominal pain 41, 42, 43
  pain 37
  rectal bleeding differential diagnosis **36**
  treatment 43
methotrexate
  Crohn's disease treatment 59
  hepatotoxicity 117
metoclopramide 65, 66
metronidazole
  bacterial overgrowth 94
  Clostridium difficile 119
  Entamoeba histolytica infection 120
  Giardia lamblia 93, 120
  H. pylori eradication 72
mineral requirements **122**
Minnesota tube 15
misoprostol 72
MLH1 mutation testing 127
morphine 41
motor neurone disease
  dysphagia 7, 8
  investigations 9
mouth ulcers in Crohn's disease 4, 18, 58
MSH2 mutation testing 127
mucosal inflammation **36**
multiple endocrine adenopathies (MEN)
  type I 72, 74, 82
mumps 75
Mycobacterium paratuberculosis 58
myelopathy 121
myocardial infarction 76

naltrexone 89
  alcoholic hepatitis 108
narcotics 118
nasogastric tube feeding 53, 54
neonates, hepatitis B 106
neuroendocrine tumours, pancreatic 82
neurological disability, progressive
  decline 53–5
nifedipine 70
nitrofurantoin autoantibodies 116
non-steroidal anti-inflammatory drugs
  (NSAIDs)
  chronic liver disease 118
  colitis 61
  enteropathy 63
  gastro-oesophageal reflux differential
    diagnosis 66
  hepatotoxicity 117
  iron-deficiency anaemia 48
  melaena 10
  oesophagitis 7
  peptic ulceration 70, 72
  rectal bleeding 37

nutrition 121–5
  acute pancreatitis 76
  artificial 55
  chronic diarrhoea 5
  chronic liver disease 112
  oesophageal carcinoma 69
  see also enteral feeding; parenteral nutrition
nutritional assessment 55
nutritional requirements for health 121
nutritional status
  assessment 121–3
  examination 121
  history 121
  investigations 122–3
nutritional support teams 125
nystagmus 25

obesity 121, 123–4
  abdominal swelling 27
  abnormal liver function tests 49–53
  epidemiology 123
  treatment 124
octreotide
  oesophageal variceal haemorrhage 15
  pancreatic neuroendocrine tumours 82
odynophagia 7
oesophageal adenocarcinoma 63, 67–9
  Barrett's disease 63, 64, 65
  endoscopic surveillance 64
  gastro-oesophageal motility 132
oesophageal carcinoma 7, 67–9
  achalasia 70
  gastro-oesophageal reflux differential
    diagnosis 66
  investigations 67–8
  palliation 68
  prevention 68
  staging 67–8
  surveillance 128
  treatment 68
oesophageal dilatation 66, 68
oesophageal manometry 9, 132
oesophageal perforation 66
oesophageal pneumatic dilatation 70
oesophageal reflux 65–7
  see also gastro-oesophageal reflux; reflux
    oesophagitis
oesophageal spasm, diffuse 70
oesophageal stents 68
oesophageal strictures 7, 8, 9
  achalasia 70
  benign 68
  malignant *68*
  management 9
  scleroderma 67
  treatment 66
  untreated reflux oesophagitis 66
oesophageal surgical myotomy 70
oesophageal tumours 67–9
oesophageal ulcer 64
oesophageal variceal haemorrhage 13–17
  alcohol use 14
  balloon tamponade 15
  band ligation 15–16, 17
  endoscopy 15–16
  examination 14
  history 14
  investigations 14
  liver disease 14
  management 14–16
  rebleeding 16, 17
  sclerotherapy 15–16, 17
oesophageal varices 13
  gastrointestinal haemorrhage 14
  haemorrhage 13–17
oesophagectomy 64
  subtotal 68

oesophagitis
  healing 66
  herpes simplex 7
    HIV infection 121
  radiation-induced 8
  radiotherapy-induced 66
  reflux 7, 65, 66, 70
oesophagogastroduodenoscopy **131**
oesophagus 63–70
  corkscrew 70
  see also achalasia; Barrett's oesophagus
onion skin fibrosis 87
ophthalmoplegia 25
opiates 81
Opisthorchis 84
oral contraceptives
  abnormal liver function tests 51
  Budd–Chiari syndrome 21
  hepatic adenoma 114, 115, 116
  hepatotoxicity 117
oral supplements, nutritional 124
orlistat 124
osteomalacia 89
osteoporosis 89

pain
  acute liver failure 46
  biliary colic 39
  Budd–Chiari syndrome 46
  cardiac 39
    gastro-oesophageal reflux differential
      diagnosis 66
  colic 41
  diverticular disease 37
  epigastric with peptic ulceration 71
  haemorrhoids 37
  liver biopsy 137
  mesenteric ischaemia 37
pain, abdominal 4, 10, 17
  bowel habit change 43
  chronic 41–3
  diarrhoea and weight loss 34
  examination 56
  factitious 55–7
  gastric carcinoma 73
  history 55–6
  Hodgkin's lymphoma 18
  investigations 56
  ischaemic colitis 99
  jaundice 20–3
  management 56–7
  pancreatic 39
  pancreatic carcinoma 80, 81
  pancreatitis 4, 32, 75
    chronic 78
  vomiting 30–2, 39–41
  weight loss 32
pancreas
  calcification 5, 40
  diseases 75–82
  endocrine/exocrine function tests 79
  imaging 82
  necrosis 40, 76, 77
  neuroendocrine tumours 82
  pain 39
pancreas divisum 75
pancreatic abscess 77
pancreatic adenocarcinoma 80
pancreatic carcinoma 20, 80–1
  biliary strictures 22
  chronic pancreatitis differential
    diagnosis 79
  imaging 80–1
  obstructive jaundice differential
    diagnosis 21
  prognosis 81
  risk 75

signs 21
  treatment 81
pancreatic enzyme replacement 79, 93
pancreatic failure 91
pancreatic insufficiency
  chronic pancreatitis 78
  weight loss 33
pancreatic lipase inhibitor 124
pancreaticobiliary investigations 129
pancreaticoduodenectomy 81
pancreatitis
  abdominal wall bruising 40
  acute 75–8
    acute liver failure 110
    aetiology 75
    choledocholithiasis 82–3
    complications 77–8
    investigation 76
    pathophysiology/pathology 75
    prognosis 78
    staging 76
    treatment 76–7
  alcohol use 4, 23
  alcoholic 24, 40, 80
  cholangiocarcinoma differential
    diagnosis 85
  chronic 40, 78–80
    alcoholic hepatitis association 108
    malabsorption 93
  hereditary 75
  idiopathic chronic 4
  investigations 5
  obstructive jaundice differential
    diagnosis 21
  pain 4, 32, 75, 78
  peptic ulceration differential diagnosis 72
  pseudocysts 40, 76, 77
paracentesis 134–5
paracetamol overdose 45, 47, 109, 110
  liver transplantation ethics 125
parenteral nutrition 124–5
parvovirus 106
peptic ulceration 10, 70–2
  acute pancreatitis differential diagnosis 76
  bacterial overgrowth 92
  chronic abdominal pain 41
    differential diagnosis 42
  chronic pancreatitis differential diagnosis 79
  disease associations 72
  H. pylori 70–2
  investigations 71
  iron-deficiency anaemia 49
  portal hypertension 13
  prevention 72
  surgery 10
  treatment 72
percutaneous enterogastrostomy feeding 53, 54
percutaneous transhepatic
  cholangiography 22, 85, 87, **129**
peripheral sensory neuropathy 108
peritonitis, bacterial 29, 112
pethidine 41
Peutz–Jeghers syndrome 95
pH monitoring 132
pharyngeal pouch 8, 9
population screening 128
portal hypertension 13, 111
  alcohol use 108
  biliary cirrhosis 89
  jaundice 25
  management 16, 17
  oesophageal variceal haemorrhage 14
  rectal bleeding 37
    differential diagnosis **36**
  therapeutic paracentesis 134
  treatment 112

portal vein thrombosis 77
portal venous pressure 16
portosystemic shunt 29
prednisolone 126
pregnancy
  abdominal swelling 27
  abnormal liver function tests 51
  ectopic 76
  hepatitis E 106
primary sclerosing cholangitis *see* sclerosing
  cholangitis, primary
proctitis in HIV infection 121
propranolol 112
protein–calorie malnutrition 123
proton pump inhibitors 9
  bacterial overgrowth 35
  Barrett's oesophagus 64
  gastrinoma 74
  gastro-oesophageal reflux disease 65
  H. pylori eradication 72
  oesophageal strictures 66
  pancreatic neuroendocrine tumours 82
  peptic ulceration 72
pyrexia of unknown origin 33
pyridoxine 25

quinolones 29

radiation injury 94
radiology of intestinal lumen 129–30, **131**
reactive metabolites 116
rebound tenderness 56
rectal biopsy 133–4
rectal bleeding 36–8
  bowel habit change 44
  colonoscopy 38
  Crohn's disease 60
  diagnosis-specific treatment **38**
  differential diagnosis **36**
  examination 37
  history 36–7
  investigations 37–8, 132–3
  management 38
  source 38
rectal ulcer, solitary 100, 101
red cell scanning **132**
reflux oesophagitis 7, 65, 66
  achalasia 70
Reiter's syndrome
  Campylobacter infection 118
  Shigella infection 119
renal failure
  acute liver failure 110
  acute pancreatitis 77
resuscitation, melaena 13
retinopathy 121
rheumatoid arthritis
  biliary cirrhosis 90
  coeliac disease associations 92
  iron-deficiency anaemia 48–9
rifampicin 89
rigid sigmoidoscopy 133–4

salmonella 118–19
sarcoidosis
  abnormal liver function tests 51
  coeliac disease associations 92
Schilling test **132**
scleroderma
  investigations 9
  reflux oesophagitis 67
sclerosing cholangitis, primary 27, 60, 63,
  86–8
  abnormal liver function tests 51
  aetiology 86
  biliary cirrhosis differential diagnosis 89
  cholangiocarcinoma 85, 114, 116

sclerosing cholangitis, primary (*continued*)
  clinical presentations 86
  complications 87–8
  disease associations 88
  investigations 86
  liver biopsy 87
  liver transplantation contraindication
    126
  pathophysiology/pathology 86
  prognosis 88
  signs 86
  treatment 87–8
sclerotherapy for oesophageal variceal
  haemorrhage 15–16, 17
screening for colorectal carcinoma 127
Sengstaken–Blakemore tube 15
sentinel loop 40
septicaemia 84
serotonergic agonists 124
Shigella infection 119
short bowel syndrome 94
sicca syndrome 90
sickle cell disease 84
sigmoid diverticula *38*
sigmoidoscopy 133–4
skin tags, Crohn's disease 37, 58
small bowel
  disease 90–4
  diverticula 35, *36*
  enema 18
  infarction 99
  obstruction 34
    vomiting 42
  strictures 35
  see also bacterial overgrowth; coeliac
    disease; duodenal *entries*;
    malabsorption
sphincter of Oddi
  acute pancreatitis 75
  balloon dilatation 84
  spasm 41
  sphincterotomy 84
sphincteroplasty 84
spironolactone 29
splenomegaly 47
steatohepatitis **51**
  drug hepatotoxicity 117
steatorrhoea
  bacterial overgrowth 93
  causes 4
  diarrhoea and weight loss 34
  gastric surgery 94
  investigations 3, 35
  tropical sprue 93
stools
  character 3
  examination 5
stroke
  dysphagia 7
  enteral feeding 53
subconjunctival haemorrhage 47
sulphamethoxazole 93
sulphasalazine 75
surgery
  Crohn's disease 60
  gastric
    bacterial overgrowth 35
    malabsorption 94
  oesophageal myotomy 70
  peptic ulceration 10
  vertical banded gastroplication 124
  see also liver transplantation
surveillance 127–8
swallowing difficulty 53–5
syncope 10
systemic lupus erythematosus (SLE) 51
systemic sclerosis 35

tacrolimus 126
terminal ileitis
  Crohn's disease *19*, 58
  Yersinia enterocolitica 120
terminal ileoscopy **131**
terminal ileum in Crohn's disease 60
tetracycline
  bacterial overgrowth 35, 93
  hepatotoxicity 117
  oesophagitis 7
  tropical sprue 93
  Yersinia enterocolitica 120
thiamine 25
  deficiency 121
Thorotrast 84
thrombophlebitis migrans 80
thyroid disease
  coeliac disease associations 92
  family history 32, 33
  hepatitis association 51
thyrotoxicosis
  bowel habit change 44
  coeliac disease differential diagnosis 91
  weight loss 32, 33
tinidazole 94
  Giardia lamblia 120
tiredness with weight loss 31–4
total body water 123
total parenteral nutrition 84
  cholestasis 90
toxic dilatation 118
toxic megacolon 60
trace elements
  deficiencies 121
  requirements 121, **122**
transglutaminase 90
transjugular intrahepatic portosystemic shunt
  (TIPSS) 16, 17
  ascites 29
trauma 75
travel, overseas
  abnormal liver function tests 51
  chronic diarrhoea 4
  traveller's diarrhoea 120
trimethoprim
  salmonella infection 119
  Whipple's disease 93
Tropheryma whippelli 93
tropical sprue 93
tuberculosis, intestinal 4, 33
  Crohn's disease differential diagnosis
    59
  weight loss 33
tumour markers for liver disease **114**
tumour necrosis factor α (TNF-α) 59

ulcerative colitis 61–3
  aetiology 61
  colectomy 128
  colonoscopy 127
  colorectal carcinoma 95
  complications 62
  Crohn's disease differential diagnosis 59
  differential diagnosis 61
  disease associations 63
  endoscopy 5, *6*
  epidemiology 61
  examination 4
  inflammatory pseudopolyps 95
  investigations 61
  management 6
  microscopic colitis differential
    diagnosis 63
  pathophysiology/pathology 61
  prevention 62
  primary sclerosing cholangitis
    association 88

  prognosis 62
  remission 62
  signs 61
  staging 61, *62*
  treatment 62
ulcerative enteritis 92
ultrasound **129**
  liver *130*
urease breath test **132**
ursodeoxycholic acid 87, 89

vancomycin 119
variceal haemorrhage 112
  chronic liver disease complications 113
varicella 106
vascular ectasia 75
vasoactive intestinal peptide (VIP) 5
vasopressin analogues 15
venous thrombosis 80
ventilation in hepatic encephalopathy 48
Verner–Morrison syndrome 82
villous atrophy 91
VIPoma 82
Virchow's node 18
  gastric carcinoma 73
visceral angiography **132**
vitamin A deficiency 121
vitamin B
  deficiency 121
  requirements **122**
vitamin B$_{12}$
  deficiency 35, 92
    gastric surgery 94
  supplementation in bacterial
    overgrowth 93
vitamin C deficiency 121
vitamin D supplementation 91
vitamin E deficiency 121
vitamin K deficiency 15, 121
vitamins, deficiencies/requirements 121
vomiting
  abdominal pain 30–2, 39–41
  abdominal swelling 27
  examination 39–40
  gastric carcinoma 73
  gastrointestinal infections 118
  history 39
  imaging 40
  investigations 40
  management 41
  melaena 10
  nutritional state 121
  pancreatic carcinoma 80
  small bowel obstruction 42

waist/hip circumference ratio 123
warfarin
  melaena 10
  rectal bleeding **36**, 37
weight loss
  alcoholics 24
  bowel habit change 44
  cholangiocarcinoma 84
  chronic abdominal pain 41, 42
  diarrhoea 34–6
  differential diagnosis 33
  examination 32–3
  gastric carcinoma 73
  history 32
  HIV infection 120
  imaging 33
  intentional 32
  investigations 33, *34*
  management 33–4
  melaena 10
  nutritional state 121
  pancreatic carcinoma 80, 81

rectal bleeding 37
   tiredness 31–4
Weil's disease 46
Werner's syndrome 82
Wernicke's encephalopathy 25, 121
   alcoholic hepatitis association 108
Whipple's disease 4, **6**
   malabsorption 93

Wilson's disease 25
   case finding 128
   haemolysis 47
   Kayser–Fleischer rings 47
   liver biopsy 52, 137
   liver failure differential diagnosis 46
   presentation **111**, 112

xenotransplantation 125
xylose excretion test **132**

Yersinia enterocolitica infection 120

Zollinger–Ellison syndrome 82